Joint Modeling of Longitudinal and Time-to-Event Data

MONOGRAPHS ON STATISTICS AND APPLIED PROBABILITY

General Editors

F. Bunea, V. Isham, N. Keiding, T. Louis, R. L. Smith, and H. Tong

1. Stochastic Population Models in Ecology and Epidemiology *M.S. Barlett* (1960)
2. Queues *D.R. Cox and W.L. Smith* (1961)
3. Monte Carlo Methods *J.M. Hammersley and D.C. Handscomb* (1964)
4. The Statistical Analysis of Series of Events *D.R. Cox and P.A.W. Lewis* (1966)
5. Population Genetics *W.J. Ewens* (1969)
6. Probability, Statistics and Time *M.S. Barlett* (1975)
7. Statistical Inference *S.D. Silvey* (1975)
8. The Analysis of Contingency Tables *B.S. Everitt* (1977)
9. Multivariate Analysis in Behavioural Research *A.E. Maxwell* (1977)
10. Stochastic Abundance Models *S. Engen* (1978)
11. Some Basic Theory for Statistical Inference *E.J.G. Pitman* (1979)
12. Point Processes *D.R. Cox and V. Isham* (1980)
13. Identification of Outliers *D.M. Hawkins* (1980)
14. Optimal Design *S.D. Silvey* (1980)
15. Finite Mixture Distributions *B.S. Everitt and D.J. Hand* (1981)
16. Classification *A.D. Gordon* (1981)
17. Distribution-Free Statistical Methods, 2nd edition *J.S. Maritz* (1995)
18. Residuals and Influence in Regression *R.D. Cook and S. Weisberg* (1982)
19. Applications of Queueing Theory, 2nd edition *G.F. Newell* (1982)
20. Risk Theory, 3rd edition *R.E. Beard, T. Pentikäinen and E. Pesonen* (1984)
21. Analysis of Survival Data *D.R. Cox and D. Oakes* (1984)
22. An Introduction to Latent Variable Models *B.S. Everitt* (1984)
23. Bandit Problems *D.A. Berry and B. Fristedt* (1985)
24. Stochastic Modelling and Control *M.H.A. Davis and R. Vinter* (1985)
25. The Statistical Analysis of Composition Data *J. Aitchison* (1986)
26. Density Estimation for Statistics and Data Analysis *B.W. Silverman* (1986)
27. Regression Analysis with Applications *G.B. Wetherill* (1986)
28. Sequential Methods in Statistics, 3rd edition *G.B. Wetherill and K.D. Glazebrook* (1986)
29. Tensor Methods in Statistics *P. McCullagh* (1987)
30. Transformation and Weighting in Regression *R.J. Carroll and D. Ruppert* (1988)
31. Asymptotic Techniques for Use in Statistics *O.E. Bandorff-Nielsen and D.R. Cox* (1989)
32. Analysis of Binary Data, 2nd edition *D.R. Cox and E.J. Snell* (1989)
33. Analysis of Infectious Disease Data *N.G. Becker* (1989)
34. Design and Analysis of Cross-Over Trials *B. Jones and M.G. Kenward* (1989)
35. Empirical Bayes Methods, 2nd edition *J.S. Maritz and T. Lwin* (1989)
36. Symmetric Multivariate and Related Distributions *K.T. Fang, S. Kotz and K.W. Ng* (1990)
37. Generalized Linear Models, 2nd edition *P. McCullagh and J.A. Nelder* (1989)
38. Cyclic and Computer Generated Designs, 2nd edition *J.A. John and E.R. Williams* (1995)
39. Analog Estimation Methods in Econometrics *C.F. Manski* (1988)
40. Subset Selection in Regression *A.J. Miller* (1990)
41. Analysis of Repeated Measures *M.J. Crowder and D.J. Hand* (1990)
42. Statistical Reasoning with Imprecise Probabilities *P. Walley* (1991)
43. Generalized Additive Models *T.J. Hastie and R.J. Tibshirani* (1990)
44. Inspection Errors for Attributes in Quality Control *N.L. Johnson, S. Kotz and X. Wu* (1991)
45. The Analysis of Contingency Tables, 2nd edition *B.S. Everitt* (1992)
46. The Analysis of Quantal Response Data *B.J.T. Morgan* (1992)
47. Longitudinal Data with Serial Correlation—A State-Space Approach *R.H. Jones* (1993)

Monographs on Statistics and Applied Probability 151

Joint Modeling of Longitudinal and Time-to-Event Data

Robert M. Elashoff, Gang Li, and Ning Li

UCLA Departments of Biostatistics and Biomathematics
Los Angeles, California, USA

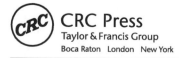

CRC Press
Taylor & Francis Group
Boca Raton   London   New York

CRC Press is an imprint of the
Taylor & Francis Group, an **informa** business
A CHAPMAN & HALL BOOK

CRC Press
Taylor & Francis Group
6000 Broken Sound Parkway NW, Suite 300
Boca Raton, FL 33487-2742

First issued in paperback 2020

Version Date: 20160607

ISBN 13: 978-0-3675-7057-6 (pbk)
ISBN 13: 978-1-4398-0782-8 (hbk)

Visit the Taylor & Francis Web site at
http://www.taylorandfrancis.com

and the CRC Press Web site at
http://www.crcpress.com

To David and Michael

- R.M.E

To Yan, Victor, Sophia and Emily

- G. L.

To Yi and Eric

- N. L.

Contents

Preface

Longitudinal data analysis and survival analysis are among the fastest expanding areas of statistics and biostatistics in the past three decades. Longitudinal data analysis generally refers to statistical techniques for analyzing repeated measurements data from a longitudinal study. Repeated measurements data include multiple observations of an outcome variable such as body mass index (BMI) that are measured over time on the same study unit during the course of follow up. The key issues for longitudinal data analysis are how to account for the within-subject correlations and how to handle missing observations. On the other hand, survival analysis deals with survival data or time-to-event data for which the outcome variable is time to the occurrence of an event. An event could be, for instance, death, relief from disease symptoms, equipment failure, or discharge from a hospital. Time-to-event data are usually incomplete, and thus cannot be handled by standard statistical tools for complete data. A typical example is *right censoring* which occurs when the survival time of interest is only known to be greater than some observed censoring time due to the end of follow up or the occurrence of early withdraw or competing events. Both types of data arise commonly in almost all scientific fields. There are numerous research papers, monographs, and text books in each subject area.

In recent years, these two seemingly different areas of statistics have crossed with the rapidly growing interest in the development of joint models for longitudinal and survival data. Interestingly, such joint models were originally introduced to address different problems in longitudinal data analysis and survival analysis independently. In longitudinal data analysis, joint models were primarily considered as a means to adjust for nonignorable missing data due to informative or outcome related dropouts which cannot be handled properly by the popularly used methods such as linear mixed effects models. In survival analysis, however, they were first proposed for Cox's proportional hazards model to deal with time-dependent covariates that are measured intermittently and/or subject to measurement error. Joint models have also become popular in medical research where both the longitudinal variable (such as a disease biomarker) and the time-to-event variable (such as the disease-free survival time) are important outcome variables to evaluate the efficacy of interventions or treatments.

This monograph is devoted to give a systematic introduction and review of state-of-the-art statistical methodology developed in recent years for joint modeling of longitudinal and survival data. We have three audiences in mind when writing the book. First, the book serves as a reference book for scientific investigators who need to analyze longitudinal and/or survival data. Secondly, it may be used as a textbook for a graduate level course in the fields of biostatistics and statistics. Thirdly, it provides mathematical statisticians some recent lines of research and some unsolved challenging issues for further methodology advancement.

The first chapter of the monograph introduces examples from biomedical studies which are used later to illustrate various joint modeling approaches. The remaining six chapters can be grouped into two themes. The first theme, composed of Chapters 2 and 3, provides an overview of statistical modeling and concepts there are fundamental to understanding joint models. Specifically, Chapter 2 introduces missing data mechanisms and surveys standard methods for longitudinal data analysis that are valid under the assumption of ignorable or non-informative missing data. Chapter 3 reviews basic concepts and models for analysis of time-to-event data. The second theme, composed of Chapters 4 to 7, is a systematic discussion of joint models for longitudinal and time-to-event data with applications in various scenarios. Specifically, Chapter 4 is the core of this monograph, providing an overview of several main areas in which joint models have been developed to address important scientific questions and issues that cannot be answered by separate analysis of longitudinal and survival data. The topics covered in this chapter include monotonic missing data in longitudinal studies caused by continuous or discrete event times, longitudinal data with both monotone and intermittent missing values, event time models with intermittently measured time-dependent covariates, longitudinal studies with informative observation times, and dynamic prediction in joint models. The next two chapters discuss extensions of the joint models to the scenario of competing risks event times (Chapter 5) and multivariate longitudinal and/or multivariate survival data (Chapter 6). Chapter 7 contains further topics including sensitivity analysis to investigate the impact of modeling assumptions on statistical inference of joint models, model diagnostics, and variable selection in joint models. Joint multistate models and cure-rate models are also discussed.

We would like to thank the many friends and colleagues who have helped us directly or indirectly during all stages of this project. We are very grateful to Donald Tashkin for selecting us to develop and carry out the data analyses for the NIH trial on Scleroderma lung disease. Our special thanks go to Peter Diggle, Michael Hughes, Mike Kenward, Zhigang Li, Cecile Proust-Lima, Dimitris Rizopoulos, Xiao Song, Jianguo Sun, Yi-Kuan Tseng, and Jane-Ling Wang for sharing with us data and programs for joint model examples. We are very grateful to Lin Du, Eric Kawaguchi, Daniel Conn, and Jennifer Leung for editing and proofreading the monograph. We extend our appreciation to

Chi-Hong Tseng, Janet Sinsheimer, and Michael Daniels for their advice and support during the course of this project. We are very grateful to the executive editor Rob Calver and the staff at Chapman & Hall/CRC for their cooperation, support, and patience. Last, but not least, we thank anonymous reviewers for reading a first draft and providing invaluable comments and suggestions that led to significant improvements of the monograph.

Robert M. Elashoff, Gang Li, and Ning Li (Los Angeles, January 2016)

Chapter 1

Introduction and Examples

1.1 Introduction

This book describes statistical methodology for joint modeling of longitudinal data and time-to-event data. Although our examples focus mostly on biomedical applications, the statistical methods we shall present are applicable to longitudinal follow-up studies in all disciplines. In the area of longitudinal data analysis, joint models were originally developed to address such issues as nonignorable missing data and informative visit times. Missing data are nonignorable when the probability of missingness is related to the missing, unobserved values; otherwise, if the probability of missingness is not related to the missing values, the missing data mechanism is ignorable. Formal definitions of the missing data mechanisms are given in Chapter 2, Section 2.2. Joint models were also studied in the area of time-to-event data analysis for Cox's (1972) proportional hazards model with time-dependent covariates that are measured intermittently and/or subject to measurement error. In addition, joint models are useful in studies where a repeatedly measured biomarker and a clinical time-to-event outcome are used as co-primary outcome variables to evaluate treatment efficacy.

This chapter introduces several data sets from longitudinal clinical studies that motivate joint analysis and are used to illustrate various modeling approaches in later chapters. All data sets introduced in this chapter are available online at http://publications.biostat.ucla.edu/gangli/jm-book.

1.1.1 Scleroderma Lung Study

The Scleroderma Lung Study, a 13-center double-blind, randomized, placebo-controlled trial sponsored by the National Institutes of Health, was designed to evaluate the effectiveness and safety of oral cyclophosphamide for one year in patients with active, symptomatic scleroderma-related interstitial lung disease [207]. The study was initiated with 158 patients, equally distributed into the

Table 1.1 *Primary variables in the scleroderma lung study.*

	Name	Data type
Primary endpoint	FVC (% predicted)	Repeated measurements
	Treatment failure or death	Time-to-event data
Baseline covariate	Baseline %FVC	
	Lung fibrosis score	
	Total lung capacity (% predicted)	
	Cough	
	Skin-thickening score	

two treatment groups and followed for a total of two years. Seventeen patients did not complete the treatment in the first 6 months, so they are excluded from the analysis. By month 24, there were 16 deaths or treatment failures and 47 dropouts. Thirty-seven of the dropouts are considered informative as they were related to patient disease condition. They are referred to as early discontinuation of treatment in the rest of the example.

Table 1.1 shows the important variables in this study. The primary endpoints of the study are FVC (forced vital capacity, % predicted) and death/failures. The baseline measure of lung fibrosis score is considered as a main confounding factor for patient response to CYC.

Figure 1.1 shows the profile plot of %FVC by randomization group. There is a large variation in baseline %FVC. We use different symbols to indicate the events that could lead to missing data in %FVC, including treatment failure or death, early discontinuation of the assigned treatment, and noninformatively censored follow up. It seems that treatment failure or death and early discontinuation of the assigned treatment are related to low %FVC scores. As is seen from the missing data patterns summarized in Table 1.2, monotone missing data occurred more frequently in the placebo group. The two types of events, treatment failure or death and early discontinuation of treatment, can be regarded as competing risks and their cumulative incidence functions are shown in Figure 1.2.

The missing data in %FVC could be nonignorable if deaths and failures are correlated with %FVC levels. Some of the dropouts may also be related to %FVC. The analysis using standard approaches such as linear mixed effects models and generalized estimating equations to compare the CYC and placebo groups would lead to biased estimates and invalid inference in the presence

Table 1.2 *Summary of completers and non-completers in the scleroderma lung study.*

	CYC group		Placebo group	
	Frequency	%	Frequency	%
Completers	47	68.1%	42	58.3%
Monotone missingness	10	14.5%	19	26.4%
Intermittent missingness	12	17.4%	11	15.3%

of nonignorable missing data. This example presents challenges for the appropriateness of %FVC modeling and evaluation of the intercorrelation between %FVC, death, and dropouts. The data set is used in Chapter 2 to illustrate the analysis of longitudinal measurements assuming ignorable missing data mechanisms, in Example 4.11 to illustrate a joint model that handles both intermittent and monotone nonignorable missing data, and in Example 5.1 for a joint analysis of longitudinal data and competing risks. It is also used to show the application of robust joint models to reduce the impact of outlying %FVC measurements in Chapter 5.

1.1.2   Stroke Study: the NINDS rt-PA trial

The National Institute of Neurological Disorders and Stroke (NINDS) rt-PA stroke study is a randomized, double-blind trial of intravenous recombinant tissue plasminogen activator (rt-PA) in patients with acute ischemic stroke (the NINDS rt-PA stroke study group, 1995 [84]). A total of 624 patients were enrolled and randomized to receive either intravenous recombinant t-PA or placebo; there were 312 patients in each treatment arm. Repeated measurements of four outcomes were recorded after randomization: the NIH stroke scale, the Barthel index, the modified Rankin scale, and the Glasgow outcome scale. In particular, the NIH stroke scale is a standardized method to measure the level of impairment in brain function due to stroke, including consciousness, vision, sensation, movement, speech, and language. The score is in the range of 0–42, with a higher value indicating a more severe impairment, and the repeated measurements are available at 2 hours post treatment, 24 hours, 7–10 days, and 3 months poststroke onset. The modified Rankin scale, which is a simplified overall assessment of function, is in an ordinal scale with six levels: no symptoms, no significant disability despite symptoms, slight disability, moderate disability, moderately severe disability, and severe disability. It was recorded at baseline, 7–10 days, 3 months, 6 months, and 12 months poststroke onset.

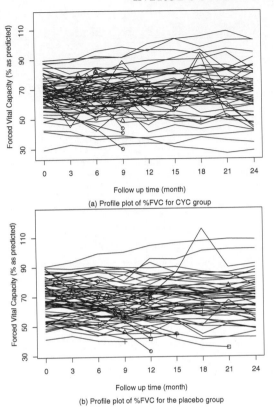

Figure 1.1 *(a)–(b) Profile plots of %FVC for CYC group vs. placebo group: ○ for treatment failure or death; + for early discontinuation of assigned treatment without %FVC measurements after the events; △ for early discontinuation of assigned treatment with %FVC measurements after the events; □ for noninformatively censored events.*

There were 25 informative dropouts before 12 months (14 in rt-PA group and 11 in the placebo) and 168 deaths (78 in rt-PA group and 90 in the placebo group, including those who died after 12 months). In addition, we observed 54 treatment failures, of which 17 died later. A treatment failure occurred if the patient remained in severe disability in two consecutive visits after treatment initiation. Table 1.3 summarizes the primary variables in this study. Treatment failure or death and informative dropout are two competing events. Figure 1.3 indicates that treatment failure or death tended to have a higher cumulative incidence rate than dropout in both groups. The average number of measurements (including the baseline) per patient is 4.2, and 30% of the data are missing in the modified Rankin scale at 12 months. As shown in Table 1.4, the placebo group had a slightly higher rate of missing data

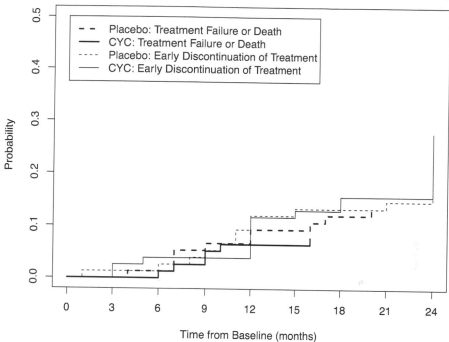

Figure 1.2 *Cumulative incidence functions for the two competing risks: (1) treatment failure or death and (2) early discontinuation of treatment in the scleroderma lung study.*

than the rt-PA group. Around 68% patients completed the study and the monotone missing data, which were caused by deaths and dropouts, are far more frequent than intermittent missingness.

The effect of rt-PA can be evaluated by comparing modified Rankin scale and/or the NIH stroke scale between the two treatment arms, but the validity of regression analysis for longitudinal measurements using available data could be compromised due to missing values following death and dropouts. Therefore, it is important to examine the missing data mechanism and its impact on statistical inference for treatment effect. The NIH stroke data are used in Chapter 2 to illustrate standard approaches to longitudinal analysis assuming ignorable missingness. The modified Rankin scale data are used in Example 5.3 to illustrate joint analysis for ordinal longitudinal data with missing values caused by competing risks. The Barthel index data are used in Example 7.5 for variable selection in joint models.

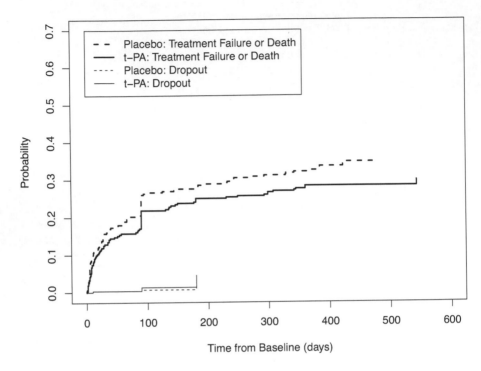

Figure 1.3 *Cumulative incidence functions for the two competing risks: (1) treatment failure or death and (2) informative dropout in the rt-PA study.*

Table 1.3 *Primary variables in the NINDS rt-PA trial.*

	Name	Data type
Primary endpoint	NIH stroke scale	Repeated measurements
	Modified Rankin scale	Repeated measurements
	Treatment failure or death	Time-to-event data
Baseline covariate	Baseline NIH stroke scale	
	Baseline modified Rankin scale	
	Small vessel occlusive disease	
	Large vessel atherosclerosis/ cardioembolic stroke	

Table 1.4 *Summary of completers and non-completers in the NINDS rt-PA trial.*

	rt-PA group		Placebo group	
	Frequency	%	Frequency	%
Completers	217	69.6%	207	66.3%
Monotone missingness	88	28.2%	96	30.8%
Intermittent missingness	7	2.2%	9	2.9%

1.1.3 ENABLE II Study

The ENABLE II study is a randomized clinical trial comparing a nurse-led, phone-based palliative care to the usual care in 322 advanced cancer patients (N = 161 in each group) [17, 16]. The main outcomes of the study included quality of life (QOL, measured by the Functional Assessment of Chronic Illness Therapy for Palliative Care), symptom intensity, and depression. Patients were enrolled in between November 2003 and May 2007, and were followed until May 2008.

Repeated measurements of QOL were recorded as baseline, 1 month, and every 3 months until death or study completion. The scores had a range of 0–184, with a higher value indicating a better QOL. The profiles of QOL shown in Figure 1.4 are truncated by either death or censoring time. Two hundred and thirty-one patients died by the end of the study. The cumulative hazard of death (Figure 1.5) suggests that a two-piece exponential distribution with a change point in the hazard rate at 13 months may provide a reasonable fit to the data.

One objective of this study is to characterize and compare the trajectories of QOL in the palliative and usual care groups over a period shortly before death. A terminal decline model, as illustrated in Example 4.7, has been developed to analyze the data.

1.1.4 Milk Protein Trial

In this study, a total of 79 cows were randomized into three diet groups, barley (N = 25), mixed barley-lupins (N = 27), and lupins (N = 27). The longitudinal outcome was protein content (measured by %) in the milk, which was recorded weekly up to 19 weeks. Dropout occurred when the cows stopped producing milk prior to the end of the study, so the missing data pattern was monotone. There were 38 (48%) dropouts, evenly distributed across groups. All dropouts took place from week 15 onward, so the response profiles shown in Figure 1.6

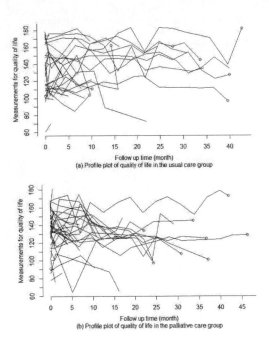

Figure 1.4 *Profile plot of QOL by treatment groups. Deaths are indicated by circles.*

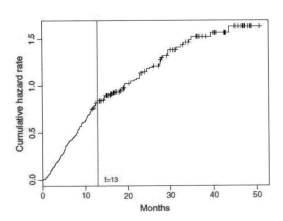

Figure 1.5 *Cumulative hazard rate of death.*

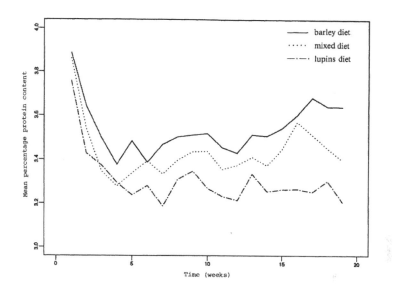

Figure 1.6 *Observed mean of the milk protein data.*

were calculated using cows still producing milk at each time point. There is clearly a nonlinear time trend in the milk production.

This data set is analyzed in Example 4.8 to examine the impact of missing data on the statistical inference of diet effect, and in Example 7.2 to illustrate the use of an index to measure the overall sensitivity of milk protein estimation in the neighborhood of a model that assumes ignorable missingness. More details of the study can be found in Verbyla and Cullis (1990)[224] and Diggle and Kenward (1994)[54].

1.1.5 ACTG study

AIDS Clinical Trials Group (ACTG) Protocol 175 is a randomized trial conducted on 2467 HIV-infected patients to compare four therapies: zidovudine alone, zidovudine + didanosine, zidovudine + zalcitabine, and didanosine alone [86]. The patients were recruited between December 1991 and October 1992, and followed until November 1994. The primary outcome of the study was time to progression to AIDS or death. Out of the 2467 patients 308 events were observed. During follow-up, absolute CD4 lymphocyte cell

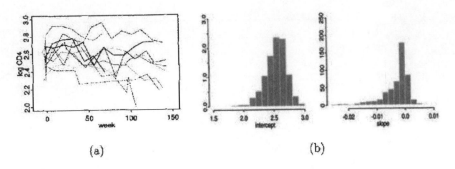

Figure 1.7 *(a) Trajectories of log$_{10}$ CD4 for 10 randomly selected subjects. (b) Histograms of subject-specific intercept and slope estimates from simple least-squares fits.*

counts were measured approximately every 12 weeks and the average number of measurements per subject was 8.2. Figure 1.7(a) shows the trajectories of log-transformed CD4 counts for 10 randomly selected patients. Subject-specific intercept and slope were empirically estimated by least-squares fit of a straight line to each individual, and the histograms of the estimated intercepts and slopes are shown in Figure 1.7(b).

Research interests focus on two questions: (1) Does progression to AIDS or death correlate with CD4 counts? (2) What is the predicted time to progression or death for a new patient given the available data? To answer these questions one usually fits Cox regression models, treating CD4 counts as a time-dependent covariate. Calculation of the partial likelihood requires that CD4 counts be available at all observed event times, which, however, can only be measured intermittently in practice. Imputing the missing data by the last observed value is not an appealing approach since it is well known that CD4 counts are highly variable and subject to measurement error.

This study is used in Example 4.12 to illustrate a joint model in which the association between CD4 counts and time to progression or death is more appropriately characterized. Since the subject-specific slope may not follow a normal distribution, as suggested by Figure 1.7(b), the joint model accommodates a flexible class of smooth densities for the subject-specific (random) intercept and slope of CD4 counts, thus relaxing the commonly used normality assumption.

1.1.6   Medfly Fecundity Data

The original study consisted of 1000 female Mediterranean fruit flies (medflies) on whom daily egg production was recorded until death [31, 212]. It is of interest to understand the longitudinal pattern of daily egg laying and its

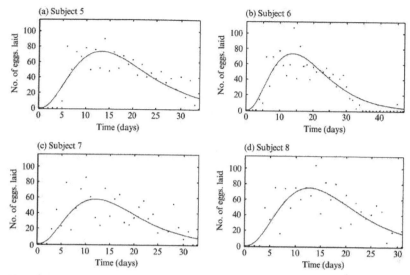

Fig. 2: Medfly data. Individual profiles are fitted by the gamma function. Number of eggs laid by (a) subject 5 is fitted by $t^{2.710}e^{-0.204t}$, (b) subject 6 by $t^{2.652}e^{-0.193t}$, (c) subject 7 by $t^{2.725}e^{-0.226t}$, and (d) subject 8 by $t^{2.803}e^{-0.221t}$. The shape and scale parameters are obtained by least squares.

Figure 1.8 *Medfly data. Individual profiles are fitted by the gamma function.*

relationship with longevity. The profile plots of the number of eggs laid each day from four individual flies are shown in Figure 1.8, where the solid curves were fitted using the Gamma function.

In the illustration given in Example 4.14, a joint analysis is used to characterize the number of eggs laid each day for a subset of most fertile medflies (N = 251). One interesting feature of the data is that the proportional hazards assumption for the survival time does not seem to be reasonable. As a result, an accelerated failure time model is used in the joint analysis. In these 251 flies, the number of observation days per medfly ranged from 22 to 99, which were also the survival times of the flies since there were no censored events or missing data. Additionally, Example 4.14 uses an artificially created incomplete data set of the same medflies population to illustrate the performance of the joint model when there are irregularly spaced, incomplete longitudinal measurements and censored survival times.

1.1.7 Bladder Cancer Study

The bladder cancer study included 85 patients with superficial bladder tumors [205]. At the study entry, the tumors were removed transurethrally. These patients received either placebo (N = 47) or thiotepa treatment (N = 38) and were followed for tumor recurrence. Data on each patient include the number

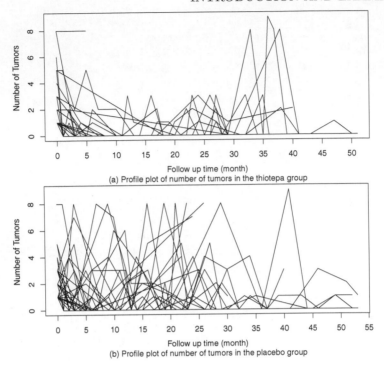

Figure 1.9 *(a)–(b) Profile plots for the number of tumors in the thiotepa group vs. the placebo group.*

of tumors at entry, the size of the largest initial tumor, the clinical visit or observation times (in months), and the number of recurrent bladder tumors between clinical visits. Many patients experienced multiple recurrences during follow-up. Note recurrent tumors were removed at clinical visits. One of the study objectives was to assess the effects of thiotepa treatment and the number of initial tumors on bladder tumor recurrence. The size of the largest initial tumor had been shown to have no effect.

There is a wide range of the number of clinical visits, with the smallest being 1 and the largest 38. The longest observation time was 53 months. Figure 1.9 displays the profile plot of the number of tumors over time for each treatment group. The observation times were irregular among individuals. The questions to address include: (1) Was the observation time (or clinical visit) related to tumor recurrence rate? If so, (2) how would it affect estimation of treatment effect on tumor recurrence rates?

The above questions cannot be answered using statistical models for repeated measurements of count data that assume the observation times are independent of tumor recurrence. When the independence assumption is violated, these methods are likely to produce biased estimates of treatment effect. In this situation, it is important to take into account the information on observation times when making inference about the tumor recurrence rate. This data set is used in Example 4.16 to illustrate a joint model for longitudinal outcomes with informative observation times.

1.1.8 Renal Graft Failure Study

In this study, 407 patients with chronic kidney disease received renal transplantations in the hospital of the Catholic University of Leuven (Belgium) between 1983 and 2000, and were followed until graft failure or being censored [186]. Time elapsed from renal transplantation to graft failure was the primary outcome. Of the 407 patients, 126 (31%) experienced a graft failure. During the study follow-up, multiple biomarkers were measured periodically to test kidney conditions: (1) *GFR*, a measure of kidney filtration rate, (2) the blood *hematocrit* level, a measure of the amount of erythropoietin produced by the kidney that regulates red blood cell production, and (3) a binary variable *proteinuria* to indicate whether the kidney was preventing important proteins from leaking into the urine. These markers are endogenous, stochastic, and measured with error. Figure 1.10 shows their trajectories on five randomly selected patients. It is apparent that there is substantial heterogeneity among subjects and the time trend is nonlinear.

The questions of interest for this study include: (1) What would be an appropriate longitudinal model to characterize the nonlinear biomarker trajectories? (2) Will improved prediction of graft failure be achieved by modeling the joint evolution of the three biomarkers? (3) Since the three biomarkers are biologically interrelated, how can the data correlation be captured in the model? This data set is used in Example 6.1 to illustrate a joint model for multivariate longitudinal outcomes and survival data.

1.1.9 PAQUID Study

This is a prospective cohort study initiated in 1988 to evaluate normal versus pathological aging among subjects 65 and older in France [130, 178]. At the study entry, 2383 subjects were free of dementia, out of whom 355 (14.9%) developed dementia during follow-up. One objective of the study is to investigate the association between cognitive decline and development of dementia. Multiple psychometric tests were conducted to measure cognitive impairment, including the Isaacs Set Test (verbal fluency), the Benton Visual Retention Test (visual memory), and the Digit Symbol Substitution Test of Wechsler (attention and logical reasoning); for all tests, lower values indicate a more severe impairment. The test scores were taken at the initial visit and then at 1, 3, 5, 8, 10, 13 years.

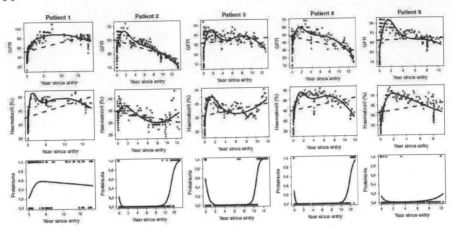

Figure 1.10 *Longitudinal response measurements for GFR, hematocrit, and protein-uria, for five randomly selected patients from the renal graft failure study. The solid lines depict the fitted subject-specific longitudinal profiles based on the multivariate joint model. The dashed lines depict the ordinary least squares fit.*

This study is used in Example 6.2 to illustrate a latent-class joint model that predicts dementia using the three cognitive measures.

1.1.10   Rat Data

Verdonck et al. (1998)[225] conducted a randomized study on male rats to evaluate the craniofacial growth after inhibiting endogenous testosterone production by cecapeptyl. Fifty Wistar rats were randomized into three groups: control (N = 18), low dose of cecapeptyl (N = 17), and high dose of cecapeptyl (N = 15). The rats started receiving treatment at the age of 45 days, and a characterization of the height of the skull was repeatedly measured every 10 days since day 50. Figure 1.11 shows individual growth curves stratified by treatment group.

Because the response was measured under anesthesia and many rats did not survive the procedure, only 22 (44%) completed all seven measurements and the data were missing in a monotone pattern. The Kaplan–Meier curve of survival time is given in Figure 1.12, which indicates that most death occurred after 70 days. The number of deaths was 10 (56%), 7 (41%), and 11 (73%) in the control, low dose, and high dose groups, respectively.

This data set is used in Example 7.1 to illustrate a local influence approach that examines the sensitivity of parameter estimation in a neighborhood of the ignorable missing data assumption.

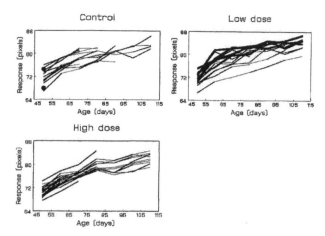

Figure 1.11 *Individual growth curves for the three treatment groups separately. Influential subjects are highlighted.*

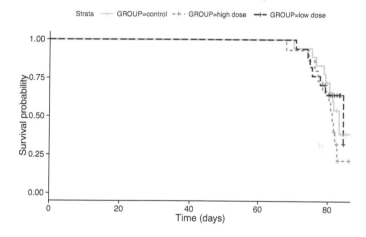

Figure 1.12 *The Kaplan–Meier survival curves for the rat study.*

1.1.11   AIDS Clinical Trial

This is a multicenter, randomized, open-label, community-based clinical trial comparing the efficacy and safety of two antiretroviral drugs, didanosine (ddI) and zalcitabine (ddC) [7, 80]. The study was initiated in December 1990 by the Terry Beirn Community Programs for Clinical Research on AIDS (the acquired immunodeficiency syndrome). In this trial, 467 HIV-infected patients who met entry conditions (either an AIDS diagnosis or two CD4 counts of 300 or fewer, and fulfilling specific criteria for zidovudine (AZT) intolerance or failure) were enrolled and randomly assigned to receive either ddI (500 mg

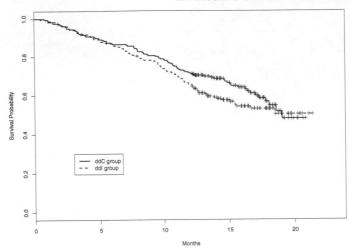

Figure 1.13 *Kaplan–Meier curves for overall survival in the AIDS study.*

per day) or ddC (2.25 mg per day), stratified by clinical unit and by AZT intolerance versus failure. Two hundred and thirty patients were randomized to receive ddI and 237 to ddC. CD4 counts were recorded at study entry, and again at the 2-, 6-, 12-, and 18-month visits.

The median follow-up was 16 months. Death occurred in 100 of 230 patients assigned to ddI and 88 of 237 patients assigned to ddC. Figure 1.13 indicates that the ddI group had a lower survival. The number of measurements for CD4 counts at the five time points was 230, 182, 153, 102, and 22 for the ddI group and 236, 186, 157, 123, and 14 for the ddC group. This sharp increase over time in missing data was due to deaths, dropouts, and missed clinic visits. Boxplots of CD4 counts for the two drug groups showed a severe skewness toward high CD4 counts, suggesting a square root transformation [85].

Data for each patient consists of survival time (months from admission to death or censoring), patient status at the follow-up time (dead = 1, alive = 0), treatment (ddI = 1, ddC = 0), gender (male = 1, female = −1), previous opportunistic infection at study entry (AIDS diagnosis = 1, no AIDS diagnosis = −1), AZT stratum (AZT failure= 1, AZT intolerance = −1), and CD4 counts at the five time points.

As we have discussed in other examples, missing data due to death could lead to biased estimates of CD4 trajectory. Furthermore, when the interest is to select important predictors for CD4 counts, the estimation bias due to missing data would compromise the validity of commonly used variable selection procedures. To address this issue, a variable selection method has been developed within the framework of joint models and the approach is illustrated in Example 7.4.

Chapter 2

Methods for Longitudinal Measurements with Ignorable Missing Data

2.1 Introduction

In longitudinal studies, multiple observations are collected over time on each subject, which is different from cross-sectional studies where a single observation is obtained. The study is said to be *balanced* if all subjects share a common set of observation times and thus have the same number of measurements. Methods for balanced data such as repeated measures ANOVA, repeated measures MANOVA, and summary measure analysis are not readily applicable to unbalanced data, which occur if the subjects have irregularly spaced observations and/or unequal numbers of measurements. In some studies, unbalanced data are caused by missing observations when some subjects miss one or more intended visits. In other cases, irregular timing of measurements arises when there is random variation of the actual measurement date around the scheduled visit, or the timing is defined relative to a subject-specific benchmark event during follow-up. Both types of unbalanced data can easily be handled using the methods reviewed in this chapter, assuming the observation times are non-informative. In Chapter 4 we discuss methods to analyze unbalanced data when the observation times are informative.

As has been noted, analysis of longitudinal data with missing observations must rely on certain missing data assumptions. This chapter reviews standard statistical techniques for longitudinal analysis with ignorable missing data. We begin with a survey of missing data mechanisms, and then review linear and generalized linear mixed effects models, generalized estimating equations, methods for multivariate longitudinal data, and missing data imputation.

2.2 Missing Data Mechanisms

The taxonomy to describe assumptions concerning missing data mechanisms was first introduced in Rubin (1976)[193]. A more systematic and comprehen-

17

sive description of missing data theory and applications is provided by Little and Rubin (2014)[153]. Diggle and Kenward (1994)[54] and Little (1995)[152] discussed missing data issues in longitudinal studies. Daniels and Hogan (2008) [49] provides a nice overview of methods for handling missing data in longitudinal studies generated by ignorable and nonignorable missingness mechanisms.

Assume the response Y is scheduled to be observed at times $t_1, \ldots, t_m$, and we denote the longitudinal observation of Y as $Y_1, \ldots, Y_m$. It is very common that one or more observations of Y are missing due to withdrawal from the study, lost to follow-up, missed visits, or death.

To study missing data mechanisms, we define an indicator R_j associated with each Y_j, $j = 1, \ldots, m$, with $R_j = 1$ if Y_j is observed and $R_j = 0$ if Y_j is missing. Here R stands for *response*. The previously mentioned two missing data patterns in longitudinal studies can be expressed in terms of R. In the case of monotone missing pattern, there exists certain $j < m$ such that $R_1 = \cdots = R_j = 1$ and $R_{j+1} = \cdots = R_m = 0$. That is, all responses are observed through time t_j and no responses are available thereafter. In the case of intermittent missing data, if $R_j = 0$ for certain $1 \le j \le m - 1$, there is an occasion k such that $R_k = 1$ and $k > j$.

Let Y_{obs} denote the observed data in the vector $Y = (Y_1, \ldots, Y_m)$ and Y_{mis} the missing components. Each element in the random vector $R = (R_1, \ldots, R_m)$ is either 1 or 0. The missing data mechanism for Y is defined by the conditional distribution of R given Y, which is classified into the following three types.

Definition 2.2.1 *Missing Completely at Random (MCAR)*
If the missingness is independent of both Y_{obs} and Y_{mis}, that is,

$$f(R|Y, X, \theta) = f(R|X, \theta) \tag{2.1}$$

for all covariates X and unknown parameters θ, then the data are called missing completely at random (MCAR).

Note that this assumption does not indicate that the missing pattern is completely random, but that the probability of missingness is not related to the response values. However, it could be dependent on the covariates X. Under the MCAR assumption, the joint distribution of Y and R is given by

$$f(Y, R|X, \phi) = f(Y|X, \phi)f(R|X, \phi),$$

where ϕ is a vector of unknown parameters and θ is a function of ϕ. In practice, an MCAR assumption is often too restrictive in longitudinal studies.

Definition 2.2.2 *Missing at Random (MAR)*
If conditional on the covariates, the missingness is dependent on Y_{obs} but not Y_{mis}, i.e.,

$$f(R|Y, X, \theta) = f(R|Y_{obs}, X, \theta), \tag{2.2}$$

then the data are missing at random (MAR).

The MAR assumption is less restrictive than MCAR, and thus is regarded as more realistic in real applications. When MAR holds, the joint distribution of Y and R can be written as

$$f(Y, R|X, \phi) = f(Y_{obs}, Y_{mis}|X, \phi)f(R|Y_{obs}, X, \phi).$$

If the parameter ϕ can be split further into two distinct components ψ and θ such that

$$f(Y, R|X, \psi, \theta) = f(Y_{obs}, Y_{mis}|X, \psi)f(R|Y_{obs}, X, \theta),$$

the likelihood for (Y_{obs}, R) is thus

$$
\begin{aligned}
f(Y_{obs}, R|X, \psi, \theta) &= \left[\int f(Y_{obs}, Y_{mis}|X, \psi)dY_{mis} \right] f(R|Y_{obs}, X, \theta) \\
&= f(Y_{obs}|X, \psi)f(R|Y_{obs}, X, \theta).
\end{aligned}
$$

Therefore, if ψ and θ are distinct, the inference for ψ based on the full likelihood $f(Y_{obs}, R|X, \psi, \theta)$ should be the same as those based on $f(Y_{obs}|X, \psi)$ since they are proportional. The MAR is thus usually called an *ignorable* missing data mechanism because valid inference about ψ can be solely based on Y_{obs} without modeling $f(R|Y_{obs})$. It is clear that an ignorable missing data mechanism includes MCAR as a special case.

Definition 2.2.3 *Missing not at Random (MNAR)*
Missing data are MNAR if R depends on both Y_{obs} and Y_{mis}, that is,

$$f(R|Y, X, \theta) = f(R|Y_{obs}, Y_{mis}, X, \theta). \qquad (2.3)$$

The missing data are *nonignorable* under MNAR. Valid inference about the population quantities of Y should be based on the full likelihood $f(Y_{obs}, R|X, \psi, \theta)$. Ignoring the missing data mechanism would cause biased estimates and misleading conclusions.

Example 2.1. *Logistic regression of R on Y has been used to model the missing data mechanism in longitudinal measurements with monotone missing patterns. A simple functional form is given by*

$$logit\ P(R_j = 1|R_{j-1} = 1, Y, X, \theta) = \theta_0 + \theta_1 y_{j-1} + \theta_2 y_j.$$

The probability that Y_j is observed at t_j is a function of the responses in the previous and current occasions. Given that this functional form is correctly specified, if $\theta_2 \neq 0$, then the missing data are MNAR. The missing mechanism is MAR if $\theta_2 = 0$ and $\theta_1 \neq 0$, and MCAR if $\theta_2 = 0$ and $\theta_1 = 0$. However, in practice the inference for θ could be affected by the assumed marginal distribution of Y. Sensitivity analysis should be conducted to investigate how sensitive the inference is in regards to modeling assumptions. This topic is discussed in Chapter 7. $\square$

2.3 Linear and Generalized Linear Mixed Effects Models

Analysis of longitudinal data can be approached in two different ways: (1) marginal models, which study the population mean of the outcome over time and covariate effects on the population mean; (2) mixed effects models, which investigate the effects of covariates on subject-specific mean response trajectories. Compared to marginal models, a distinctive aspect of the mixed effects models is that the mean response on a particular subject consists of population characteristics which are shared by all subjects (fixed effects) and subject-specific effects which are unique to each subject (random effects). Mixed effects models have become popular because of the following appealing features. First, mixed effects models explicitly formulate the between-subject and within-subject sources of variation, which enables prediction of response trajectories over time at individual level. Second, all or part of data correlation is induced by random effects. The covariance matrix can be a function of time with a distinctive random effects structure, but usually requires less parameters. Third, mixed effects models are flexible in accommodating unbalanced longitudinal data with different sets of measurement occasions and different lengths of sequences.

In this section we review two main classes of models, starting with linear mixed effects models (LMM) for normally distributed longitudinal data. We then take a look at generalized linear mixed effects models, which is an extension of LMM to exponential families.

2.3.1 Linear Mixed Effects Models

Linear mixed effects models (LMMs) have been a standard approach to analyze normally distributed longitudinal outcome variables. Harville (1976, 1977)[90, 91] introduced the general concept of linear mixed effects models in the context of repeated measures and growth curves. Laird and Ware (1982)[125], Jennrich and Schluchter (1986)[109], and Diggle (1988)[55], among others, proposed the general form of the models for longitudinal data. The asymptotic properties of maximum likelihood estimates and restricted maximum likelihood estimates are provided in Miller (1977)[164], Richardson and Welsh (1994)[182], Jiang (1998)[110], and Chapter 6 of Verbeke and Molenberghs (2001)[223]. This section reviews the general form of LMMs and inference procedures.

General Form of Linear Mixed Effects Models

The linear mixed effects model assumes

$$Y_i = X_i\beta + Z_ib_i + \epsilon_i, \tag{2.4}$$

where Y_i is the outcome vector for subject i with dimension n_i, and X_i and Z_i are $n_i \times p$ and $n_i \times q$ matrices of known covariates, $i = 1, \ldots, n$. Let $N = \sum_{i=1}^{n} n_i$. Usually the columns of Z_i are a subset of the columns in X_i such that $q \leq p$. The parameter β is a p-dimensional vector of regression coefficients called the fixed effects, and b_i is a q-dimensional vector called the subject-specific random effects. It is assumed that $b_i \sim N_q(0, D)$, which is a q-dimension normal variable with zero mean and variance-covariance matrix D. The error term ϵ_i is assumed to follow a n_i-dimension normal distribution $N_{n_i}(0, \Omega_i)$. The matrix Ω_i, together with D, is determined by a set of unknown parameters θ. For example, if b_i is a random intercept and the error terms are assumed to be mutually independent, we can then write $D = \sigma_b^2$ and $\Omega_i = \sigma_\epsilon^2 I_{n_i}$, where I_{n_i} is the identity matrix of dimension n_i. It follows that $\theta = (\sigma_b^2, \sigma_\epsilon^2)$, or it can be reparameterized as (σ_b^2, ρ), where the intra-class correlation coefficient ρ is defined as $\sigma_b^2 / (\sigma_b^2 + \sigma_\epsilon^2)$.

Equation (2.4) can be regarded as a linear regression model in which some regression coefficients are subject-specific (b_i) and others are not (β). The model implies that, marginally, Y_i follows a normal distribution with mean $X_i \beta$ and variance-covariance matrix $V_i = Z_i D Z_i^T + \Omega_i$. The random effects b_i can be interpreted as residuals to express unit-specific trends deviating from the population mean. The simplest form of Ω_i is $\sigma^2 I_{n_i}$.

We drop the index i and rewrite the model as $Y = X\beta + Zb + \epsilon$, where X and Z are block diagonal matrices with blocks X_i and Z_i, respectively, and together with vectors Y, b, and ϵ, they represent the matrices and vectors that collect information from all study subjects. The variance-covariance matrix of Y is $V = ZDZ^T + \Omega$, where D and Ω are block diagonal matrices with blocks D and Ω_i, respectively.

Estimation and Inference

Statistical estimation and inference for linear mixed models can be based on likelihood approaches. Here we focus on two methods: maximum likelihood (ML) and restricted maximum likelihood (REML), both of which assume that the missing data in Y are missing at random. These two methods are implemented in standard statistical packages such as SAS, R, and STATA.

A classical approach to obtain the ML and REML estimates of β and θ is based on the marginal distribution of the longitudinal outcome. The difference between ML and REML essentially stems from maximization of different objective functions with respect to θ, the unknown parameters in D and Ω. The ML estimate of θ, denoted as $\hat{\theta}_M$, is obtained by maximizing

$$l(\theta) = -\frac{1}{2}log|V| - \frac{1}{2}r^T V^{-1} r - \frac{N}{2}log(2\pi), \qquad (2.5)$$

where $r = Y - X(X^T V^{-1} X)^- X^T V^{-1} Y$. This is the log-likelihood function based on the marginal distribution of the longitudinal outcome after profiling out the fixed effects β.

Maximizing (2.5) provides $\hat{\theta}_M$, and thus $\hat{D}$ and $\hat{\Omega}$, the maximum likelihood estimates of θ, D, and Ω. Then $\hat{\beta}$ and $\hat{b}$ can be obtained by solving the linear equations

$$
\begin{bmatrix} X^T \hat{\Omega}^{-1} X & X^T \hat{\Omega}^{-1} Z \\ Z^T \hat{\Omega}^{-1} X & \hat{D}^{-1} + Z^T \hat{\Omega}^{-1} Z \end{bmatrix} \begin{bmatrix} \beta \\ b \end{bmatrix} = \begin{bmatrix} X^T \hat{\Omega}^{-1} Y \\ Z^T \hat{\Omega}^{-1} Y \end{bmatrix},
$$

and the solutions are

$$
\begin{aligned}
\hat{\beta} &= (X^T \hat{V}^{-1} X)^- X^T \hat{V}^{-1} Y \\
\hat{b} &= \hat{D} Z^T \hat{V}^{-1} (Y - X\hat{\beta}),
\end{aligned} \tag{2.6}
$$

where $\hat{b}$ is known as the empirical "best linear unbiased predictor" (empirical BLUP). Since $\hat{b} = E[b|Y, \hat{\beta}, \hat{\theta}]$, it is also an empirical Bayes estimate of b. The standard error of $\hat{\beta}$ is derived from

$$
Var(\hat{\beta}) = (X^T \hat{V}^{-1} X)^-. \tag{2.7}
$$

We denote A^- as an arbitrary generalized inverse of A.

However, $\hat{\theta}_M$ derived from (2.5) is a biased estimator of θ under finite samples since it does not take into account the loss in degrees of freedom from estimating β. The REML method is proposed to correct this bias:

$$
l_R(\theta) = -\frac{1}{2} log|V| - \frac{1}{2} log|X^T V^{-1} X| - \frac{1}{2} r^T V^{-1} r - \frac{N - p}{2} log(2\pi). \tag{2.8}
$$

We denote the resulting estimator of θ as $\hat{\theta}_R$. The estimate of β and b under REML will then be obtained by following the similar approach as outlined for ML.

Statistical inference concerning β and θ can be carried out using Wald's tests or likelihood ratio tests. The asymptotic standard error of $\hat{\theta}$ is derived from the Hessian of the likelihood function. It has been shown that the REML estimate of θ obtained from (2.8) is jointly asymptotic normal with $\hat{\beta}$ in (2.6). In addition, the empirical distribution of the estimated random effects by (2.6) converges to their true distribution.

Assuming the functional form of the likelihood is correctly specified, likelihood-based methods using observed data are valid if the missing data are MAR and the response model parameters and missing data mechanism parameters are distinct. In the presence of nonignorable missing data, these methods would produce biased estimates.

Note that linear mixed effects models as presented above assume a normal distribution for the measurement error term ϵ_i in (2.4), which may not be robust when ϵ_i has longer than normal tails or there is other form of deviations from normality. In the first case, a t-distribution can be used to obtain robust inference [127]. This generalization of linear mixed effects models can also be applied to the random effects b_i. Alternatively, nonparametric approaches can be employed to deal with other non-normal features such as multimodality or skewness [131]. This topic will be revisited in joint models discussed in Chapters 4 and 5.

After fitting a linear mixed effects model, it is necessary to identify outliers and assess the adequacy of model fit. Different from regression models with independent observations, residuals derived from linear mixed effects models are correlated because of within-subject dependence among the measurements. However, residual analysis developed for independent observations can, in principle, be applied to longitudinal settings using transformed residuals, which are calculated as $r_i^* = L_i^{-1} r_i = L_i^{-1}(Y_i - X_i \hat{\beta})$ where L_i is a lower triangular matrix obtained from the Cholesky decomposition that satisfies $L_i L_i^T = \hat{V}_i$. Another method called *semivariogram* can be used to check the model fit for assumptions in data variances and correlations. Further information on residual diagnostics in longitudinal studies can be found in Waternaux et al. (1989)[231] and Waternaux and Ware (1992)[232]; also see Chapter 3 of Diggle et al.[56] for the use of semivariogram.

Example 2.2. *The Scleroderma Lung Study*

We illustrate linear mixed effects models using the scleroderma lung study [207]. Procedure MIXED in SAS was used to analyze the data. As introduced in Chapter 1, the scleroderma lung study is a double-blinded, randomized clinical trial to evaluate effectiveness of oral cyclophosphamide (CYC) versus placebo in the treatment of lung disease due to scleroderma. One hundred and fifty-eight patients were randomized to receive either CYC (2 mg/kg) (79 patients) or an identical-appearing placebo (79 patients) for 12 months. A second year of follow-up was performed to determine if the CYC effect persisted after stopping treatment.

The primary outcome was forced vital capacity (FVC, as % predicted), determined at 3-month intervals from baseline. The %FVC measurements were unbalanced due to skipped visits, dropout before completion, or death. The average number of visits per patient was 7.3 in the two-year follow-up period (including the baseline visit). Because of the dose-escalation protocol for CYC in the first 6 months and the anticipated delay in treatment effect, %FVC measured at 6–24 months was used in the analysis.

Our preliminary analysis revealed that change in %FVC over time was highly influenced by its baseline value FVC_0 and degree of lung fibrosis FIB_0 (also measured at baseline). We calculated the %FVC score at 6 - 24 months adjusted for baseline %FVC and fibrosis. The calculation was based on a regression model that used FVC_0, FIB_0, and cubic splines for time to predict the longitudinal measurements %FVC. As shown in Figure 2.1, the CYC group

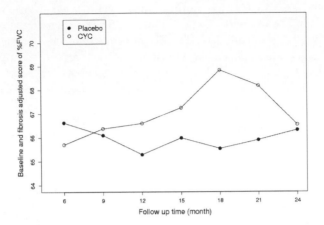

Figure 2.1 *Mean of adjusted %FVC scores in each group.*

had a steady increase up to 18 months, followed by a fast decline from 18 months to 24 months. This indicates that the effect of CYC persisted for half a year after the treatment was stopped. On the other hand, the placebo group had no substantial change in %FVC.

Based on the above observation, in our analysis we considered the following linear mixed model with piecewise linear splines to characterize the change in %FVC:

$$
\begin{aligned}
\%FVC_{ij} = \ & \beta_0 + \beta_1 FVC_{0i} + \beta_2 FIB_{0i} + \beta_3 CYC_i + \beta_4 CYC_i \times FIB_{0i} \\
& + \beta_5 t_{ij} + \beta_6 (t_{ij} - 18)_+ + \beta_7 CYC_i \times t_{ij} + \beta_8 CYC_i \times (t_{ij} \\
& - 18)_+ + b_{1i} + b_{2i} t_{ij} + b_{3i} (t_{ij} - 18)_+ + \epsilon_{ij}, \quad\quad (2.9)
\end{aligned}
$$

where CYC_i is a binary group indicator, $(t_{ij} - 18)_+ = t_{ij} - 18$ if $t_{ij} > 18$ and $(t_{ij} - 18)_+ = 0$ if $t_{ij} \leq 18$, $b_i = (b_{1i}, b_{2i}, b_{3i})$ are random effects, and ϵ_{ij} are assumed to be i.i.d. random errors. We did not include a random intercept because FVC_0 explained most of data variation at baseline. The co-variates FVC_{0i} and FIB_{0i} were centered at their means. This model also tests interaction between FIB_0 and treatment. In the placebo group, the mean slope in %FVC from baseline to 18 months is β_5, and is $\beta_5 + \beta_6$ after 18 months. The mean slope is $\beta_5 + \beta_7$ before 18 months in the CYC group, and is $\beta_5 + \beta_6 + \beta_7 + \beta_8$ 18 to 24 months.

Table 2.1 shows the REML estimates for the fixed and random effects. %FVC scores were highly correlated with the baseline value and lung fibrosis. The Wald's test statistic for the null hypothesis $H_0 : \beta_3 = \beta_4 = \beta_7 = \beta_8 = 0$ was 6.62 with 4 degrees of freedom ($p = 0.16$), indicating that CYC did not have a significant effect on %FVC. The test for between-group difference in the linear slopes ($H_0 : \beta_7 = \beta_8 = 0$) yielded a p-value of 0.20. The second part of the *table shows estimated variances and covariances for the random effects. There was a larger variation in the slope of %FVC from 18 to 24 months relative to 0–18 months.*

Table 2.1 *Estimated fixed and random effects for %FVC.*

Parameter	Estimate	SE	p-value
Fixed Effects			
$Intercept$	66.523	0.912	<0.0001
FVC_0	0.971	0.039	<0.0001
FIB_0	−1.623	0.601	0.0072
CYC_i	−1.290	1.288	0.3170
$CYC_i \times FIB_0$	1.556	0.866	0.0730
t_{ij}	−0.108	0.102	0.2901
$(t_{ij} - 18)_+$	−0.030	0.209	0.8861
$CYC_i \times t_{ij}$	0.239	0.143	0.0950
$CYC_i \times (t_{ij} - 18)_+$	−0.485	0.292	0.0975
$H_0 : \beta_3 = \beta_4 = \beta_7 = \beta_8 = 0$			0.1574
Random Effects			
$Var(b_{1i})$	22.717		
$Var(b_{2i})$	0.433		
$Var(b_{3i})$	1.091		
$Cov(b_{1i}, b_{2i})$	−1.724		
$Cov(b_{1i}, b_{3i})$	1.608		
$Cov(b_{2i}, b_{3i})$	−0.516		
$Var(\epsilon_{ij})$	15.947		

Note that the model assumes the missing data in %FVC are MAR, which could be violated due to death and disease-related dropout. Analyses under the MNAR assumption are conducted in Chapter 5 via the joint model approach. □

Example 2.3. *The NINDS rt-PA Stroke Study*

The NINDS rt-PA trial of intravenous recombinant tissue plasminogen activator (rt-PA) recruited a total of 624 patients with acute ischemic stroke and randomized them into either rt-PA or placebo group. One primary endpoint was the NIH storke scale (NIHSS), which was recorded at 2 hours post-treatment, and 24 hours, 7–10 days, and 3 months poststroke onset. Due to death and dropout during study follow-up, we observed around 20% missing data at 3 months. Data were square-root transformed to reduce skewness.

The following covariates were considered in the analysis: treatment group (rt-PA or placebo), NIH stroke scale at baseline, and three subtypes of acute stroke (small vessel occlusive disease, large vessel atherosclerosis or cardioembolic stroke, and unknown reasons). An unstructured time trend was assumed. The model included three dummy variables, timehr24, timeday710, and timem3, for measurements at 24 hours, 7–10 days, and 3 months poststroke onset. Specifically, the model is given by

$$
\begin{aligned}
\%NIHSS_{ij} = \ & \beta_0 + \beta_1 NIHSS_{0i} + \beta_2 small_i + \beta_3 large_i + \beta_4 timehr24 \\
& + \beta_5 timeday710 + \beta_6 timem3 + \beta_7 group_i + \beta_8 group_i \\
& \times small_i + \beta_9 group_i \times large_i + b_{1i} timehr24 \\
& + b_{2i} timeday710 + b_{3i} timem3 + \epsilon_{ij},
\end{aligned} \tag{2.10}
$$

where random effects b_{1i}, b_{2i}, and b_{3i} were used to capture between-subject variation at the three time points. Interaction between treatment and disease subtype was included as suggested by the preliminary analysis.

Table 2.2 shows estimated parameters for model (2.10). NIHSS scores were significantly correlated with baseline measurements and decreased significantly over time. The average square-root transformed NIHSS scores were 0.183 lower at 24 hours post stroke onset compared to that at 2 hours, and were 0.543 and 0.999 lower at 7–10 days and 3 months, respectively. The treatment was not as effective for large vessel or cardioembolic stroke patients as for patients with unknown reasons, and there was no significant difference in the treatment effects between patients with small vessel and those with unknown reasons. For patients with unknown reasons, the average square-root transformed NIHSS was 0.523 lower (p < 0.0001) comparing the rt-PA group to placebo. In contrast, among the large vessel or cardioembolic stroke patients, the between-group difference reduced to $0.523 - 0.303 = 0.220$ (p = 0.0011). The overall treatment effect was tested by $H_0 : \beta_7 = \beta_8 = \beta_9 = 0$, which yielded a p < 0.0001. □

2.3.2 Generalized Linear Mixed Effects Models

Generalized linear mixed effects models (GLMMs) are an extension of generalized linear models by incorporating random regression coefficients to characterize within-subject correlations in longitudinal or clustered data. GLMMs also extend linear mixed effects models to a rich class of distributions, which can be generally expressed in the form of exponential families conditional on random coefficients. A distinctive feature of GLMMs is that the fixed effects may no longer have a marginal interpretation. In addition, the computational burden increases substantially in GLMMs. References for generalized linear mixed models include Williams (1982)[235], Wong and Mason (1985)[237], Schall (1991)[197], and Breslow and Clayton (1993)[24].

Table 2.2 *Estimated fixed effects and covariance of the random effects for NIH stroke scale (square root transformed).*

Parameter	Estimate	SE	p-value
Fixed Effects			
$Intercept$	3.536	0.074	<0.0001
$NIHSS_0$	0.964	0.029	<0.0001
$small\ vessel$	−0.119	0.138	0.3904
$large\ vessel$	−0.045	0.086	0.6022
$timehr24$	−0.183	0.057	0.0014
$timeday710$	−0.543	0.066	<0.0001
$timem3$	−0.999	0.065	<0.0001
$group$	−0.523	0.102	<0.0001
$group \times small\ vessel$	0.261	0.193	0.1776
$group \times large\ vessel$	0.303	0.122	0.0131
$H_0 : \beta_7 = \beta_8 = \beta_9 = 0$			<0.0001
Random Effects			
$Var(b_{1i})$	0.635		
$Var(b_{2i})$	1.202		
$Var(b_{3i})$	1.011		
$Cov(b_{1i}, b_{2i})$	1.231		
$Cov(b_{1i}, b_{3i})$	0.967		
$Cov(b_{2i}, b_{3i})$	1.410		
$Var(\epsilon_{ij})$	0.636		

Model Assumptions

We assume each subject is associated with a vector of random coefficients (effects) b_i. Let Y_{ij} denote the observation on subject i at occasion j, $j = 1, \ldots, n_i$, $i = 1, \ldots, n$. Conditional on the random effects b_i, Y_{ij} are assumed to follow a distribution in the exponential family with probability density function

$$f(y_{ij}|b_i, \beta, \phi) = exp\{[y_{ij}\theta_{ij} - a(\theta_{ij}) + c(y_{ij})]\phi\},$$

where θ_{ij} and ϕ are parameters and $a(\cdot)$ and $c(\cdot)$ are known functions. Based on the theory of exponential families, the conditional mean and variance of Y_{ij} are $\mu_{ij} = E(Y_{ij}|b_i, \beta, \phi) = a'(\theta_{ij})$ and $v_{ij} = var(Y_{ij}|b_i, \beta, \phi) = a''(\theta_{ij})/\phi$, respectively. Here we use $a'(\cdot)$ and $a''(\cdot)$ to denote the first and second derivatives of $a(\cdot)$.

Difference from linear mixed effects models, GLMMs model the mean of Y through a one-to-one continuous differentiable transformation $\eta_{ij} = g(\mu_{ij})$ and assume that the transformed mean is characterized by a linear model, i.e., $\eta_{ij} = x_{ij}^T\beta + z_{ij}^T b_i$, where η_{ij} is the *linear predictor* and $g(\cdot)$ is the *link function*. Similar to linear mixed effects models, the parameter β represents fixed effects of x_{ij}, and the random coefficients b_i are subject-specific effects of z_{ij} to account for between-subject heterogeneity and within-subject correlations. The random effects b_i are usually assumed to follow a multivariate normal distribution with zero mean and variance-covariance matrix D and, moreover, are assumed to be independent of the covariates.

Special cases of exponential families include normal, binomial, Poisson, exponential, gamma, and inverse Gaussian distributions. For example, the dispersion parameter ϕ equals 1 for binomial distributions and the link function $g(\mu_{ij})$ is $log\frac{\mu_{ij}}{1-\mu_{ij}}$. For the normal distribution $Y_{ij} \sim N(\mu_{ij}, \sigma^2)$, we have $\phi = 1/\sigma^2$ and $g(\mu_{ij}) = \mu_{ij}$. When the linear predictor η_{ij} equals the canonical parameter θ_{ij}, the corresponding link function is called a *canonical link*. Identity function is the canonical link for normal distributions and logit is the canonical link for binomial distributions.

Therefore, linear mixed effects models are a special case of GLMMs, in which β has a marginal interpretation because $E(Y_{ij}|\beta) = E\{E(Y_{ij}|b_i,\beta)\} = E(x_{ij}^T\beta + z_{ij}^T b_i) = x_{ij}^T\beta$ given that $E(b_i) = 0$. This indicates that the marginal mean of Y is a linear model with respect to β. However, this relationship is not generally true when the link function $g(\cdot)$ is nonlinear. For other distributions in GLMMs, β is generally interpreted as the impact of covariates on the mean response of a specific subject conditional on the random effects.

Estimation and Inference

In GLMMs, the marginal distribution of Y in general does not have a closed form expression. The likelihood function of β, ϕ, and D is evaluated by integrating the conditional probability distribution over b_i. Specifically, we have

$$L(\beta,\phi,D) = \prod_{i=1}^{n} \int f(Y_i|b_i)f(b_i)db_i$$

$$= \prod_{i=1}^{n} \int \prod_{j=1}^{n_i} f(Y_{ij}|b_i)f(b_i)db_i. \qquad (2.11)$$

Maximum likelihood estimates can be obtained by maximizing (2.11). Because the integration is intractable, several numerical procedures have been proposed to approximate the integral. For example, the Gaussian quadrature approximates the integral as a weighted sum:

$$L(\beta,\phi,D) \approx \prod_{i=1}^{n} \sum_{k=1}^{K} f(Y_i|b_i)f(b_i = v_k)w_k,$$

where v_k and w_k are predetermined evaluation points and weights to provide the approximation at a certain level of accuracy. One can always achieve a higher degree of accuracy by increasing the number of quadrature points K, but at the price of an exponential growth rate of the computational burden. It is recommended to use the minimum K for all parameter estimates and standard errors to be numerically stable. After the likelihood function is approximated at a satisfactory level of accuracy, optimization procedures are carried out to obtain maximum likelihood estimates, and standard errors can be derived in the regular way. Alternative approximation methods other than Gaussian quadrature for estimation in generalized linear mixed models include penalized quasi-likelihood proposed by Stiratelli et al. (1984)[202] and higher-order Laplace approximations described in Breslow and Lin(1995)[25] and Lin and Breslow (1996)[150].

An appealing feature of numerical approximation is that one can do likelihood ratio tests among nested models and compute fit-statistics that are defined based on likelihood functions. However, these methods generally require the dimension of random effects be relatively small for the sake of practical feasibility. This problem is overcomed by linearizing the model via Taylor series expansion. Compared to numerical approximation methods, the linearization-based approaches have the advantage of easy implementation and are capable of dealing with complex random effects structures in a large dimension. However, there could be potential bias in parameter estimates caused by the linearization approximation. Details of estimation and inference are not provided here. We refer the reader to Wolfinger and O'Connell (1993)[236].

2.4 Generalized Estimating Equations

When research interests focus on the marginal mean of longitudinal measurements, so-called generalized estimating equations (GEE) can be used as an alternative to GLMMs. Closely related to qausi-likelihood, the GEE method does not require specification of the full joint distribution of multiple measurements within subjects. Instead, it relies on correct specification of the univariate marginal distribution and adopts a *working* assumption for the correlation structure. Therefore, the GEE method avoids invalid inference about mean parameters resulting from misspecification of the correlation structure, which is an appealing feature compared to fully parametric approaches such as GLMMs. On the other hand, since GEE is an extension of quasi-likelihood methods, it requires the missing data to be MCAR. The method was proposed by Liang and Zeger (1986)[142] and Zeger and Liang (1986)[247]; also see Liang, Zeger, and Qaqish (1992)[144] and Liang and Zeger(1995)[143]. A review of this method is provided by Geys et al.(2002)[8] and Fitzmaurice et al.(2012)[70].

2.4.1   General Theory

For the jth observation on the ith subject Y_{ij}, $j = 1, \ldots, n_i$, $i = 1, \ldots, n$, the marginal density is assumed to take the form of an exponential family

$$f(y_{ij}|\beta, \phi) = exp\{[y_{ij}\theta_{ij} - a(\theta_{ij}) + c(y_{ij})]\phi\}, \tag{2.12}$$

where θ_{ij} is a function of μ_{ij}, the marginal mean of Y_{ij}. The linear predictor $\eta_{ij} = g(\mu_{ij}) = x_{ij}^T \beta$. Denote $Y_i = (Y_{i1}, \ldots, Y_{in_i})^T$ and $\mu_i = (\mu_{i1}, \ldots, \mu_{in_i})^T$. In the setting of generalized linear models that assume independence among all observations, the score equation to estimate the maximum likelihood estimate of β is

$$\sum_{i=1}^{n} (\frac{\partial \mu_i}{\partial \beta})^T (A_i^{1/2} I_{n_i} A_i^{1/2})^{-1} (Y_i - \mu_i) = 0, \tag{2.13}$$

where A_i is a diagonal matrix with v_{ij}, the marginal variance of Y_{ij}, as the diagonal elements and I_{ni} is the n_i dimensional identity matrix. By adopting a *working* correlation matrix G_i, the GEE method extends equation (2.13) to account for association within subjects:

$$\sum_{i=1}^{n} (\frac{\partial \mu_i}{\partial \beta})^T (A_i^{1/2} G_i A_i^{1/2})^{-1} (Y_i - \mu_i) = 0. \tag{2.14}$$

The working covariance matrix is thus $V_i = A_i^{1/2} G_i A_i^{1/2}$. Denote α the vector of unknown parameters in the correlation matrix G_i.

Under mild regularity conditions, the estimator $\hat{\beta}$ obtained by solving (2.14) is asymptotically normal with mean β and covariance matrix

$$[\sum_{i=1}^{n} (\frac{\partial \mu_i}{\partial \beta})^T V_i^{-1} \frac{\partial \mu_i}{\partial \beta}]^{-1} [\sum_{i=1}^{n} (\frac{\partial \mu_i}{\partial \beta})^T V_i^{-1} Var(Y_i) V_i^{-1} \frac{\partial \mu_i}{\partial \beta}]$$

$$\times [\sum_{i=1}^{n} (\frac{\partial \mu_i}{\partial \beta})^T V_i^{-1} \frac{\partial \mu_i}{\partial \beta}]^{-1}. \tag{2.15}$$

Valid statistical inference for β requires correct model assumptions for the first order moments of Y, but not the correlation matrix G. However, the choice of G could affect the efficiency of $\hat{\beta}$.

In real applications, the estimates $\hat{\beta}$, $\hat{\alpha}$, and $\hat{\phi}$ can be obtained from an iterative procedure. Given current estimates of α and ϕ, β can be updated from modified Fisher scoring:

$$\hat{\beta}^{t+1} = \hat{\beta}^t + [\sum_{i=1}^{n} (\frac{\partial \mu_i}{\partial \beta})^T |_{\beta = \hat{\beta}^t} V_i^{-1}(\hat{\beta}^t) (\frac{\partial \mu_i}{\partial \beta}) |_{\beta = \hat{\beta}^t}]^{-1}$$

$$\cdot [\sum_{i=1}^{n} (\frac{\partial \mu_i}{\partial \beta})^T |_{\beta = \hat{\beta}^t} V_i^{-1}(\hat{\beta}^t) (Y_i - \mu_i(\hat{\beta}^t)]. \tag{2.16}$$

Given the current estimate of β, Pearson residuals are calculated by

$$\hat{r}_{ij} = (Y_{ij} - \hat{\mu}_{ij})/\sqrt{\hat{v}_{ij}}.$$

Let $N = \sum_{i=1}^{n} n_i$, then ϕ is estimated by

$$\hat{\phi}^{-1} = \sum_{i=1}^{n} \sum_{j=1}^{n_i} \hat{r}_{ij}^2 / (N - p).$$

When $G(\alpha)$ is unspecified, it can be estimated by

$$\frac{\hat{\phi}}{n} \sum_{i=1}^{n} \hat{A}_i^{-1/2} (Y_i - \hat{\mu}_i)(Y_i - \hat{\mu}_i)^T \hat{A}_i^{-1/2}.$$

The estimator of α for specific correlation structures, such as the exchangeable correlation and AR(1), can be found in Liang and Zeger (1986)[142]. After α and ϕ are updated, β will then be recalculated using equation (2.16). The iteration is repeated until convergence. The standard error of $\hat{\beta}$ can be estimated using (2.15) by replacing $Var(Y_i)$ with $\frac{1}{n-1}(Y_i - \hat{\mu}_i)(Y_i - \hat{\mu}_i)^T$. This estimation procedure is implemented in SAS Proc GENMOD.

Although the working correlation matrix G does not have to be correctly specified in order to obtain consistent estimates of β, the choice of correlation structure could influence estimation efficiency. Therefore, one needs to specify a working correlation matrix that seems reasonable for a given study. A second order extension of the GEE method by incorporating marginal pairwise association is nearly fully efficient (the so-called GEE2), but similar to GLMMs, misspecification of the association structure in GEE2 could lead to biased estimates.

Example 2.4. *The Scleroderma Lung Study (continued)*

%FVC scores at 6–24 months were analyzed using the GEE method, assuming the same mean structure as in model (2.9). The working correlation matrix was posited to be a stationary m-dependent structure with m = 6, which provided the best fit among the available correlation structures in Proc GENMOD. Note that for normally distributed longitudinal outcomes, the marginal effects are the same as the fixed effects in linear mixed effects models, which makes it feasible to compare the results with those reported in Table 2.1. As we can see, significant interaction effects $CYC_i \times FIB_0$ and $CYC_i \times t_{ij}$ are obtained by the GEE method (Table 2.3). This discrepancy may be the result of different missing data assumptions in the GEE and linear mixed effects models. In this study, MAR seems more reasonable since the missing data were caused by disease-related dropout and death. □

Example 2.5. *The rt-PA Stroke Study (continued)*

A GEE model with the same mean function as specified in (2.10) was fit to the repeated measurements of NIHSS. The working correlation matrix was specified to be AR(1). Table 2.4 indicates that, for most parameters, the point estimates from the GEE method were quite close to those obtained using the linear mixed effects model (Table 2.2). However, the GEE method tends to produce smaller standard errors for the time trend parameters and, at the same time, slightly larger standard errors for the other parameters, so the interaction between treatment and large vessel disease subtype became boundary significant. □

Table 2.3 *Analysis of longitudinal %FVC scores using GEE method with MDEP(6) working correlation matrix.*

Parameter	Estimate	SE	p-value
Intercept	66.452	0.857	<0.0001
FVC_0	1.009	0.053	<0.0001
FIB_0	−1.304	0.604	0.0309
CYC_i	−1.767	1.319	0.1804
$CYC_i \times FIB_0$	2.030	0.901	0.0242
t_{ij}	−0.074	0.090	0.4153
$(t_{ij}\text{-}18)_+$	−0.058	0.172	0.7362
$CYC_i \times t_{ij}$	0.280	0.131	0.0332
$CYC_i \times (t_{ij}\text{-}18)_+$	−0.483	0.292	0.0984

Table 2.4 *Analysis of NIH stroke scale (square root transformed) using the GEE method with AR(1) working correlation matrix.*

Parameter	Estimate	SE	p-value
Intercept	3.530	0.091	<0.0001
$NIHSS_0$	0.959	0.041	<0.0001
small vessel	−0.122	0.159	0.4422
large vessel	−0.054	0.111	0.6293
timehr24	−0.182	0.038	<0.0001
timeday710	−0.559	0.047	<0.0001
timem3	−1.014	0.050	<0.0001
group	−0.533	0.169	0.0016
group × *small vessel*	0.298	0.260	0.2520
group × *large vessel*	0.351	0.192	0.0682

2.4.2   Weighted Generalized Estimating Equations

Weighted generalized estimating equations (weighted GEE) relax the MCAR assumption to allow MAR. This is achieved by incorporating the probability of nonresponse into GEE [189]. Consider monotone missing patterns in the longitudinal measurements $Y_i = (Y_{i1}, \ldots, Y_{in_i})^T$. A vector of indicators $R_i = (R_{i1}, \ldots, R_{in_i})^T$ are defined such that $R_{ij} = 1$ if Y_{ij} is observed, and $R_{ij} = 0$ if Y_{ij} is missing, $j = 1, \ldots, n_i$. Monotone missing patterns imply that if $R_{ij} = 0$ then $R_{ik} = 0$, $k = j+1, \ldots, n_i$. Denote $\bar{W}_{ij} = (X_i, Z_{i0}, Y_{i0}, \ldots, Z_{i(j-1)}, Y_{i(j-1)})$ that collect data information on the entire path right before occasion j, where Z_{ij} is a vector of time-dependent covariates and $X_i = (x_{i1}, \ldots, x_{in_i})^T$. Assume X_i is completely observed even if Y_i is missing for some j. The GEE method described previously relies on the assumption that, given X_i, the missing mechanism does not depend on either the observed or missing (Y_{ij}, Z_{ij}). In what follows, we show how this method can be extended to MAR.

Under the monotone missing pattern, the MAR assumption implies that

$$P(R_{ij} = 1 | R_{i(j-1)} = 1, \bar{W}_{i(m+1)}) = P(R_{ij} = 1 | R_{i(j-1)} = 1, \bar{W}_{ij}), \quad (2.17)$$

where m is the maximum number of occasions per subject. Therefore, when equation (2.17) holds,

$$P(R_{ij} = 1 | R_{i(j-1)} = 1, \bar{W}_{ij}, Y_i) = P(R_{ij} = 1 | R_{i(j-1)} = 1, \bar{W}_{ij}), \quad (2.18)$$

which implies that, given $\bar{W}_{ij}$, among subjects observed at occasion $j-1$, the probability of nonresponse at occasion j is unrelated to the current and future observations of Y.

Let $\bar{\lambda}_{ij} = P(R_{ij} = 1 | R_{i(j-1)} = 1, \bar{W}_{ij})$, and assume there exists a known function of γ and $\bar{W}_{ij}$ such that

$$\bar{\lambda}_{ij} = \bar{\lambda}_{ij}(\gamma). \quad (2.19)$$

The partial maximum likelihood estimator of γ is denoted as $\hat{\gamma}$, which maximizes

$$L(\gamma) = \prod_{i=1}^{n} \prod_{j=1}^{m} \{\bar{\lambda}_{ij}(\gamma)^{R_{ij}} [1 - \bar{\lambda}_{ij}(\gamma)]^{1-R_{ij}}\}^{R_{i(j-1)}}.$$

Note that $\bar{\lambda}_{ij}(\gamma)$ is usually chosen to be a logistic function.

Further define $\bar{\pi}_{ij}(\gamma) = \bar{\lambda}_{i1}(\gamma) \times \cdots \times \bar{\lambda}_{ij}(\gamma)$. Under the MAR assumption in (2.17), $\bar{\pi}_{ij}(\gamma)$ is the conditional probability of observing Y_{ij} given $\bar{W}_{i(m+1)}$. Define a $m \times m$ diagonal matrix $\Delta_i(\gamma)$ with the diagonal elements $\Delta_{ij}(\gamma)$ being $\bar{\pi}_{ij}(\gamma)^{-1} R_{ij}$. The weighted estimating equation is then given by

$$\sum_{i=1}^{n} (\frac{\partial \mu_i}{\partial \beta})^T (A_i^{1/2} G_i A_i^{1/2})^{-1} \Delta_i(\gamma)(Y_i - \mu_i) = 0. \quad (2.20)$$

Compared to (2.14), incorporating $\Delta_i(\gamma)$ is equivalent to weighting each observed residual $Y_{ij} - \mu_{ij}$ by $\bar{\pi}_{ij}(\gamma)^{-1}$. Let $\hat{\beta}$ denote the root of (2.20) in which γ is replaced by its partial maximum likelihood estimate $\hat{\gamma}$. Assuming that $P(R_{ij} = 1 | R_{i(j-1)} = 1, \bar{W}_{ij})$ is bounded away from zero, under (2.12), (2.18), and (2.19), $\hat{\beta}$ is a consistent estimator of the true value β_0 and asymptotically normal.

The above results can be extended to arbitrary missing patterns. More details can be found in Robins, Rotnitzky, and Zhao (1995)[189].

2.5   Further topics

This section briefly reviews three additional topics that are relevant to longitudinal analysis, which include multivariate longitudinal data, pseudo-likelihood methods, and missing data imputation. More details can be found in the references for each topic. Some of the approaches will be revisited later in the context of joint models.

2.5.1   Multivariate Longitudinal Data Analysis

We have focused our discussion on two major approaches, mixed effects models and GEE methods, in the analysis of a univariate longitudinal outcome. However, in medical and social science studies it is commonplace to observe multiple outcomes at each follow-up visit. Collecting information on more than one outcome allows a comprehensive understanding of the effects of important factors and at the same time enables one to study the joint evolution of the outcomes over time. Two sources of correlations need particular attention when formulating the model: the correlation among multiple outcomes at each observation time and the correlation within each outcome over time.

Approaches to modeling multivariate longitudinal data include (1) data dimension reduction, replacing the multiple outcomes using a single summary score, and (2) simultaneous analysis of the outcomes via more sophisticated methods such as GEE or mixed effects models. The missing data mechanism in these methods is either MCAR or MAR, similar to single outcome analyses. Each method has its own pros and cons. A review is provided by Bandyopadhyay et al. (2011)[18].

2.5.2   Pseudo-Likelihood Methods for Longitudinal Data

Pseudo-likelihood methods were initially introduced to overcome estimation and computation difficulty in full likelihood approaches involving nuisance parameters. Their applications include, but are not limited to, longitudinal analysis in which the focus is to make statistical inference about the mean of longitudinal measurements. In a general setting, denote the full likelihood function as $L(\theta, \phi)$, where θ is the parameter of interest and ϕ is a nuisance parameter. The pseudo-likelihood MLE of θ is then obtained by maximizing $L(\theta, \hat{\phi})$, where $\hat{\phi}$ is a convenient estimator of ϕ derived using an approach other than maximum likelihood estimation. In the context of longitudinal analysis, the pseudo-likelihood approach relies on the fact that θ, the parameter concerning the mean of Y, is the focus of statistical inference and estimation of inter-correlations among multiple measurements within subject is of little interest. A pseudo-likelihood for the available data (ignoring missing observations) can then be constructed by treating Y_{ij} as independent observations, forcing the within-subject correlation to be zero. It has been shown that $\hat{\theta}$ obtained from such a pseudo-likelihood is consistent and asymptotically normal if the missingness mechanism is MCAR. The variance of $\hat{\theta}$ can be estimated using the *sandwich* variance estimator. Theoretical results for pseudo-likelihood methods are given in Gong and Samaniego (1991)[81] and Liang and Self (1996)[141].

2.5.3 Missing Data Imputation

In longitudinal analysis, the simplest way to handle missing data is to carry out the analysis using complete cases only, i.e., individuals who complete all prescheduled measurements. This method omits all incomplete longitudinal sequences, and, when the number of incomplete cases is high, there is substantial information loss. As a consequence, complete case analysis is often criticized for lower precision and power. Moreover, biased estimates may arise when the missing data are not MCAR.

Alternatively, imputation has been proposed to "fill in" the missing values. Various methods are surveyed in Rubin (2004)[194], Little and Rubin (2014)[153], Schafer (1997)[196], Molenberghs et al.(2004)[167], and the references therein. There are two main types of imputation: single imputation and multiple imputation. In single imputation, only one value is imputed for each missing response, whereas in multiple imputation, $K \geq 2$ plausible values are imputed for each missing response to take into account imputation uncertainty. Usually $5 \leq K \leq 10$ is adequate. Imputation generally relies on a predictive distribution from which we obtain the mean or a random draw. The predictive distribution can either be based on an explicit statistical model or an algorithm which implies an underlying model. Standard statistical methods for complete data can then be applied to the imputed data sets. In the case of multiple imputation, it is necessary to combine the results from multiple imputed data sets to calculate the final estimates. In particular, suppose m complete data sets are created by multiple imputation. From the ith imputed data set, $i = 1, \ldots, m$, we obtain the point and covariance estimates of β, which are denoted as $\hat{\beta}^{(i)}$ and $\hat{Cov}(\hat{\beta}^{(i)})$, respectively. The point estimate of

β based on all m imputed data sets is then given by

$$\bar{\beta} = \frac{1}{m} \sum_{i=1}^{m} \hat{\beta}^{(i)},$$

and the covariance of $\bar{\beta}$ is estimated by

$$\frac{1}{m} \sum_{i=1}^{m} \hat{Cov}(\hat{\beta}^{(i)}) + (1 + \frac{1}{m})\frac{1}{m-1} \sum_{i=1}^{m} (\hat{\beta}^{(i)} - \bar{\beta})(\hat{\beta}^{(i)} - \bar{\beta})^T.$$

Notice that both the within- and between-imputation variances are considered when constructing the overall estimated variance of $\bar{\beta}$.

Last observation carried forward (LOCF), as a special case of single impu-tation, is often used in medical studies in which missing values are imputed by the last observation in record. The method can be applied to dropout or intermittent missing patterns. In the case of dropout, it asserts the strong assumption that longitudinal measurements remain unchanged after dropout. This is probably unrealistic if an individual drops out because the disease con-dition keeps worsening due to low treatment (or intervention) efficacy. Thus, LOCF will likely result in biased estimates. Another danger of using LOCF is that, similar to other single imputation methods, it artificially increases the amount of information without accounting for imputation uncertainty, and as a consequence leads to underestimated standard errors and invalid statistical inference.

When the missing pattern is monotone, one can use the propensity score method or predictive mean matching technique to draw values of Y_{mis} sequen-tially from $f(Y_{mis}|Y_{obs}, X)$. The propensity score method assumes a model for the propensity of dropout which leads to monotone missing data. The method then imputes missing values from the subjects who have a similar dropout propensity but have not dropped out. One example for the model of dropout propensity is

$$logit\{Pr(R_{ij} = 0|R_{ij-1} = 1, Y_{i1}, \ldots, Y_{ij})\} = \theta_1 + \theta_2 Y_{ij-1}.$$

In predictive mean matching methods, when the longitudinal outcome is continuous, a sequence of linear regression models can be fit for Y_{ij} given $Y_{i1}, \ldots, Y_{ij-1}$ using subjects who have not dropped out by occasion j. Let $\hat{\gamma}$ and $\hat{\sigma}^2$ denote the estimated regression coefficients and variance of the error term. The predictive values can be calculated from

$$\gamma_1^* + \gamma_2^* Y_{i1} + \cdots + \gamma_j^* Y_{ij-1} + \sigma^* e_i,$$

where γ^* and σ^* are random draws from the distributions of γ and σ, re-spectively, and e_i is generated from the standard normal distribution. The missing values are then imputed using the observed data that have the best match with the predicted values. This method can be generalized to other forms of longitudinal outcomes, i.e., binary or count data, using generalized linear models with link function g:

$$g\{E(Y_{ij})\} = \gamma_1 + \gamma_2 Y_{i1} + \cdots + \gamma_j Y_{ij-1}.$$

For longitudinal data with arbitrary missing patterns, the Markov chain Monte Carlo (MCMC) method can be used to implement multiple imputations. It assumes that Y follows a multivariate normal distribution and the missing data mechanism is MAR. The procedure involves iterations between two steps, the imputation step (I-step) and the posterior step (P-step). In the I-step, $Y_{mis}^{(t+1)}$ are randomly drawn from a conditional distribution $f(Y_{mis}|Y_{obs}, \mu^{(t)}, \Sigma^{(t)})$, where $\mu^{(t)}$ and $\Sigma^{(t)}$ are the current estimates for the mean and variance-covariance matrix. In the P-step, $\mu^{(t+1)}$ and $\Sigma^{(t+1)}$ are generated from $f(\mu, \Sigma|Y_{obs}, Y_{mis}^{(t+1)})$. Thus, the algorithm creates a Markov chain $(Y_{mis}^{(1)}, \mu^{(1)}, \Sigma^{(1)})$, $(Y_{mis}^{(2)}, \mu^{(2)}, \Sigma^{(2)})$, ..., which converges to $f(Y_{mis}, \mu, \Sigma|Y_{obs})$. Approximately independent samples of Y_{mis} are obtained from this distribution and used as the imputed values.

In general, imputation should be used with caution because it will give rise to biased estimates when the imputation model is wrong. Some imputation methods assume MCAR, which is a restrictive assumption in reality. It is common practice to carry out longitudinal analysis via likelihood-based methods or generalized estimating equations using available data without imputation. Likelihood-based methods include linear and generalized linear mixed effects models, which are essentially MAR types of analyses. The GEE method assumes MCAR, but its extended version, weighted generalized estimation equations, relaxes the assumption to MAR.

Example 2.6. *The Scleroderma Lung Study (continued)*

A complete-case analysis of %FVC scores measured at 6–24 months was conducted; that is, patients with missing data in %FVC during this time period were excluded. The subsample contained 90 subjects (48 in CYC group and 42 in the placebo group), which were analyzed using linear mixed effects model (2.9). Table 2.5 shows the estimated fixed effects and covariance parameters. In this analysis, the fixed effects tended to have larger standard errors compared to those obtained in the available-case analysis (Table 2.1). Similar to the results from the GEE method (Table 2.3), the interactions $CYC_i \times FIB_0$ and $CYC_i \times t_{ij}$ were significant. However, the complete-case analysis revealed a faster decrease in %FVC scores after 18 months in the CYC group ($\beta_8 = -0.71$, p = 0.0184). In addition, the estimated residual variance was smaller, which could be the result of a less "diverse" sample after excluding the non-completers. This analysis assumes that the missing data are MCAR, which is unlikely to be true in the presence of disease-related dropout and death and thus makes the results questionable.

Table 2.5 *Estimated fixed effects and covariance parameters for %FVC using complete-case analysis.*

Parameter	Estimate	SE	p-value
Fixed Effects			
$Intercept$	67.587	1.098	<0.0001
FVC_0	1.013	0.041	<0.0001
FIB_0	−1.298	0.619	0.0368
CYC_i	−2.017	1.505	0.1812
$CYC_i \times FIB_0$	1.912	0.900	0.0342
t_{ij}	−0.042	0.104	0.6886
$(t_{ij} - 18)_+$	−0.032	0.219	0.8829
$CYC_i \times t_{ij}$	0.302	0.143	0.0354
$CYC_i \times (t_{ij} - 18)_+$	−0.711	0.300	0.0184
Random Effects			
$Var(b_{1i})$	24.475		
$Var(b_{2i})$	0.304		
$Var(b_{3i})$	0.865		
$Cov(b_{1i}, b_{2i})$	−1.851		
$Cov(b_{1i}, b_{3i})$	1.977		
$Cov(b_{2i}, b_{3i})$	−0.354		
$Var(\epsilon_{ij})$	14.857		

In a second analysis, the MCMC method implemented in SAS Proc MI was used to impute the missing data in %FVC scores. As indicated in Figure 2.1, the two treatment groups had different time trends over time. Thus, the missing data were imputed for each group separately (with a repetition of 6), and the data were analyzed using linear mixed effects model (2.9). Estimated effects from each of the six imputed data sets were combined to obtain the final results (Table 2.6). Overall, the conclusion is similar to that in Table 2.1, which is conceivable since both methods assume the missing data to be MAR. □

Example 2.7. *The rt-PA Stroke Study (continued)*

A linear mixed effects model was fit to the longitudinal measurements of NIHSS scores on patients who had complete measurements at the four time points: 2 hours post-treatment, 24 hours, 7–10 days, and 3 months poststroke onset. The analysis included 461 patients: 237 in the rt-PA group and 224 in the placebo group. As is shown in Table 2.7, the standard errors for all the mean structure parameters are larger than those in the available-case analysis (Table 2.2), but the variation of random time trend effects and residuals is reduced after

Table 2.6 *Estimated fixed effects for %FVC after multiple imputation.*

Parameter	Estimate	SE	p-value
$Intercept$	66.550	0.936	<0.0001
FVC_0	0.963	0.041	<0.0001
FIB_0	−1.567	0.619	0.0113
CYC_i	−1.845	1.547	0.2409
$CYC_i \times FIB_0$	1.461	0.891	0.1010
t_{ij}	−0.115	0.098	0.2427
$(t_{ij} - 18)_+$	−0.081	0.204	0.6922
$CYC_i \times t_{ij}$	0.317	0.172	0.0782
$CYC_i \times (t_{ij} - 18)_+$	−0.537	0.349	0.1386

excluding the non-completers. There are also considerable changes in the point estimates of the fixed effects, especially small vessel and time trend, suggesting that the completers are not a random sample from the original cohort and that the missing data in NIHSS do not appear to be MCAR. □

Table 2.7 *Estimated fixed effects and covariance parameters for NIHSS (square root transformed) using complete-case analysis.*

Parameter	Estimate	SE	p-value
Fixed Effects			
Intercept	3.403	0.084	<0.0001
NIH_0	0.906	0.033	<0.0001
small vessel	−0.036	0.151	0.8099
large vessel	0.027	0.097	0.7838
timehr24	−0.285	0.063	<0.0001
timeday710	−0.740	0.069	<0.0001
timem3	−1.131	0.067	<0.0001
group	−0.543	0.111	<0.0001
group × *small vessel*	0.336	0.204	0.1005
group × *large vessel*	0.288	0.133	0.0314
Random Effects			
$Var(b_{1i})$	0.589		
$Var(b_{2i})$	0.947		
$Var(b_{3i})$	0.860		
$Cov(b_{1i}, b_{2i})$	1.098		
$Cov(b_{1i}, b_{3i})$	0.853		
$Cov(b_{2i}, b_{3i})$	1.188		
$Var(\epsilon_{ij})$	0.610		

Chapter 3

Methods for Time-to-Event Data

This chapter gives an introduction to the key elements of survival analysis or time-to-event data analysis.

Survival analysis, or time-to-event data analysis, refers to statistical methods for time-to-event data. An event time, or survival time, is defined as the time from an initial event such as diagnosis of a disease to the occurrence of an event of interest such as death. Time-to-event data arise commonly in clinical trials and other follow-up studies. For example, *time to death or treatment failures* is a primary clinical outcome variable to evaluate the effectiveness of oral cyclophosphamide as a treatment for patients with scleroderma-related lung disease in the Scleroderma Lung Study discussed in Section 1.1.1. For convenience, we will use the words *event*, *failure*, and *death* interchangeably.

A common phenomena associated with time-to-event data is *censoring*, which refers to a situation where the event time of interest is only partially known. There are many types of censoring including right-censoring, left-censoring, interval censoring, and double censoring [119]. In this chapter, we will confine our attention to *right censoring* when the event time is not observed due to the occurrence of a competing censoring event such as the end of a study, but is known to be greater than the observed censoring time.

3.1 Right Censoring

Let T be a nonnegative random variable representing the event time of interest. The event time T is said to be right–censored by a censoring time C if T is not observed, but is known to be greater than C which is observed. Mathematically, instead of observing T, one observes $\tilde{T} = \min\{T, C\}$, the observation time that equals either the survival time T or the censoring time C whichever occurs first, and an event indicator $\delta = I(T \leq C)$ (1=uncensored and 0=censored).

Throughout this chapter we will assume that T and C are independent, or conditionally independent given a set of covariates in a regression setting. This assumption is referred to as the *noninformative censoring* assumption since under such an assumption the censoring distribution is factored out of the likelihood and thus knowledge of the censoring distribution would not contribute to the inference for T.

3.2   Survival Function and Hazard Function

Commonly used quantities to characterize an event time T include the survival function and hazard function defined by:

Survival function: $S(t) = P(T > t)$,

Hazard function: $\lambda(t) = \lim_{\Delta t \searrow 0} \dfrac{P(t \leq T < t + \Delta t | T \geq t)}{\Delta t}$.

For any t, $S(t) = P(T > t)$ is the probability that the event will occur after time t (or survival beyond time t). The hazard $\lambda(t)$ is the instantaneous failure rate at time t, indicating how likely a subject who has not experienced the event prior to time t will experience the event in the next instant.

One can easily verify the following properties.

Property 3.1. *If T is a nonnegative continuous random variable with probability density function $f(t)$, then*

$$S(t) = \int_0^t f(s)ds,$$

$$\lambda(t) = f(t)/S(t) = -\frac{d\ln S(t)}{dt},$$

$$S(t) = \exp\{-\Lambda(t)\},$$

where $\Lambda(t) = \int_0^t \lambda(s)ds$ is called the "cumulative hazard function" of T.

Property 3.2. *If T is a discrete random variable with support $0 < t_1 < t_2 < \cdots$ and probability mass function $p_i = P(T = t_i)$, $i = 1, \ldots$, where $p_i > 0$ and $\sum_i p(t_i) = 1$, then*

$$S(t) = \sum_{i:t_i>t} p_i,$$

$$\lambda(t_i) = \frac{S(t_{i-1}) - S(t_i)}{S(t_{i-1})}, \quad \text{for } i = 1,2,\ldots, \text{ and } t_0 \equiv 0,$$

$$S(t) = \prod_{i:t_i>t} \{1 - \lambda(t_i)\}. \quad \text{(Product-limit representation)} \quad (3.1)$$

Equation (3.1) is often referred to as the *product-limit representation* of a discrete survival function.

3.3 Estimation of a Survival Function

Assume that one observes a randomly right–censored event time data consisting of n independent and identically distributed (i.i.d.) replicates $(\tilde{T}_1, \delta_1), \ldots, (\tilde{T}_n, \delta_n)$ of $\tilde{T}, \delta$, where $\tilde{T} = \min\{T, C\}$ and $\delta = I(T \leq C)$.

3.3.1 The Kaplan–Meier Estimate

The survival function $S(t) = P(T > t)$ of T can be estimated consistently by the well-known Kaplan–Meier estimate [114]:

$$\widehat{S}(t) = \begin{cases} 1, & 0 \leq t < t_1, \\ \prod_{t_j \leq t} \left(1 - \frac{d_j}{r_j}\right), & t > t_1, \end{cases} \tag{3.2}$$

where $0 < t_1 < \ldots < t_D$ denote the distinct uncensored event times, $r_j = \sum_{i=1}^{n} I(\tilde{T}_i \geq t_j)$ is the number of subjects who are "at risk" just prior to time t_j, and $d_j = \sum_{i=1}^{n} I(\tilde{T}_i \leq t_j, \delta_i = 1)$ is the number of uncensored events at t_j. Note that $\widehat{S}(t)$ is a proper survival function only if the largest observation time is uncensored.

It can be shown that $\widehat{S}(t)$ is the nonparametric maximum likelihood estimate (NPMLE) of $S(t)$ that maximizes the likelihood

$$L(S) = \prod_{i=1}^{n} [S(T_i - 0) - S(T_i)]^{\delta_i} S(T_i)^{1-\delta_i} \tag{3.3}$$

over the space of all survival functions S [114].

From the product-limit representation (3.1), it is seen that the Kaplan–Meier estimate $\widehat{S}(t)$ is a discrete survival function with hazard d_j/r_j at time t_j, $j = 1, \ldots, D$. Its corresponding cumulative hazard function is

$$\widehat{\Lambda}(t) = \sum_{t_j \leq t} \frac{d_j}{r_j}, \tag{3.4}$$

the Nelson–Aalen estimate of $\Lambda(t) = -\ln S(t)$.

Remark. Counting process notation. It is useful to study the Kaplan–Meier estimate under the counting process setting [1, 12, 73]. Let $N_i(t) = I(\tilde{T}_i \leq t, \delta_i = 1)$ be the counting process for the number of observed events by time t for subject i and $Y_i(t) = I(\tilde{T}_i \geq t)$ the at-risk process indicating by the value 1 that subject i is at risk just prior to time t. Then the Nelson–Aalen estimate defined by (3.4) can be rewritten as

$$\widehat{\Lambda}(t) = \int_0^t \frac{dN(s)}{Y(s)}, \tag{3.5}$$

where $N(t) = \sum_{i=1}^{n} N_i(t)$ and $Y(t) = \sum_{i=1}^{n} Y_i(t)$. Note that the Nelson–Aalen estimate in (3.5) can be derived as a moment estimate from the fact that $E\{dN(t)|$history up to $t-\} = Y(t)d\Lambda(t)$. Furthermore, the Kaplan–Meier estimate defined by (3.2) can be reexpressed as

$$\widehat{S}(t) = \prod_{s \leq t} \{1 - d\widehat{\Lambda}(s)\}, \tag{3.6}$$

where $d\widehat{\Lambda}(s) = \widehat{\Lambda}(s) - \widehat{\Lambda}(s-)$.

3.3.2 Asymptotic Inference

Breslow and Crowley [22] first established the asymptotic theory for the Kaplan–Meier estimate. Aalen [2] formally introduced the now popular counting process model for event time data. Under some regularity conditions, it can be shown that $\widehat{S}(t)$ is asymptotically normal with mean $S(t)$. Its variance is consistently estimated by Greenwood's formula [83]:

$$\widehat{Var}(\widehat{S}(t)) = [\widehat{S}(t)]^2 \sum_{t_j \leq t} \frac{d_j}{r_j(r_j - d_j)}.$$

Confidence Intervals for $S(t)$

The asymptotic normal theory enables one to draw large-sample inference for $S(t)$. For example, an approximate $1 - \alpha$ confidence interval for $S(t)$ is given by

$$\widehat{S}(t) \pm z_{1-\alpha/2}\widehat{S}(t)\sqrt{\sum_{t_j \leq t} \frac{d_j}{r_j(r_j - d_j)}}, \tag{3.7}$$

where $z_{1-\alpha/2}$ is the $1 - \alpha/2$ percentile of the standard normal distribution.

Transformation-Based Confidence Intervals for $S(t)$

It is worth noting that $S(t)$ is a survival probability between 0 and 1. However, a confidence interval produced by (3.7) could include values outside the range [0,1]. To address this problem one can use a transformation-based method. Specifically, let $g(t)$ be a differentiable monotonically increasing function. By the delta-method, $g(\widehat{S}(t))$ is asymptotically normal with mean $g(S(t))$ and estimated variance

$$\{g'(\hat{S}(t))\}^2\widehat{Var}(\widehat{S}(t)).$$

Thus, a $1 - \alpha$ confidence interval for $g(S(t))$ is given by

$$[L, U] = g(\hat{S}(t)) \pm z_{1-\alpha/2}\sqrt{\{g'(\hat{S}(t))\}^2\widehat{Var}(\widehat{S}(t))}.$$

Consequently,

$$[g^{-1}(L), g^{-1}(U)] \tag{3.8}$$

gives a $1 - \alpha$ confidence interval for $S(t)$.

Nonparametric Likelihood Ratio Confidence Intervals for $S(t)$

A more appealing solution is to construct a likelihood-ratio based confidence interval for $S(t)$ [208, 132, 169]. For $t > 0$ and $0 < p < 1$, define the following likelihood ratio

$$R(t, p) = \frac{\sup_S \{L(S) : S(t) = p\}}{\sup_S \{L(S)\}},$$

for testing $H_0 : S(t) = p$, where $L(S)$ is defined in (3.3). Clearly a large value of $R(t, p)$ indicates evidence in favor of H_0. A confidence interval for $S(t)$ is then obtained as the set of values p for which H_0 is not rejected by a likelihood ratio test based on $R(t, p)$. Specifically, a $(1 - \alpha)$ likelihood ratio confidence interval $[p_L, p_U]$ for $S(t)$ is given by

$$p_L = \prod_{t_j \leq t} \left(1 - \frac{d_j}{r_j + \lambda_L} \right),$$

$$p_U = \prod_{t_j \leq t} \left(1 - \frac{d_j}{r_j + \lambda_U} \right),$$

where λ_L and λ_U are the unique solutions of

$$-2 \sum_{t_j \leq t} \left\{ (r_j - d_j) \log \left(1 + \frac{\lambda}{r_j - d_j} \right) - r_j \log \left(1 + \frac{\lambda}{r_j} \right) \right\} = \chi_1^2 (1 - \alpha)$$

on the intervals $(D = \max_{t_j \leq t} \{d_j - r_j\}, 0)$ and $(0, \infty)$, respectively.

3.4   Cox's Semiparametric Multiplicative Hazards Model

In this section we discuss the popular Cox semiparametric multiplicative hazards model [42] for regression analysis of right–censored time-to-event data. A survival regression model describes the relationship between a survival time and a set of predictors. It is useful to 1) study the effects of a variable on the event time adjusted for possible confounders, 2) select important prognostic predictors, and 3) make a prognostic prediction for a new subject.

Assume that one observes a randomly right–censored regression data consisting of n independent and identically distributed triples $(\tilde{T}_1, \delta_1, \mathbf{Z}_1), \ldots,$ $(\tilde{T}_n, \delta_n, \mathbf{Z}_n)$, where for the ith subject, $\tilde{T}_i = \min\{T_i, C_i\}$ is the observation time that equals either the survival time T_i or the censoring time C_i whichever occurs first, $\delta_i = I(T_i \le C_i)$ is an event indicator (1=uncensored and 0=censored), and $\boldsymbol{Z}_i$ is a vector of p covariates that are observed on $[0, \tilde{T}_i]$.

A covariate is called *time-independent, time-invariant, or fixed* if it does not change over time, and *time-dependent or time-varying* otherwise.

3.4.1 Model Formulation

Let $\lambda(t|\boldsymbol{Z}(t))$ be the conditional hazard of T at time t given the covariate history up to t. The Cox (1972) semiparametric multiplicative hazards model postulates that

$$\lambda(t|\boldsymbol{Z}(t)) = \lambda_0(t) \exp(\boldsymbol{\beta}^T \boldsymbol{Z}(t)), \tag{3.9}$$

where $\boldsymbol{\beta} = (\beta_1, \dots, \beta_p)^T$ is a vector of regression coefficients and $\lambda_0(t)$ is an unspecified baseline hazard function.

Model (3.9) can also be written as

$$\Lambda(t|\boldsymbol{Z}(t)) = \int_0^t \exp(\boldsymbol{\beta}^T \boldsymbol{Z}(s)) d\Lambda_0(s), \tag{3.10}$$

or

$$S(t|\boldsymbol{Z}(t)) = \exp\left[-\int_0^t \exp\{\boldsymbol{\beta}^T \boldsymbol{Z}(s)\} d\Lambda_0(s) \right], \tag{3.11}$$

where $\Lambda(t|\boldsymbol{Z}(t))$ and $S(t|\boldsymbol{Z}(t))$ are the conditional cumulative hazard function and conditional survival function given the covariate history up to t, and $\Lambda_0(t)$ is an unspecified baseline cumulative hazard function.

Example 3.1. *Two-sample problem; proportional hazards model. Suppose that there is only one binary covariate Z, $p = 1$, an indicator variable for two samples. Then model (3.9) implies that the hazards in samples 0 and 1 are $\lambda_0(t)$ and $e^\beta \lambda_0(t)$. In other words, the two hazards are proportional with hazard ratio e^β. Similarly, the two cumulative hazards are proportional with $\Lambda(t|Z = 0) = \Lambda_0(t)$ and $\Lambda(t|Z = 1) = e^\beta \Lambda_0(t)$. Finally, $S(t|Z = 1) = \{S_0(t)\}^{\exp\{\beta\}}$ and $S_0(t) = \exp\{-H_0(t)\}$.*

Example 3.2. *Two-sample problem; two-piece proportional hazards model. Let Z_1 be the indicator variable of example 1. In addition, define $Z_2 = I(t > \tau)Z_1$ for a some fixed $\tau > 0$. Then model (3.9) with $p = 2$ implies that the hazard in sample 1 is $e^{\beta_1}\lambda_0(t)$ for $t \le \tau$, and $e^{\beta_1+\beta_2}\lambda_0(t)$ for $t > \tau$. In other words, the hazard ratio (sample 1 relative to sample 0) is e^{β_1} on the time interval $[0, \tau]$ and $e^{\beta_1+\beta_2}$ on (τ, ∞).*

Example 3.3. *Regression problem with time-dependent covariate. Suppose that $T =$ time to death and $Z(t) = CD4$ count at time t. Then the Cox model (3.9) can be used to study how CD4 count monitored over time is related to the clinical outcome T.*

3.4.2 Partial Likelihood

A commonly used method for making inference on $\boldsymbol{\beta}$ is the *partial likelihood* method [43, 44]. The partial likelihood for $\boldsymbol{\beta}$ defined as

$$L(\boldsymbol{\beta}) = \prod_{i=1}^{n} \left\{ \frac{\exp(\boldsymbol{\beta}^T \boldsymbol{Z}_i(\tilde{T}_i))}{\sum_{j \in R(\tilde{T}_i)} \exp(\boldsymbol{\beta}^T \boldsymbol{Z}_j(\tilde{T}_i))} \right\}^{\delta_i}, \tag{3.12}$$

where $R(t) = \{i : \tilde{T}_i \geq t\}$ is the risk set at time $t-$, the set of individuals who are *at risk* or *alive* just prior to time t.

The partial likelihood in (3.12) can also be interpreted as a profile likelihood [112] obtained by maximizing a joint likelihood of $\boldsymbol{\beta}$ and Λ_0

$$L(\boldsymbol{\beta}, \Lambda_0) = \prod_{i=1}^{n} \left[\{d\Lambda_0(\tilde{T}_i)\} \exp(\boldsymbol{\beta}^T \boldsymbol{Z}_i(\tilde{T}_i)) \right]^{\delta_i} \exp\left[-\int_0^{\tilde{T}_i} \exp(\boldsymbol{\beta}^T \boldsymbol{Z}_i(s)) d\Lambda_0(s) \right]$$

with respect to Λ_0 for a fixed $\boldsymbol{\beta}$. For simplicity, assume that there are no ties in the observed event times. It can be seen that to maximize $L(\boldsymbol{\beta}, \Lambda_0)$ with respect to the cumulative hazard function Λ_0, it suffices to consider only right-continuous step functions Λ_0 with positive jumps only at the uncensored event times $t_1 < \cdots < t_D$. Let (j) denote the individual failing at t_j and write $\Lambda_0(t) = \sum_{t_j \leq t} \lambda_{0j}$ where λ_{0j} denotes the jump size of Λ_0 at t_j. Then

$$
\begin{aligned}
L(\boldsymbol{\beta}, \Lambda_0) &= \left[\prod_{j=1}^{D} \lambda_{0j} \exp(\boldsymbol{\beta}^T \boldsymbol{Z}_{(j)}(t_j)) \right] \exp\left[-\sum_{i=1}^{n} \sum_{j:t_j \leq \tilde{T}_i} \lambda_{0j} \exp(\boldsymbol{\beta}^T \boldsymbol{Z}_i(t_j)) \right] \\
&= \left[\prod_{j=1}^{D} \lambda_{0j} \exp(\boldsymbol{\beta}^T \boldsymbol{Z}_{(j)}(t_j)) \right] \exp\left[-\sum_{j=1}^{D} \lambda_{0j} \sum_{i:\tilde{T}_i \geq t_j} \exp(\boldsymbol{\beta}^T \boldsymbol{Z}_i(t_j)) \right].
\end{aligned}
\tag{3.13}
$$

Taking partial derivative of $\log L(\boldsymbol{\beta}, \Lambda_0)$ with respect to λ_{0j} and setting it to zero, we have

$$\frac{1}{\lambda_{0j}} - \sum_{i \in R(t_j)} \exp(\boldsymbol{\beta}^T \boldsymbol{Z}_i(t_j)) = 0, \quad j = 1, ..., D,$$

which lead to the following estimates:

$$\widehat{\lambda_{0j}} = \frac{1}{\sum_{i \in R(t_j)} \exp(\boldsymbol{\beta}^T \boldsymbol{Z}_i(t_j))}, \quad j = 1, \ldots, D,$$

and

$$\widehat{\Lambda}_0^{(\boldsymbol{\beta})}(t) = \sum_{t_j \leq t} \frac{1}{\sum_{i \in R(t_j)} \exp(\boldsymbol{\beta}^T \boldsymbol{Z}_i(t_j))}. \tag{3.14}$$

Substituting Λ_0 by $\widehat{\Lambda}_0^{(\beta)}$ in (3.13) yields the profile likelihood of β:

$$L(\beta, \widehat{\Lambda}_0^{(\beta)}) = \prod_{j=1}^{D} \frac{\exp(\beta^T Z_{(j)}(t_j))}{\sum_{i \in R(t_j)} \exp(\beta^T Z_i(t_j))} \exp(-1),$$

which is proportional to the partial likelihood defined in (3.12).

3.4.3 Estimation of β and $\Lambda_0(t) = \int_0^t \lambda_0(s)ds$

It can be shown that under certain regularity conditions, the partial likelihood function in (3.12) is strictly concave [108]. Define

$$\hat{\beta} = \arg\max_{\beta} L(\beta)$$

to be the maximum partial likelihood estimate of β. Then $\hat{\beta}$ can be obtained by solving the score equation

$$U(\beta) = 0,$$

where the score function is given by

$$U(\beta) = \frac{\partial \log L(\beta)}{\partial \beta} = \sum_{i=1}^{n} \delta_i \left[Z_i(\tilde{T}_i) - \frac{\sum_{j \in R(\tilde{T}_i)} Z_j(\tilde{T}_i) \exp(\beta^T Z_j(\tilde{T}_i))}{\sum_{j \in R(\tilde{T}_i)} \exp\{\beta^T Z_j(\tilde{T}_i)\}} \right].$$

Partial likelihood inference for β is made in the same manner as the usual maximum likelihood method. In particular, the sampling distribution of $\hat{\beta}$ can be approximated by a normal distribution with mean β and variance $I^{-1}(\hat{\beta})$ [13, 214], where

$$I(\beta) = -\frac{1}{n} \frac{\partial^2 \log L(\beta)}{\partial \beta \partial \beta^T}.$$

It follows from (3.14) that the baseline cumulative hazard function Λ_0 is estimated by

$$\widehat{\Lambda}_0(t) = \widehat{\Lambda}_0^{(\hat{\beta})}(t) = \sum_{\tilde{T}_i \leq t} \frac{\delta_i}{\sum_{j \in R(\tilde{T}_i)} \exp(\hat{\beta}^T Z_j(\tilde{T}_i))}, \tag{3.15}$$

which is referred to as the Breslow estimator [23, 21]. Its consistency and asymptotic normality can be found in [13].

3.4.4 Prediction of a Conditional Survival Function

Time-Independent Covariates

Suppose that $\mathbf{Z}$ is time-independent. The survival function $S(t|\mathbf{Z})$ of a subject with covariate $\mathbf{Z}$ can be predicted from the Cox model [11]. Let

$$\widehat{S}(t|\mathbf{Z}) = \exp\left\{-\widehat{\Lambda}_0(t)\exp(\hat{\boldsymbol{\beta}}^T\mathbf{Z})\right\}. \tag{3.16}$$

Then $\widehat{S}(t|\mathbf{Z})$ can be approximated by a normal distribution with mean $S(t|\mathbf{Z})$ and variance

$$\widehat{Var}\{\hat{S}(t|Z)\} = \{\hat{S}(t|Z)\}^2 \left\{\sum_{\tilde{T}_i \leq t} \frac{\delta_i}{[\sum_{j \in R(\tilde{T}_i)} \exp\{\hat{\boldsymbol{\beta}}^T\mathbf{Z}_j(\tilde{T}_i)\}]^2} + Q^T F^{-1} Q\right\}, \tag{3.17}$$

where

$$Q = \sum_{\tilde{T}_i \leq t} \delta_i \frac{\sum_{j \in R(\tilde{T}_i)}\mathbf{Z}_j(\tilde{T}_i)\exp\{\hat{\boldsymbol{\beta}}^T\mathbf{Z}_j(\tilde{T}_i)\}}{[\sum_{j \in R(\tilde{T}_i)}\exp\{\hat{\boldsymbol{\beta}}^T\mathbf{Z}_j(\tilde{T}_i)\}]^2} - \widehat{\Lambda}_0(t)\mathbf{Z},$$

$$F = \sum_{i=1}^n \delta_i \left[\frac{\sum_{j \in R(\tilde{T}_i)}\mathbf{Z}_j(\tilde{T}_i)\mathbf{Z}_j(\tilde{T}_i)^T\exp\{\hat{\boldsymbol{\beta}}^T\mathbf{Z}_j(\tilde{T}_i)\}}{\sum_{j \in R(\tilde{T}_i)}\exp\{\hat{\boldsymbol{\beta}}^T\mathbf{Z}_j(\tilde{T}_i)\}}\right.$$

$$\left. - \frac{[\sum_{j \in R(\tilde{T}_i)}\mathbf{Z}_j(\tilde{T}_i)\exp\{\hat{\boldsymbol{\beta}}^T\mathbf{Z}_j(\tilde{T}_i)\}][\sum_{j \in R(\tilde{T}_i)}\mathbf{Z}_j(\tilde{T}_i)\exp\{\hat{\boldsymbol{\beta}}^T\mathbf{Z}_j(\tilde{T}_i)\}]^T}{[\sum_{j \in R(\tilde{T}_i)}\exp\{\hat{\boldsymbol{\beta}}^T\mathbf{Z}_j(\tilde{T}_i)\}]^2}\right].$$

The methods described in Section 3.3.2 can be applied to construct confidence intervals for $S(t|\mathbf{Z})$.

Time-Dependent Covariates

With time-dependent covariates $\mathbf{Z}(t)$, the conditional survival function $S(t|\mathbf{Z}(t))$ can be estimated by either

$$\widehat{S}(t|\mathbf{Z}(t)) = \exp\left[-\int_0^t \exp\{\hat{\boldsymbol{\beta}}^T\mathbf{Z}(s)\}d\widehat{\Lambda}_0(s)\right], \tag{3.18}$$

or the product-limit version

$$\tilde{S}(t|\mathbf{Z}(t)) = \prod_{s \leq t}\left[1 - \exp\{\hat{\boldsymbol{\beta}}^T\mathbf{Z}(s)\}d\widehat{\Lambda}_0(s)\right]. \tag{3.19}$$

It is nontrivial to obtain an analytical variance estimate of $\widehat{S}(t|\mathbf{Z}(t))$ or $\tilde{S}(t|\mathbf{Z}(t))$. In this case, the bootstrap method can be used. We refer the reader to [58, 59, 60] for the bootstrap method with right–censored data.

3.4.5   Remark on Cox's Model with Intermittently Measured
Time-Dependent Covariates and Measurement Error

Note that the partial likelihood in (3.12) requires measurement of $Z_i(t_j)$ at every uncensored event time for every subject i. However, it is more often in practice that a subject's covariate is observed only intermittently over time. For example, the CD4 count of a patient in Example 3.3 of this section is usually measured only at scheduled visits. The observed CD4 count could also be subject to measurement error. In this case, the partial likelihood method is not applicable. In Chapter 4, we will discuss how to address these issues by jointly modeling the survival time and the covariate trajectory.

3.5   Accelerated Failure Time Models with Time-Independent Covariates

An accelerated failure time (AFT) model relates the survival time T of a subject with time-independent covariate $\boldsymbol{Z}$ to a baseline time variable T_0 that corresponds to the condition $\boldsymbol{Z} = 0$ by

$$T_0 = T \exp(\boldsymbol{\beta}^T \boldsymbol{Z}), \tag{3.20}$$

where T_0 is independent of $\boldsymbol{Z}$.

Model (3.20) implies that a subject with covariate $\boldsymbol{Z}$ fails on a contracted or expanded time scale relative to the baseline time scale by a factor of $\exp\{-\boldsymbol{\beta}^T \boldsymbol{Z}\}$ [43]. One may also imagine that the survival time is determined by an underlying "biological clock" such that a faster clock leads to a shorter survival. Then model (3.20) implies that the biological clock of a subject with covariate $\boldsymbol{Z}$ is accelerated by a factor of $\exp(\boldsymbol{\beta}^T \boldsymbol{Z})$ compared to a subject with covariate $\boldsymbol{Z} = 0$.

Alternatively, model (3.20) can be written as

$$S(t|\boldsymbol{Z}) = S_0 \left\{ t \exp(\boldsymbol{\beta}^T \boldsymbol{Z}) \right\}, \tag{3.21}$$

or

$$\lambda(t|\boldsymbol{Z}) = \lambda_0 \left\{ t \exp(\boldsymbol{\beta}^T \boldsymbol{Z}) \right\} \exp\{\boldsymbol{\beta}^T \boldsymbol{Z}\}, \tag{3.22}$$

where $S(t|\boldsymbol{Z})$ and $\lambda(t|\boldsymbol{Z}(t))$ are the conditional survival function and conditional hazard of a subject with covariate $\boldsymbol{Z}$ and $S_0(t)$ and $\lambda_0(t)$ are the survival function and baseline hazard function of the baseline time T_0.

The AFT model (3.20) can also be expressed as a linear model of the logarithm of the survival time T on $\boldsymbol{Z}$:

$$\log(T) = \gamma_0 + \boldsymbol{\gamma}^T \boldsymbol{Z} + \epsilon, \tag{3.23}$$

where $\boldsymbol{\gamma} = -\boldsymbol{\beta}$, $E(\epsilon) = 0$, $\exp(\epsilon + \gamma_0) \sim S_0$, and ϵ and $\boldsymbol{Z}$ are independent.

3.5.1 Parametric AFT Models

A parametric AFT model assumes that the error term ϵ in (3.23) follows a parametric distribution. Below are some common parametric AFT models.

Example 3.4. *Exponential AFT model. The exponential AFT model assumes that*

$$\log(T) = \gamma_0 + \boldsymbol{\gamma}^T \boldsymbol{Z} + \epsilon, \tag{3.24}$$

where ϵ is independent of $\boldsymbol{Z}$ and follows the standard extreme-value distribution or the standard Gumbel distribution with survival function $P(\epsilon > x) = \exp\{-\exp(x)\}$.

Model (3.24) is equivalent to

$$S(t|\boldsymbol{Z}) = S_0\{t \exp(\boldsymbol{\beta}^T \boldsymbol{Z})\}, \tag{3.25}$$

where $S_0(t) = \exp\{-\lambda t\}$, $\lambda = \exp(-\gamma_0)$, and $\boldsymbol{\beta} = -\boldsymbol{\gamma}$.

It is easy to see that the exponential AFT model (3.24) or (3.25) satisfies the proportional hazards assumption

$$\lambda(t|\boldsymbol{Z}) = \lambda_0(t) \exp(\boldsymbol{\beta}^T \boldsymbol{Z}), \tag{3.26}$$

with an exponential baseline hazard $\lambda_0(t) = \lambda$.

Example 3.5. *Weibull AFT model. The Weibull AFT model assumes that*

$$\log(T) = \gamma_0 + \boldsymbol{\gamma}^T \boldsymbol{Z} + \sigma\epsilon, \tag{3.27}$$

where $\sigma > 0$ is a scale parameter, and ϵ is independent of $\boldsymbol{Z}$ and follows the standard extreme-value distribution or the standard Gumbel distribution with survival function $P(\epsilon > x) = \exp\{-\exp(x)\}$.

Model (3.27) is equivalent to

$$S(t|\boldsymbol{Z}) = S_0\{t \exp(\boldsymbol{\beta}^T \boldsymbol{Z})\}, \tag{3.28}$$

where $S_0(t) = \exp(-\lambda t^\alpha)$, $\lambda = \exp(-\gamma_0/\sigma)$, $\alpha = 1/\sigma$, and $\boldsymbol{\beta} = -\boldsymbol{\gamma}$.

The Weibull AFT model (3.28) is also a proportional hazards model

$$\lambda(t|\boldsymbol{Z}) = \lambda_0(t) \exp(\alpha\boldsymbol{\beta}^T \boldsymbol{Z}) \tag{3.29}$$

where the baseline hazard is $\lambda_0(t) = \lambda\alpha t^{\alpha-1}$.

Finally, the Weibull AFT model reduces to the exponential AFT model when $\alpha = 1$.

Example 3.6. *Log-normal AFT model. The log-normal AFT model assumes that*

$$\log(T) = \gamma_0 + \boldsymbol{\gamma}^T \boldsymbol{Z} + \epsilon, \tag{3.30}$$

where ϵ is independent of $\boldsymbol{Z}$ and follows a normal distribution with mean 0 and variance σ^2.

Model (3.30) is equivalent to

$$S(t|\boldsymbol{Z}) = 1 - \Phi\left\{\frac{\log(t) - (\gamma_0 - \boldsymbol{\beta}^T \boldsymbol{Z})}{\sigma}\right\}, \tag{3.31}$$

where $S_0(t) = 1 - \Phi\{\frac{\log(t) - \gamma_0}{\sigma}\}$ and $\boldsymbol{\beta} = -\boldsymbol{\gamma}$.

The usual parametric maximum likelihood method can be used to draw inference under a parametric AFT model. Let $\theta = (\gamma_0, \boldsymbol{\gamma}^T, \boldsymbol{\eta}^T)^T$, where γ_0 and $\boldsymbol{\gamma}$ are the intercept and slope parameters in model (3.30) and η represents parameters in the error distribution. The right–censored data likelihood for a parameter AFT model is

$$L(\theta) = \prod_{i=1}^{n} \lambda(\tilde{T}_i|\boldsymbol{Z}_i)^{\delta_i}) S(\tilde{T}_i|\boldsymbol{Z}_i).$$

Define

$$\hat{\theta} = \arg\max_{\theta} L(\theta).$$

Then, under some regularity conditions, $\hat{\theta}$ can be approximated by the normal distribution with mean θ and variance

$$I(\hat{\theta}) = -\left.\frac{\partial^2 logL(\theta)}{\partial\theta\partial\theta^T}\right|_{\theta=\hat{\theta}}.$$

The above result, combined with the delta-method, can be used to draw inference on any smooth function $\psi(\theta)$ of θ. Specifically, assume that $\psi(\theta)$ is a column vector of q parameters. Then $\psi(\hat{\theta})$ can be approximated by a normal distribution with mean $\psi(\theta)$ and variance

$$\psi'(\hat{\theta})I^{-1}(\hat{\theta})\{\psi'(\hat{\theta})\}^T,$$

where $\psi'(\theta) = \frac{\partial\psi(\theta)}{\partial\theta^T}$.

3.5.2   Semiparametric AFT Model

Assume the following model

$$Y = \gamma_0 + \boldsymbol{\gamma}^T \boldsymbol{Z} + \epsilon, \tag{3.32}$$

where Y is a known monotone increasing transformation of a survival time, ϵ is independent of $\boldsymbol{Z}$, and its distribution is completely unspecified. To make γ_0 identifiable, assume further that $E(\epsilon) = 0$. Alternatively, one may rewrite (3.32) as

$$Y = \boldsymbol{\gamma}^T \boldsymbol{Z} + e, \qquad (3.33)$$

where $e = \epsilon + \gamma_0$.

Suppose that one observes a right–censored data consisting of n independent and identically distributed triplets $(\tilde{Y}_i, \delta_i, \boldsymbol{Z}_i)$, where for subject i, $\tilde{Y}_i = \min\{Y_i, C_i\}$ is the minimum of the survival time Y_i and its associated censoring time C_i, $\delta_i = I(Y_i \leq C_i)$, and $\boldsymbol{Z}_i$ is a vector of p time-independent covariates.

A number of estimation methods have been developed for the semiparametric AFT model (3.32), which include the synthetic data methods [203, 252, 253, 124, 134, 181, 229], generalization of the least squares method [29, 165], rank-based methods [176, 234, 215, 111, 243], least absolute deviation method [175], and M-estimation [254], among others. Below we describe a synthetic data method, the Buckley-James method, and a linear rank method.

Synthetic Data Method

We first discuss a synthetic data method developed by Koul et al. [121].

Define a synthetic variable

$$Y_{iG} = \frac{\delta_i \tilde{Y}_i}{G(Y_i-)},$$

where $G(x) = P(C_i > x)$ is the survival function of the censoring time C_i. Then it can be shown that

$$E(Y_{iG}|\boldsymbol{Z}_i) = E(Y_i|\boldsymbol{Z}_i) = \gamma_0 + \boldsymbol{\gamma}^T \boldsymbol{Z},$$

provided that C_i is independent of $\boldsymbol{Z}_i$ and Y_i. Thus it is natural to estimate the regression parameters by minimizing

$$\sum_{i=1}^{n} \{Y_{i\hat{G}} - (\gamma_0 + \boldsymbol{\gamma}^T \boldsymbol{Z}_i)\}^2,$$

where $\hat{G}$ is the Kaplan–Meier estimate of G. This leads to the following estimates

$$\hat{\boldsymbol{\gamma}} = \left\{ \sum_{i=1}^{n} (\boldsymbol{Z}_i - \bar{\boldsymbol{Z}})(\boldsymbol{Z}_i - \bar{\boldsymbol{Z}})^T \right\}^{-1} \sum_{i=1}^{n} (\boldsymbol{Z}_i - \bar{\boldsymbol{Z}}) Y_{i\hat{G}}, \qquad (3.34)$$

$$\hat{\gamma}_0 = \bar{Y}_{\hat{G}} - \hat{\boldsymbol{\gamma}}^T \bar{\boldsymbol{Z}}, \qquad (3.35)$$

where $\bar{Z} = n^{-1} \sum_{i=1}^{n} Z_i$ and $\bar{Y}_{\hat{G}} = n^{-1} \sum_{i=1}^{n} Y_{i\hat{G}}$.

The asymptotic normality and estimated variance of $(\hat{\gamma}_0, \hat{\gamma})$ are given in [121, 201].

Remark 3.1. *The synthetic data estimate* $(\hat{\gamma}_0, \hat{\gamma})$ *may be highly biased and unstable for small samples, especially in the presence of heavy censoring. We refer the reader to [203, 252, 253, 124, 134, 181, 229] among others for improved inference procedures and alternative synthetic data methods.*

The Buckley–James Method

Buckley and James [29] introduced an extension of the least squares estimation method to right–censored data by iteratively imputing the censored survival times.

Define

$$
\begin{aligned}
Y_{iF,\gamma}^* &= E(Y_i | \tilde{Y}_i, \delta_i, Z_i) \\
&= \delta_i \tilde{Y}_i + (1 - \delta_i) \left\{ \gamma^T Z_i + \frac{1}{1 - F(\tilde{e}_i)} \int_{\tilde{e}_i}^{\infty} x dF(x) \right\}, \quad (3.36)
\end{aligned}
$$

where $\tilde{e}_i(\gamma) = \tilde{Y}_i - \gamma^T Z_i$ and F is the distribution function of $e_i = Y_i - \gamma^T Z_i = \gamma_0 + \epsilon_i$.

By the double expectation theorem,

$$
E(Y_{iF,\gamma}^* | Z_i) = E(Y_i | Z_i) = \gamma_0 + \gamma^T Z_i.
$$

If $Y_{iF,\gamma}^*$ were known for all i, then the least squares estimates of γ_0 and γ are given by

$$
\begin{aligned}
\tilde{\gamma}(F, \gamma) &= \left\{ \sum_{i=1}^{n} (Z_i - \bar{Z})(Z_i - \bar{Z})^T \right\}^{-1} \sum_{i=1}^{n} (Z_i - \bar{Z}) Y_{iF,\gamma}^*, \quad (3.37) \\
\tilde{\gamma}_0(F, \gamma) &= \bar{Y}_{F,\gamma}^* - \hat{\gamma}^T \bar{Z}, \quad (3.38)
\end{aligned}
$$

where $\bar{Z} = n^{-1} \sum_{i=1}^{n} Z_i$ and $\bar{Y}_{F,\gamma}^* = n^{-1} \sum_{i=1}^{n} Y_{iF,\gamma}^*$.

Because $Y_{iF,\gamma}^*$ depends on γ and F that are unknown, Buckley and James [29] proposed the following iterative estimation algorithm for γ.

Step 1. Let $\hat{\gamma}^{(0)}$ be an initial estimate of γ.

Step 2. For $k = 1, 2, \ldots$, update $\hat{\gamma}^{(k-1)}$ by

$$
\hat{\gamma}^{(k)} = \tilde{\gamma}(\hat{F}^{(k-1)}, \hat{\gamma}^{(k-1)})
$$

where $\hat{F}^{(k-1)}$ is the Kaplan–Meier estimate based on the right–censored residuals $(\tilde{e}_i(\hat{\gamma}^{(k-1)}), \delta_i)$, $i = 1, \ldots, n$.

The Buckley-James estimates of γ_0 and γ are defined as

$$\hat{\gamma} = \lim_{k \to \infty} \hat{\gamma}^{(k)}, \qquad (3.39)$$

$$\hat{\gamma}_0 = \bar{Y}^*_{\hat{F},\hat{\gamma}} - \hat{\gamma}^T \bar{Z}, \qquad (3.40)$$

where $\hat{F}$ is the Kaplan–Meier estimate based on the right–censored residuals $(\tilde{e}_i(\hat{\gamma}), \delta_i)$, $i = 1, ..., n$. Note that $\hat{\gamma}_0$ is simply the mean of $\hat{F}$.

The Buckley–James estimates are consistent and asymptotically normal under certain regularity conditions [123, 183]. The asymptotic variance of $\hat{\gamma}$ involves the unknown hazard function of F and its derivative [183]. Although the hazard function and its derivative can be estimated nonparametrically using smoothing techniques, the resulting variance estimate is unstable. In practice, the bootstrap method can be used for variance estimation by resampling the triplets $\{(\tilde{Y}_i, \delta_i, \mathbf{Z}_i)\}_{i=1}^n$ with replacement. An alternative is to use the empirical likelihood method [255].

Linear Rank Method

For the ease of presentation, we will focus on estimation of γ.

Define

$$S(W_n, \gamma) = \sum_{i=1}^n \int W_n(u, \gamma)\{\mathbf{Z}_i - \bar{\mathbf{Z}}(u, \gamma)\}dN_i(u), \qquad (3.41)$$

where $W_n(u, \gamma)$ is a weight function, $N_i(u) = I(\tilde{e}_i(\gamma) \leq u, \delta_i = 1)$, $Y_i(u) = I(\tilde{e}_i(\gamma) \geq u)$, and

$$\bar{\mathbf{Z}}(u, \gamma) = \frac{\sum_{i=1}^n Y_i(u)Z_i}{\sum_{i=1}^n Y_i(u)}$$

is the sample average of the covariate $\mathbf{Z}$ over the subjects who are at risk prior to u on the error time scale.

Note that $S(W_n, \gamma_0)$ is a linear rank test statistic for $H_0 : \gamma = \gamma_0$ or for the hypothesis that $\mathbf{Z}$ and e are independent. Furthermore, it is centered at 0 under H_0. Therefore

$$S(W_n, \gamma) = 0 \qquad (3.42)$$

can be used as an estimation equation for γ.

Let $\hat{\gamma}(W_n)$ be a solution of (3.42). It has been shown that $\hat{\gamma}(W_n)$ is consistent and asymptotically normal [215]. Similar to the Buckley–James estimate, it is difficult to obtain a reliable estimate of the variance of $\hat{\gamma}(W_n)$ analytically because its asymptotic variance involves the unknown hazard function of the error e. Jin et al. [111] proposed a resampling method through a perturbed objective function. An alternative approach is to use the bootstrap method by resampling the triplets $\{(\tilde{Y}_i, \delta_i, \mathbf{Z}_i)\}_{i=1}^n$ with replacement.

Remark 3.2. *Choice of the weight function $W_n(u, \gamma)$. If $W_n(u, \gamma) \equiv 1$, the $S(W_n, \gamma)$ corresponds to the log-rank statistic [160]. It is optimal under the exponential AFT model. If $W_n(u, \gamma) = \sum_{i=1}^{n} Y_i(u)$, then $S(W_n, \gamma)$ corresponds to the Gehan statistic [76]. Other common weight functions include Prentice–Wilcoxon [176] and the general class of Harrington and Fleming [89].*

Remark 3.3. *Computation of the rank estimate. Note that the estimating functions in (3.42) are step functions of the regression parameters. Thus the estimating equations (3.42) may have multiple roots. Jin et al. [111] showed that the Gehan-type rank can be obtained by minimizing a convex objective function using a standard linear programming method and that non-monotone weighted log-rank estimating equations can be solved by an iterative algorithm with the Gehan estimator as an initial value.*

Remark 3.4. *Asymptotic normality. Note that*

$$S(W_n, \gamma) = \sum_{i=1}^{n} \int W_n(u, \gamma)\{\boldsymbol{Z}_i - \bar{\boldsymbol{Z}}(u, \gamma)\}dM_i(u), \qquad (3.43)$$

where $M_i(t) = N_i(t) - \int_0^t Y_i(u)\lambda_0(u)du$ is a martingale and $\lambda_0(u)$ is the hazard function of e. Assume $W_n(u, \gamma)$ and $\boldsymbol{Z}_i$'s are predictable, then $S(W_n, \gamma)$ is a martingale and its asymptotic normality follows directly from the martingale central limit theorem. Applying the Taylor series expansion gives the asymptotic normality of $\hat{\gamma}$.

3.6 Accelerated Failure Time Model with Time-Dependent Covariates

3.6.1 Model Formulation

An accelerated failure time (AFT) model relates the survival time T of a subject with a time-dependent covariate $\boldsymbol{Z}$ to a baseline time variable T_0 that corresponds to the condition $\boldsymbol{Z} = 0$ by

$$T_0 = \int_0^T \exp\{\boldsymbol{\beta}^T \boldsymbol{Z}(s)\}ds, \qquad (3.44)$$

where T_0 is assumed to be independent of $\boldsymbol{Z}$. Equivalently, model (3.44) can be written as

$$S(t|\boldsymbol{Z}(t)) = S_0\left[\int_0^t \exp\{\boldsymbol{\beta}^T \boldsymbol{Z}(s)\}ds\right], \qquad (3.45)$$

where $S(t|\boldsymbol{Z}(t))$ is the conditional survival function of a subject given $Z(s), (0 < s \leq t)$, the covariate history up to time t, and $S_0(t)$ is the survival function of T_0 [45, 188, 147]. It implies that subjects with covariate $\boldsymbol{Z}$ fail on a contracted or expanded time scale $\int_0^t \exp\{\boldsymbol{\beta}^T \boldsymbol{Z}(s)\}ds$. Under this model, the biological clock of a subject with covariate history $\{Z(s), 0 \leq s \leq t\}$ is accelerated by a factor of $\exp\{\beta^T Z(t)\}$ at time t relative to the baseline clock.

Model (3.44) can also be written as

$$\lambda(t|Z(t)) = \lambda_0 \left[\int_0^t \exp\{\beta^T Z(s)\} ds \right] \exp\{\beta^T Z(t)\}, \qquad (3.46)$$

where $\lambda(t|Z(t))$ is the conditional hazard of T at time t given the covariate history up to t and $\lambda_0(t)$ is a baseline hazard function.

Note that the AFT model (3.46) allows the entire covariate history to influence the subject specific hazard. In contrast, the Cox model (3.9) assumes that the conditional hazard given the past covariate history is influenced only by covariate value at the current time.

Example 3.7. *Consider a simple situation with one binary covariate ($p = 1$) where $Z(t) = 0$ before an intermittent event such as development of graft-versus-host disease in a bone marrow transplant patient, and 1 after the intermittent event. Then model (3.44) implies that the survival function $S(t|Z(t))$ is $S_0(t)$ before the intermittent event and $S_0\{\tau + e^\beta(t - \tau)\}$ after the intermittent event, where τ is the time at which the intermittent event occurs. In other words, the "biological clock" of the patient is accelerated by a factor of e^β after the occurrence intermittent event.*

Example 3.8. *Suppose that $p = 1$ and $Z(t)$ is a time-dependent indicator of exposure such that $Z(t) = 1$ if the subject is exposed at time t and 0 otherwise. Then model (3.44) implies that the "biological clock" of the subject is accelerated by a factor of e^β during times of exposure. In particular, under constant exposure ($Z(t) = 1$ for all t), the survival time is contracted by a factor of $e^{-\beta}$, or $T = e^{-\beta}T_0$.*

Example 3.9. *Suppose that one is interested in studying the effects of a continuously monitored biomarker $Z(t)$ such as CD4 count or PSA on an event time such as time to death. The model (3.44) implies that at time t, the "biological clock" of the subject is accelerated by a factor of $e^{\beta Z(t)}$. So the biological clock of the subject is being adjusted continuously according to its current biomarker level.*

3.6.2 Rank-Based Estimation

We now describe a rank-based method for the AFT model (3.44) with time-dependent covariate [147, 188].

Let

$$h_i(t, b) = \int_0^t \exp\{b^T Z_i(s) ds\}, \quad \tilde{X}_i(b) = h_i(\tilde{T}_i, b), \quad \tilde{Z}_i(t, b) = Z_i\{h_i^{-1}(t, b)\},$$

$$N(t, b) = \sum_{i=1}^n I\{\tilde{X}_i(b) \leq, \delta_i = 1\}, \quad Y_i = I\{\tilde{X}_i(b) \geq t),$$

where $h_i^{-1}(t, b)$ is an inverse function of h_i with b being fixed.

The parameter β can be estimated from the following estimating equation

$$U(b) = 0,$$

where

$$U(b) = \int_0^\infty \left\{ \tilde{Z}_i(t, b) - \frac{\sum_{i=1}^n \tilde{Z}_i(t, b) Y_i(t, b)}{\sum_{i=1}^n Y_i(t, b)} \right\} dN(t, b)$$

is the log rank statistic based on $\{\tilde{X}_i(b), \Delta_i, \tilde{Z}_i\}$, $i = 1, \ldots, n$, derived from the likelihood score function under model (3.44) [147].

Let

$$\hat{\beta} = \arg\min_b \|U(b)\|.$$

Under certain regularity conditions, it can be shown that $\hat{\beta}$ is asymptotically normal. However, its asymptotic variance involves the unknown hazard of S_0 which is difficult to estimate in practice. Below we describe an inference procedure that does not involve hazard estimation [147].

Suppose one wishes to test $H_0 : \beta^{(1)} = \beta_0^{(1)}$, where $\beta^{(1)}$ is a $q \times 1$ subvector of β. Define the minimum dispersion statistic

$$G(\beta_0^{(1)}) = \inf_{b^{(1)} = \beta_0^{(1)}, \|b^{(2)} - \beta_0^{(2)}\| \leq B} U(b)^T V^{-1}(\hat{\beta}) U(\beta),$$

where $B > 0$ is any given constant. Then, under appropriate conditions, $G(\beta_0^{(1)})$ has an asymptotic χ_q^2 distribution. Therefore, we reject H_0 at level α if $G(\beta_0^{(1)}) > \chi_q^2(\alpha)$, where $\chi_q^2(\alpha)$ is the upper α-quantitle of the χ_q^2 distribution. Consequently, an $(1 - \alpha)$ confidence interval for $\beta_0^{(1)}$ is given by $\{\phi : G(\phi) \leq \chi_q^2\}$.

Alternatively, the bootstrap method can be used to draw inference for β.

3.7   Methods for Competing Risks Data

Competing risks survival data are encountered frequently in clinical trials, reliability testing, and other studies. It occurs when there are multiple types of failure and exactly one type of failure is observed for each subject. Specifically, the outcome is composed of a pair of random variables (T, D), where T is a continuous event time and D denotes the failure type taking values in $\{1, \ldots, K\}$ for some integer $K \geq 1$.

Example 3.10. *In a clinical trial, one may be interested in time to death due to a particular disease, but a patient may also die from other competing diseases. Here T is time to death and D is the disease type. The competing diseases are potentially positively correlated.*

Example 3.11. *In a kidney transplantation program, patients who are ineligible for transplantation due to reasons, such as being overweight, are put on a waiting list until they become eligible (see, e.g., [195]). An important outcome variable is the waiting time to become eligible for transplantation. In this example, death before becoming eligible for transplantation is a competing risk event that is potentially negatively correlated with the waiting time.*

Example 3.12. *In economics studies, it is often of interest to study the effects of the level and length of unemployment insurance (UI) benefits on unemployment duration. There are several causes for ending unemployment including taking a new job, recall to a previous job, and withdrawal from the labor force. The competing risks model is useful to study unemployment duration data.*

For more examples of competing risks failure time data we refer the reader to [177, 174, 78, 180], and the references therein.

3.7.1 Basic Quantities for Competing Risks Data

Let

$$Q(t, s) = P(T \leq t, D \leq s) \tag{3.47}$$

be the joint distribution function of (T, D).

Definition 3.1. *For each $k \in \{1, ..., K\}$, define*

$$\lambda_k(t) = \lim_{\Delta t \downarrow 0} \frac{P(t \leq T < t + \Delta t, D = k | T \geq t)}{\Delta t}, \quad t > 0, \tag{3.48}$$

to be the cause-specific hazard function *for failure type k. The cause-specific hazard is also referred to as the "crude" hazard.*

Definition 3.2. *For each $k \in \{1, ..., K\}$, define $F_k(t) = P(T \leq t, D = k) = Q(t, k) - Q(t, k - 1)$ to be the cumulative incidence function for failure type k.*

Let $\Lambda_k(t) = \int_0^t \lambda_k(s)ds$ be the cumulative cause-specific hazard function for failure type k. Denote by $\lambda(t)$, $\Lambda(t)$, and $S(t)$ the hazard function, cumulative hazard function, and survival function of T. Then

$$\lambda(t) = \sum_{k=1}^{K} \lambda_k(t), \tag{3.49}$$

$$\Lambda(t) = \sum_{k=1}^{K} \Lambda_k(t), \tag{3.50}$$

$$S(t) = e^{-\Lambda(t)}, \tag{3.51}$$

$$F_k(t) = \int_0^t S(s-)\lambda_k(s)ds, \quad k = 1, \ldots, K. \tag{3.52}$$

Clearly, the joint distribution of (T, D) is fully characterized either by $\{F_1(t), \ldots, F_K(t)\}$, or by $\{\lambda_1(t), \ldots, \lambda_K(t)\}$.

It is worth noting from (3.52) that for a fixed k, the cumulative incidence function F_k depends not only on the kth cause-specific hazard λ_k, but also on other cause-specific hazards functions through the overall survival function $S(t)$.

3.7.2 Latent Variable Representation of Competing Risks Data

We now describe a latent variable representation of competing risks data.

Proposition 3.1. *Assume that (T, D) is a pair of competing risk outcomes with a joint distribution function $Q(t, s)$ as defined in (3.47).*

(a) *Then, there exist K independent latent random variables $T^{(1)}, \ldots, T^{(K)}$ such that (T^*, D^*) has the same joint distribution $Q(t, s)$ as (T, D), where $T^* = \min\{T^{(1)}, \ldots, T^{(K)}\}$ and D^* is defined by $T^{(D^*)} = T^*$.*

(b) *Furthermore, the type k cause-specific hazard of T defined by (3.48) is identical to the marginal hazard function of $T^{(k)}$, $k = 1, \ldots, K$.*

Part (a) of Proposition 3.47 was established by Tsiatis [213]. To understand part (b) of Proposition 3.47, we consider the simple case $K = 2$. Let $f_k(t)$ and $S_k(t)$ be the density function and survival function of $T^{(k)}$, $k = 1, 2$. By part (a), the type 1 cause-specific hazard of T is

$$
\begin{aligned}
\lambda_1(t) &= \lim_{\Delta t \downarrow 0} \frac{P(t \leq T^* < t + \Delta t, D^* = 1 | T^* \geq t)}{\Delta t} \\
&= \lim_{\Delta t \downarrow 0} \frac{P(t \leq T^{(1)} < t + \Delta t, T^{(1)} < T^{(2)} | T^{(1)} \geq t, T^{(2)} \geq t)}{\Delta t} \\
&= \lim_{\Delta t \downarrow 0} \frac{P(t \leq T^{(1)} < t + \Delta t, T^{(1)} < T^{(2)}, T^{(2)} \geq t)}{\Delta t P(T^{(1)} \geq t, T^{(2)} \geq t)} \\
&= \lim_{\Delta t \downarrow 0} \frac{\int_t^{t+\Delta t} \int_u^\infty f_1(u) f_2(v) dv du)}{\Delta t S_1(t) S_2(t)} \\
&= \lim_{\Delta t \downarrow 0} \frac{\int_t^{t+\Delta t} f_1(u) S_2(v) du)}{\Delta t S_1(t) S_2(t)} \\
&= \frac{f_1(t) S_2(t)}{S_1(t) S_2(t)} \\
&= \frac{f_1(t)}{S_1(t)} = \text{marginal hazard function of } T^{(1)}.
\end{aligned}
$$

An example of competing risk data with independent risks is the failure time T of a serial system consisting of K independently operated components under which the system fails if one of its components fails.

Remark 3.5. *For competing risks data with dependent risks, Proposition 3.1 implies that there is always a hypothetical working model with independent risks that gives the same distribution as the observed competing risks data. Furthermore, for a given k, inference on type k cause-specific hazard can be made using the methods in the previous sections for a single failure time by treating other risks as independent censoring.*

Remark 3.6. *Although the latent time model provides a convenient working model for drawing inference on a cause-specific hazard, the latent variables $T^{(1)}, \ldots, T^{(K)}$ do not always have plausible practical interpretations. Furthermore, without the independence assumption, the joint distribution and the marginal distribution of $T^{(1)}, \ldots, T^{(K)}$ are not identifiable from the observed competing risks data.*

3.7.3 Estimation of the Cumulative Cause-Specific Hazard and Cumulative Incidence

Suppose that one observes a right–censored competing risks failure time data consisting of n i.i.d. triples $\{(\tilde{T}_i, \delta_i), i = 1, \ldots, n\}$, where $\tilde{T}_i = \min(T_i, C_i)$ and $\delta_i = D_i I(T_i \leq C_i)$, where for subject i, T_i, D_i, and C_i denote the continuous failure time, failure type, and censoring time, respectively.

Let $N_k(t) = \sum_{i=1}^{n} I(\tilde{T}_i \leq t, \delta_i = k)$ be the counting process of the number of observed type k failures by time t, and $Y(t) = \sum_{i=1}^{n} I\{\tilde{T}_i \geq t\}$ be the at-risk process indicating the number of subjects who are at risk for any type of failure prior to time t.

The type k cumulative cause-specific hazard function $\Lambda_k(t)$ is estimated by the Nelson–Aalen type estimate

$$\hat{\Lambda}_k(t) = \int_0^t \frac{dN_k(s)}{Y(s)}, \quad k = 1, \ldots, K. \tag{3.53}$$

Although the competing risks may be correlated, it follow from Remark 3.5 that for any k, $\hat{\Lambda}_k(t)$ has the same properties as the usual Nelson–Aalen estimate obtained by treating other causes as independent censoring.

It follows from (3.52) that the type k cumulative incidence function $F_k(t)$ is estimated by

$$\hat{F}_k(t) = \int_0^t \hat{S}(s-)d\hat{\Lambda}_k(t), \quad k = 1, \ldots, K, \tag{3.54}$$

where $\hat{S}(t)$ is the Kaplan–Meier estimate of $S(t)$.

Consistency and weak convergence results of (3.53) and (3.54) can be found in [1, 5, 72, 71, 79, 166].

3.7.4 Regression Models for a Cause-Specific Hazard

As discussed in Remark 3.5, the hazard regression models for a single failure time with right–censored data discussed in the previous sections can be adopted to study the relationship between a cause-specific hazard and a set of covariates by treating other risks as independent censoring.

Multiplicative Cause-Specific Hazards Model

The multiplicative cause-specific hazards model for type k failure is given by

$$\lambda_k(t|\boldsymbol{Z}(t)) = \lambda_{k0}(t)\exp(\boldsymbol{\beta}_k^T\boldsymbol{Z}(t)), \tag{3.55}$$

where $\lambda_k(t|\boldsymbol{Z}(t))$ is the type-k conditional cause-specific hazard of T at time t given the covariate history up to t, $\boldsymbol{\beta}_k$ is a vector of regression coefficients, and $\lambda_{k0}(t)$ is an unspecified baseline cause-specific hazard function.

Define the score function for $\boldsymbol{\beta}_k$ as

$$\boldsymbol{U}_k(\boldsymbol{\beta}_k) = \sum_{i=1}^n \int_0^\infty \left\{\boldsymbol{Z}_i(s) - \bar{\boldsymbol{Z}}(\boldsymbol{\beta}_k, s)\right\} dN_{ik}(s), \tag{3.56}$$

where $N_{ik}(t) = I(\tilde{T}_i \leq t, D_i = k)$, $Y_i(t) = I(\tilde{T}_i \geq t)$, and

$$\bar{\boldsymbol{Z}}(\boldsymbol{\beta}, t) = \frac{\sum_{l=1}^n Y_l(t)\boldsymbol{Z}_l \exp(\boldsymbol{\beta}^T\boldsymbol{Z}_l(t))}{\sum_{l=1}^n Y_l(t) \exp(\boldsymbol{\beta}^T\boldsymbol{Z}_l(t))}.$$

Let $\hat{\boldsymbol{\beta}}_k$ be the solution of the score equation

$$\boldsymbol{U}_k(\boldsymbol{\beta}_k) = 0.$$

Then $n^{1/2}(\hat{\boldsymbol{\beta}}_k - \boldsymbol{\beta}_k)$ is approximately normally distributed with mean zero and variance $\hat{\Omega}_k^{-1}$, where

$$\hat{\Omega}_k = \frac{1}{n}\sum_{i=1}^n \int_0^\infty \left[\frac{\sum_{l=1}^n Y_l(s)\boldsymbol{Z}_l(s)^{\otimes 2}\exp(\hat{\boldsymbol{\beta}}_k^T\boldsymbol{Z}_l(s))}{\sum_{l=1}^n Y_l(s)\exp(\hat{\boldsymbol{\beta}}_k^T\boldsymbol{Z}_l(s))} - \bar{\boldsymbol{Z}}(\boldsymbol{\beta}_k, s)^{\otimes 2}\right] dN_{ik}(s).$$

Note that the above inference method for $\boldsymbol{\beta}_k$ is equivalent to applying the standard partial likelihood method to type k failure by treating other risks as independent censoring [177, 122, 96, 45, 128, 156].

Accelerated Failure Time Model

Similarly, the accelerated failure time model (3.44) can also be used to model a cause-specific hazard

$$\lambda_k(t|\boldsymbol{Z}(t)) = \lambda_{k0} \left[\int_0^t \exp\{\boldsymbol{\beta}_k^T \boldsymbol{Z}(s)\} ds \right] \exp\{\boldsymbol{\beta}_k^T \boldsymbol{Z}(t)\}, \qquad (3.57)$$

where $\lambda_k(t|\boldsymbol{Z}(t))$ is the type k conditional cause-specific hazard of T at time t given the covariate history up to t and $\lambda_{k0}(t)$ is a corresponding baseline cause-specific hazard function. Inference for a specific $\boldsymbol{\beta}_k$ can be made using the methods described in Sections 3.5 and 3.6 by regarding other causes as independently censored.

3.7.5 Regression Models for Cumulative Incidence

To study the effects of a covariate on the cumulative incidence function of a particular failure type, say, type 1, one could model the cause-specific functions of different failure types using the proportional hazards type models, and then combine estimates from these models to obtain an estimate of the conditional cumulative incidence function $F_1(t|z)$ using (3.52). However, the effect of a covariate on the cause-specific hazard function of type 1 may be very different from the effect of the covariate on the corresponding cumulative incidence function [82, 68, 173, 135]. Various methods have been proposed to directly model the relationship between a cumulative incidence function and a set of covariates using different models such as the multiplicative subdistribution hazards model [68], transformation models [66, 69, 67, 118, 77], quantile regression [172], and additive models [117]. Below we describe the Fine and Gray [68] multiplicative subdistribution hazards model for the cumulative incidence function.

Multiplicative Subdistribution Hazards Model

For each $1 \le k \le K$, define

$$\begin{aligned}
\tilde{\lambda}_k(t) &= \lim_{dt\downarrow 0} P(t \le T < t + dt, D = k | T \ge t \cup (T < t \cap D \ne k))/dt \\
&= -d\log\{1 - F_k(t)\}/dt
\end{aligned}$$

to be the *subdistribution* hazard function for type k failure. Clearly $\tilde{\lambda}_k(\cdot)$ and $F_k(\cdot)$ uniquely determine each other.

The proportional subdistribution hazards model for type k failure postulates that

$$\tilde{\lambda}_k(t|\boldsymbol{Z}(t)) = \tilde{\lambda}_{k0}(t) \exp(\boldsymbol{\gamma}_k^T \boldsymbol{Z}(t)), \qquad (3.58)$$

where $\tilde{\lambda}_k(t|\boldsymbol{Z}(t))$ is the type k conditional subdistribution hazard of T at time t given the covariate history up to t and $\tilde{\lambda}_{k0}(t)$ is an unknown baseline subdistribution hazard.

Note that the risk set for the subdistribution is rather unnatural because subjects who have failed from causes other than k are still considered being at risk for type k failure. However, it is easy to see that the proportional subdistribution hazards model is equivalent to the following transformation model

$$log(-log(F_k(t|\boldsymbol{Z}))) = h_0(t) + \boldsymbol{\gamma}_k^T \boldsymbol{Z},$$

where $h_{k0}(t) = \log \int_0^t \tilde{\lambda}_{k0}(u)du$. Therefore, $\boldsymbol{\gamma}$ has a straightforward interpretation for F_k that does not depend on the probabilistic interpretation of the subdistribution hazard.

For uncensored competing risks data, estimation of parameters in model (3.58) is done by performing a standard Cox regression analysis of a modified data set where individuals failing from causes other than k are given a censored observation time of ∞ (or a censored time larger than the largest observed cause k failure time).

For censored competing risks data, an inverse probability weighting method can be used to derive estimation equations for $\boldsymbol{\gamma}$. Specifically, the score function for γ_k is defined as

$$\tilde{\boldsymbol{U}}_k(\boldsymbol{\gamma}_k) = \sum_{i=1}^n \int_0^\infty \left\{ \boldsymbol{Z}_i(s) - \bar{\boldsymbol{Z}}_{k,\omega}(\boldsymbol{\gamma}_k, s) \right\} \omega_i(s) d\tilde{N}_{ik}(s), \qquad (3.59)$$

where

$$\bar{\boldsymbol{Z}}_{k,\omega}(\boldsymbol{\gamma}, t) = \frac{\sum_{l=1}^n \omega_l(t)\tilde{Y}_{lk}(t)\boldsymbol{Z}_l \exp(\boldsymbol{\gamma}^T \boldsymbol{Z}_l(t))}{\sum_{l=1}^n \omega_l(t)\tilde{Y}_{lk}(t) \exp(\boldsymbol{\gamma}^T \boldsymbol{Z}_l(t))},$$

$\tilde{N}_{ik}(t) = I(T_i \leq t, D_i = k)$, $\tilde{Y}_{ik}(t) = 1 - \tilde{N}_{ik}(t-)$, $\omega_i(t) = I(C_i \geq T_i \wedge t)\hat{G}^c(t)/\hat{G}^c(X_i \wedge t)$, and $\hat{G}^c$ is the Kaplan–Meier estimate of the survival function G^c of the censoring variable C. Note that although $\tilde{N}_{ik}(t)$ may not be always be observed, $\omega_i(t)\tilde{N}_{ik}(t)$ is always computable from the observed data.

Let $\hat{\boldsymbol{\gamma}}_k$ be the solution of the score equation

$$\tilde{\boldsymbol{U}}_k(\boldsymbol{\gamma}_k) = 0.$$

The distribution of $n^{1/2}(\hat{\boldsymbol{\gamma}}_k - \boldsymbol{\gamma}_k)$ can be approximated by a normal distribution with mean zero and variance $\hat{\Omega}_k^{-1}\hat{\Sigma}_k\hat{\Omega}_k^{-1}$, where

$$\hat{\Omega}_k = \frac{1}{n}\sum_{i=1}^n \left\{ \frac{\tilde{S}_k^{(2)}(\hat{\boldsymbol{\gamma}}_k, \tilde{T}_i)}{\tilde{S}_k^{(0)}(\hat{\boldsymbol{\gamma}}_k, \tilde{T}_i)} - \bar{\boldsymbol{Z}}_k(\hat{\boldsymbol{\gamma}}_k, \tilde{T}_i)^{\otimes 2} \right\} I(\delta_i = 1),$$

$$\hat{\Sigma}_k = \frac{1}{n}\sum_{i=1}^{n}(\hat{\boldsymbol{\eta}}_i + \hat{\boldsymbol{\psi}}_i)^{\otimes 2},$$

$$\bar{\boldsymbol{Z}}_k(\boldsymbol{\gamma}, t) = \frac{\tilde{S}_k^{(1)}(\boldsymbol{\gamma}, t)}{\tilde{S}_k^{(0)}(\boldsymbol{\gamma}, t)},$$

$$\tilde{S}_k^{(l)}(\boldsymbol{\gamma}, t) = \frac{1}{n}\sum_{i=1}^{n}\omega_i(t)\tilde{Y}_{ik}(t)\boldsymbol{Z}_i(t)^{\otimes l}\exp(\boldsymbol{\gamma}^T\boldsymbol{Z}_i(t)), \quad l = 0,1,2,$$

$$\hat{\boldsymbol{\eta}}_i = \int_0^\infty \left\{\boldsymbol{Z}_i(s) - \bar{\boldsymbol{Z}}_k(\hat{\boldsymbol{\gamma}}_k, s)\right\}\omega_i(s)d\hat{\tilde{M}}_{ik}(s),$$

$$\hat{\tilde{M}}_{ik}(t) = \tilde{N}_{ik}(t) - \int_0^t \tilde{Y}_{ik}(s)\exp(\hat{\boldsymbol{\gamma}}_k^T\boldsymbol{Z}_i(s))d\hat{\tilde{\Lambda}}_{k0}(s),$$

$$\hat{\tilde{\Lambda}}_{k0}(t) = \frac{1}{n}\sum_{i=1}^{n}\int_0^t \{\tilde{S}_k^{(0)}(\boldsymbol{\gamma}, s)\}^{-1}\omega_i(s)d\tilde{N}_{ik}(s),$$

$$\hat{\boldsymbol{\psi}}_i = \int_0^\infty \frac{\hat{\boldsymbol{q}}(s)}{\hat{\pi}(s)}d\hat{M}_i^c(s),$$

$$\hat{\boldsymbol{q}}(t) = -n^{-1}\sum_{i=1}^{n}\int_0^\infty \left\{\boldsymbol{Z}_i(s) - \bar{\boldsymbol{Z}}_k(\hat{\boldsymbol{\gamma}}_k, s)\right\}I(s \geq t > \tilde{T}_i)\omega_i(s)d\hat{\tilde{M}}_{i1}(s),$$

$$\hat{\pi}(t) = n^{-1}\sum_{i=1}^{n}I(\tilde{T}_i \geq t),$$

$$\hat{M}_i^c(t) = I(\tilde{T}_i \leq t, \delta_i = 0) - \int_0^t I(\tilde{T}_i \geq s)d\hat{\Lambda}^c(s),$$

$$\hat{\Lambda}^c(t) = \int_0^t \frac{\sum_{i=1}^{n}d\{I(\tilde{T}_i \leq s, \delta_i = 0)\}}{n\hat{\pi}(s)}.$$

3.7.6 Joint Inference of Cause-Specific Hazard and Cumulative Incidence

When studying the effects of a variable on a specific type of failure, say type 1 failure, it is not sufficient to consider either the cause-specific hazard function $\lambda_1(t)$ alone, or the cumulative incidence function $F_1(t)$ alone since 1) $\lambda_1(t)$ and $F_1(t)$ describe different characteristics of type 1 failure, 2) they do not uniquely determine each other, and 3) the effects of a variable on the two functions can be different and one often does not know which effects are to be expected. Instead, it would be important to draw joint inference on multiple quantities such as $\lambda_1(t)$ together with $F_1(t)$ for competing risks data. We refer the reader to [135] for various joint inference procedures to study the effects of a variable with competing risks data.

3.8 Further Topics

Most of the survival analysis methods discussed in this chapter can be implemented using standard statistical software such as SAS, Stata, SPSS, and R. For example, there are an abundance of books of event time data analysis with a software such as SAS [10] and R [26]. A survival analysis R package is available at https://cran.r-project.org/web/packages/survival/index.html.

In addition to the Cox model and the accelerated failure time models discussed in Sections 3.4, 3.5, and 3.6, there are available other regression models for right–censored survival data. Useful alternative models include additive risks models [3, 105, 4, 146, 162], transformation models [38, 32, 48, 39, 35, 250], partly linear models [36, 229, 159], frailty models [120, 170, 168, 97, 98, 161, 4, 151], and nonparametric regression methods [20, 46, 47, 163, 62, 133, 220, 221] .

There are additional important topics such as multistate models, multivariate survival analysis, cure models, and model diagnostics methods that are not discussed in this chapter. Interested readers are referred to [12, 45, 73, 113, 119], among many other excellent monographs, for more comprehensive and in-depth coverage of survival analysis methods.

Chapter 4

Overview of Joint Models for Longitudinal and Time-to-Event Data

This chapter is the core of this monograph, providing an overview of several main areas in which joint models have been developed to address statistical issues that cannot be handled in separate analysis of longitudinal and survival data. Specifically, in the first three sections, we discuss joint models that are used as a tool to tackle the nonignorable missing data problem in longitudinal studies. The topics include monotone missing data caused by continuous or discrete event times, and longitudinal measurements with both monotone and intermittent missing values.

An important area that fosters development of joint models is survival analysis with time-dependent covariates. Joint analysis is an elegant approach to model the association between time-dependent covariates and the event of interest when the covariate trajectory is not completely observed and subject to measurement error and/or biological variation. Research in this area is discussed in Section 4.4.

Other important topics, including longitudinal studies with informative observation times and dynamic prediction in joint models, are reviewed in Sections 4.5 and 4.6.

4.1 Joint Models of Longitudinal Data and an Event Time

This section introduces joint modeling of longitudinal measurements and time-to-event data, focusing on methods for joint analysis with a longitudinal outcome Y and an event time T from a single failure type. Two general types of models, selection models and mixture models, have been proposed in the literature to address various research interests in real applications. In a selection model, the joint distribution $f(Y, T)$ is decomposed into the marginal distribution of Y, $f(Y)$, and the conditional distribution of T given Y, $f(T|Y)$. The marginal distribution of Y is usually characterized by a linear mixed model or a generalized linear mixed model, and the conditional distribution $f(T|Y)$ is specified via a regression model for T in which Y or characteristics of $f(Y)$, such as random effects, are included as covariates. However, in a mixture model, the joint distribution is characterized by first conditioning on T, that is, $f(Y,T) = f(Y|T)f(T)$. Therefore, the marginal density of Y can be viewed as a mixture of distributions specified by T. Note that both joint models assume non-informative censorship for the event time. In what follows we discuss and compare the two different approaches in more detail.

4.1.1   Selection Models

Consider a sample of n subjects. The longitudinal measurements Y_{ij} are collected on each subject at times t_{ij}, $i = 1, \ldots, n$, $j = 1, \ldots, n_i$, in which n_i is the number of measurements on subject i. Write $Y_i = (Y_{i1}, \ldots, Y_{in_i})$. Let T_i be the event time for subject i, which is subject to right censoring by C_i. Assume non-informative censorship, so that C_i is independent of T_i given covariates X_i. The observed event time data for subject i are $\tilde{T}_i = min(T_i, C_i)$ and $\Delta_i = I(T_i \leq C_i)$, such that $\Delta_i = 1$ if $T_i \leq C_i$ and $\Delta_i = 0$ if $T_i > C_i$.

In selection models, one needs to specify the marginal distribution of Y_i. It is common to use linear or generalized linear mixed effects models in which the within-subject correlations are modeled by latent random effects b_i. One appealing interpretation of b_i in the context of joint models is that b_i or a function of b_i, $f(b_i)$, reflects the underlying trajectory/trend in Y_i. In some applications, this is assumed to be the characteristic that is closely related to T_i. If b_i is used to link together Y_i and T_i, then the missing data in Y are nonignorable. Definitions of ignorable and nonignorable missing data are given in Chapter 2 (Section 2.2). Little (1995)[152], Hogan and Laird (1997)[95], Tsiatis and Davidian (2004)[217], and Ibrahim (2009)[107] provide comprehensive overviews of selection models.

Shared Parameter Models

Under the framework of linear mixed effects models, the distribution of Y_{ij} is specified as

$$Y_{ij} = X_{ij}^{(1)T}\beta_1 + \tilde{X}_{ij}^{(1)T}b_i + \epsilon_{ij}, \tag{4.1}$$

where $X_{ij}^{(1)}$ and $\tilde{X}_{ij}^{(1)}$ are vectors of possibly time-varying covariates, β_1 is a vector of fixed effects, $b_i \sim N(0, \Sigma_b)$ is a vector of random effects, and $\epsilon_{ij} \sim N(0, \sigma^2)$ is the error term. Assume $\epsilon_{ij} \perp b_i$. More generally, for distributions in exponential families, a generalized linear mixed effects model can be used:

$$g\{E(Y_{ij}|b_i)\} = X_{ij}^{(1)T}\beta_1 + \tilde{X}_{ij}^{(1)T}b_i,$$

in which $g(\cdot)$ is a link function. In the case of linear mixed models, g is the identity function. When the mean of Y_{ij} cannot be fully captured by linear functions, nonlinear mixed effects models have also been considered [238, 239].

In selection models, the event time is associated with the longitudinal data through Y_i or the random effects b_i. When b_i is used to link together Y_i and T_i, the approach is referred to as *shared parameter* models, although b_i is a covariate, not a parameter, in the model for T_i. The "shared random effects" assumption may appear restrictive, but it reflects an intuitive and appealing idea that the same set of random effects induces the interdependence between longitudinal and survival processes. This approach provides a useful tool in practice when the unobserved factors that affect the longitudinal response are believed to affect the risk of failures as well.

In the joint model literature, T_i is usually characterized using parametric or Cox-type semiparametric models. A parametric model can be specified as

$$g\{E(T_i|b_i)\} = X_i^{(2)T}\beta_2 + \nu b_i, \tag{4.2}$$

where $X_i^{(2)}$ is a vector of covariates that are associated with the event process, and $g(\cdot)$ is a known link function. In the analysis of AIDS data, a generalized linear model of form (4.2) with the identity link function has been used to characterize the survival time [51]. Under the Cox regression framework the hazard of T_i is specified as

$$\lambda_i(t|b_i) = \lambda_0(t)exp(X_i^{(2)T}\beta_2 + \nu b_i), \tag{4.3}$$

where $\lambda_0(t)$ is a parametric or completely unspecified baseline hazard function. If $b_i = (b_{0i}, b_{1i})$ contains the random intercept and slope for Y_i, then the model assumes that the subject-specific starting value and time trend in the underlying trajectory of Y_i affect the event risk. A natural extension is that a function of b_i, e.g., $b_{0i} + b_{1i}t$, is treated as a time-dependent covariate in model (4.3). This approach and its application will be discussed in more detail later. Note that, in (4.2) and (4.3), ν is a key parameter to model the association between Y and T, and the joint model reduces to separate analysis when $\nu = 0$.

Missingness in Y

The joint distribution of Y and T is completely specified by models (4.1)–(4.3), assuming they are independent given the random effects and covariates. If the event causes missing data in Y, such as death or dropout, then models (4.1)–(4.3) implicitly assume that the data are missing not at random (MNAR) when $\nu \neq 0$. Let $Y_{i(obs)}$ and $Y_{i(mis)}$ denote the observed and missing components in $\tilde{Y}_i$, respectively, where $\tilde{Y}_i$ is a complete sequence of measurements of Y_i when there are no missing data. It can be shown that

$$f(T_i|Y_{i(obs)}, Y_{i(mis)}) \tag{4.4}$$

$$= \int_{b_i} f(T_i|b_i, Y_{i(obs)}, Y_{i(mis)}) f(b_i|Y_{i(obs)}, Y_{i(mis)}) db_i$$

$$= \int_{b_i} f(T_i|b_i) f(b_i|Y_{i(obs)}, Y_{i(mis)}) db_i,$$

which indicates that the distribution of T_i is dependent on the missing data $Y_{i(mis)}$ because $f(b_i|Y_{i(obs)}, Y_{i(mis)})$ involves $Y_{i(mis)}$ when $\nu \neq 0$.

Extensions of Shared Parameter Models

The above joint model can be extended to allow an additional source of variation at the survival endpoint that cannot be explained by the longitudinal data. Specifically, a separate random variable u_i can be introduced into model (4.3), so that we have

$$\lambda_i(t|b_i, u_i) = \lambda_0(t) exp(X_i^{(2)T} \beta_2 + \nu b_i + u_i). \tag{4.5}$$

Usually u_i is assumed to follow a zero-mean normal distribution. Equations (4.1) and (4.5) are no longer a shared parameter model because u_i is not shared by the longitudinal data. This joint model includes (4.3) as a special case when the variance of u_i shrinks to zero. Alternatively, the survival model can be specified as

$$\lambda_i(t|u_i) = \lambda_0(t) exp(X_i^{(2)T} \beta_2 + u_i), \tag{4.6}$$

and u_i and b_i are assumed to have a multivariate normal distribution with variance-covariance matrix

$$\Sigma = \begin{pmatrix} \Sigma_{bb} & \Sigma_{bu}^T \\ \Sigma_{bu} & \sigma_u^2 \end{pmatrix}.$$

The joint model reduces to a separate analysis of the two endpoints when $b_i \perp u_i$, that is, $\Sigma_{bu} = 0$, and the missing data are ignorable in this case.

A more general extension of shared parameter models is proposed by Henderson et al. (2000)[93], in which a latent zero-mean bivariate Gaussian process $W_i(t) = \{W_{1i}(t), W_{2i}(t)\}$ is used to characterize the association between Y and T. In particular, the model is given by

$$Y_{ij} = X_{ij}^{(1)T} \beta_1 + W_{1i}(t_{ij}) + \epsilon_{ij}, \tag{4.7}$$

and

$$\lambda_i(t|W_2) = \lambda_0(t) exp\{X_i^{(2)T} \beta_2 + W_{2i}(t)\}. \tag{4.8}$$

Various functional forms have been proposed for the latent processes $W_{1i}(t)$ and $W_{2i}(t)$. For example, $W_{1i}(t)$ can be b_{0i} or $b_{0i} + b_{1i}t$, where b_{0i} and b_{1i} are random intercept and slope, respectively, and $W_{2i}(t)$ can be $\gamma W_{1i}(t)$, $\gamma_1 b_{0i} + \gamma_2 b_{1i} + \gamma_2 W_{1i}(t)$, or $\gamma_1 b_{0i} + \gamma_2 b_{1i} + \gamma_2 W_{1i}(t) + u_i$, where u_i is a frailty term that cannot be explained by Y. Even more flexibly, a stochastic Gaussian process $V_i(t)$ which is independent of b_i can be incorporated into $W_{1i}(t)$ and then shared with $W_{2i}(t)$. Specifically, $V_i(t) \sim N(0, \sigma_v^2)$ and $Corr(V_i(t), V_i(t - s)) = r(s; \phi)$. A typical example of $r(s; \phi)$ is $\exp(-|s|^v/\phi)$, where v and ϕ are unknown parameters to be estimated from the data.

Likelihood and Parameter Estimation

For the joint models discussed above, the observed-data likelihood can be easily written out based on the conditional independence assumption of Y and T given the random effects and covariates. For example, the likelihood for model (4.1) and (4.6) is

$$
\begin{aligned}
L(\Psi) &= \prod_{i=1}^{n} f(Y_i, \tilde{T}_i, \Delta_i | \Psi) \\
&= \prod_{i=1}^{n} \int f(Y_i | b_i, \Psi) f(\tilde{T}_i, \Delta_i | u_i, \Psi) f(b_i, u_i | \Psi) db_i du_i \\
&= \prod_{i=1}^{n} \int f(Y_i | b_i, \Psi) [f(\tilde{T}_i | u_i, \Psi)^{\Delta_i} (1 - F(\tilde{T}_i | u_i, \Psi))^{1-\Delta_i}] \\
&\qquad\qquad \times f(b_i, u_i | \Psi) db_i du_i,
\end{aligned}
\tag{4.9}
$$

where Ψ denotes a vector that contains all parameters for the joint model. The complete-data likelihood function $L(\Psi; Y, T, b, u)$ is defined based on (4.9) assuming b_i and u_i are known.

Write $\Psi = (\psi, \Lambda_0)$ where $\Lambda_0(t) = \int_0^t \lambda_0(u) du$ and ψ collects the remaining parameters. The goal is to calculate $\hat{\Psi}$, the maximum likelihood estimate of Ψ, over a space in which ψ belongs to a bounded set and Λ_0 is in a space consisting of all increasing functions in t with $\Lambda_0(0) = 0$. The likelihood function (4.9) is difficult to maximize in the presence of integration, but $\hat{\Psi}$ can be obtained through an expectation-maximization (EM) algorithm which iterates between an *Expectation* step (E-step) and a *Maximization* step (M-step) [52, 61]. The E-step evaluates the expected value of the complete-data log-likelihood with respect to b_i and u_i, conditional on $(Y, \tilde{T}, \Delta, \Psi^{(m)})$ where $\Psi^{(m)}$ is the current estimate of Ψ and $m = 0, 1, \ldots$ is the iteration index. Specifically, for any function $h(\cdot)$ of b_i and u_i, its expectation can be evaluated by

$$
E\{h(b_i, u_i) | Y_i, \tilde{T}_i, \Delta_i, \Psi^{(m)}\} = \int h(b_i, u_i) f(b_i, u_i | Y_i, \tilde{T}_i, \Delta_i, \Psi^{(m)}) db_i du_i
$$

$$= \frac{\int h(b_i, u_i) f(b_i, u_i, Y_i, \tilde{T}_i, \Delta_i | \Psi^{(m)}) db_i du_i}{f(Y_i, \tilde{T}_i, \Delta_i | \Psi^{(m)})}$$

$$= \frac{\int h(b_i, u_i) f(Y_i, \tilde{T}_i, \Delta_i | b_i, u_i, \Psi^{(m)}) f(b_i, u_i | \Psi^{(m)}) db_i du_i}{\int f(Y_i, \tilde{T}_i, \Delta_i | b_i, u_i, \Psi^{(m)}) f(b_i, u_i | \Psi^{(m)}) db_i du_i}.$$

In the M-step, Ψ is updated using

$$\Psi^{(m+1)} = argmax_\Psi \, Q(\Psi; \Psi^{(m)}),$$

where $Q(\Psi; \Psi^{(m)}) = E_{b,u|Y,\tilde{T},\Delta_i,\Psi^{(m)}}(\log L(\Psi; Y, \tilde{T}, \Delta_i, b, u))$. Estimation for the joint model (4.7)–(4.8) can proceed in a similar way.

Note that the above E-step involves integration of the complete-data log-likelihood function with respect to the posterior distribution of (b_i, u_i) given the observed data and current parameter estimates. When (b_i, u_i) is in a low dimension, the integral can be evaluated via Gaussian quadrature, which approximates the integral by a weighted sum of the target function evaluated at prespecified sample points [226]. Note that the computational burden increases exponentially with the dimension of (b_i, u_i). When the dimension is greater than three, it is demanding to calculate the integrals with satisfactory approximation accuracy. To solve this problem, a so-called Monte Carlo EM algorithm (MCEM) has been employed for joint models [233]. It works differently than the EM algorithm in that the expectation is computed numerically through Monte Carlo simulations by repeatedly drawing random (b_i, u_i) samples from its posterior distribution via Gibbs or Metropolis–Hastings samplers. When implementing MCEM, one needs to pay particular attention to the choice of Monte Carlo sample size and algorithms to obtain Markov chain Monte Carlo (MCMC) samples.

An alternative strategy to reduce the computational burden was proposed by Tseng et al. (2012)[211], in which adaptive Gaussian–Hermite quadrature and Taylor series expansion are used to approximate the integrals based on moment estimates of random effects. The method is discussed in detail in Section 4.3.

Standard Error Estimation

Under the likelihood framework, standard errors of estimated parameters in fully parametric joint models can be estimated using the inverse of the observed information matrix [155]. For joint models that involve non-parametric baseline hazards, standard errors can be derived in the following three ways which are generally applicable to the likelihood-based semiparametric joint models surveyed in Chapters 4–7.

One difficulty in calculating standard errors in joint models with non-parametric baseline hazards lies in the fact that the dimension of the parameter space increases as the sample size grows. In view of this problem, it has been proposed to approximate the variance of parameter estimates based on profile likelihood function where the baseline hazards are profiled out [249, 248, 148].

Standard errors may also be derived using the inverse of the observed information matrix, but the matrix would be in a large size when the number of distinct event times (and thus the dimension of $\lambda_0(t)$) is high. Let Λ denote baseline hazards and Ω the remaining model parameters whose dimension does not change with sample size. It has been reported that standard error estimates obtained from the observed information matrix when keeping $\hat{\lambda}_0(t)$ fixed are close to those calculated using the whole matrix, suggesting that Ω and Λ are nearly orthogonal [199].

Alternatively, standard errors can be estimated via bootstrap [99]. In the first step, B bootstrap samples ($B = 200$–500) are generated from the original data. Then the maximum likelihood estimate of Ψ is obtained on each sample. The standard deviation of each parameter over the B bootstrap samples can be used to approximate the standard error. Although simple in concept, this approach is computationally demanding in general, especially for large samples.

Bayesian Approaches

Statistical inference in selection models can also be done via Bayesian methods (Daniels and Hogan, 2008 [49]; Ibrahim and Molenberghs, 2009 [107]; and the references therein). Compared to likelihood approaches, Bayesian methods, in principle, are relatively straightforward to implement. In addition, in Bayesian joint models, the variance-covariance matrix of model parameters can be estimated as a by-product of the sampling procedure, so there is no extra burden to compute standard errors. In general, Bayesian methods are computationally more efficient when b_i has a high dimension.

However, there are some issues one should be aware of when fitting a Bayesian joint model: (1) The posterior distribution may be improper when improper priors are used, especially in the nonignorable missing data setting; (2) The model could be weakly identifiable when a nonignorable missing data mechanism is assumed and thus the inference is quite sensitive to the choice of hyperparameters. Careful considerations are needed when specifying priors to avoid dominating the likelihood. (3) The computation is usually intensive and MCMC convergence may not be easily achieved. A detailed discussion of these issues is provided in Ibrahim and Molenberghs (2009)[107].

Nonparametric Distributions for Random Effects in Joint Models

In selection models, the longitudinal data are often characterized by mixed effects models in which normally distributed random effects are assumed to capture the correlation within longitudinal data and their relation to event times. Normality of random effects, though easy to understand and interpret, may lead to invalid statistical estimation and inference when this assumption is violated. Simulated studies have showed biased parameter estimates at the survival endpoint and shrinkage in standard error estimation under heavily skewed random effects distributions, and thus questioned the robustness of the normality assumption. This section presents a class of robust joint models in which the random effects distribution is completely unspecified (Tsonaka, Verbeke, and Lesaffre, 2009[219]; Li, Elashoff, Li, and Tseng, 2012[139]).

Assume the longitudinal model is characterized using equation (4.1) and the distribution of survival time T is specified via the Cox regression model (4.3), in which the baseline hazard function $\lambda_0(t)$ is left unspecified. The reason for choosing a shared random-effects formulation is that a distinct random effect at the survival endpoint could make the survival sub-model unidentifiable because both baseline hazard and random effect are nonparametric.

In the joint model (4.1) and (4.3), the only constraint for b_i is that $E(b_i) = 0$. Assume that $b_i \sim F_b$ with $F_b \in \Omega_M$, where Ω_M is the set of all distribution functions with mean zero on the parameter space M of b_i. Let Ψ denote the joint model parameters. Note that the distribution F_b can be continuous or discrete. The density function for subject i is

$$f(Y_i, \tilde{T}_i, \Delta_i | F_b, \Psi) = \int_{\Omega_M} f(Y_i | b_i, \Psi) f(\tilde{T}_i, \Delta_i | b_i, \Psi) dF_b(b_i). \qquad (4.10)$$

It has been shown that the nonparametric maximum likelihood estimate of F_b is discrete with the number of support points not greater than the number of distinct contributions in the likelihood function. Let $\mu = (\mu_1, \mu_2, \ldots)$ be the support points and $\pi = (\pi_1, \pi_2, \ldots)$ the corresponding weights. An iterative procedure can be implemented to obtain the nonparametric maximum likelihood estimate of F_b: at each iteration, μ (or π) is updated conditional on the current estimate of π (or μ). The iterations continue until convergence is obtained. However, it has been noted that the improvement from updating μ is minimal, so a simplified version of the algorithm that omits the step of updating μ is recommended. Therefore, π can be estimated conditional on a fixed grid $\mu_1, \ldots, \mu_L$, where L is the total number of support points.

Adopting a fixed μ, the density (4.10) reduces to

$$f(Y_i, \tilde{T}_i, \Delta_i | F_b, \Psi) = \sum_{l=1}^{L} \pi_l f(Y_i | \mu_l, \Psi) f(\tilde{T}_i, \Delta_i | \mu_l, \Psi),$$

where $l = 1, \ldots, L$. Conditional on Ψ, this marginal density can be maximized by a modified version of the Vertex Exchange Method (VEM). The maximum likelihood estimates of Ψ and π can be obtained via the VEM in conjunction with an Expectation-Maximization (EM) algorithm.

It is not straightforward to estimate standard errors for this joint model because of the nonparametric feature of random effects and baseline hazard. In addition, there is no closed-form profile likelihood from which we could draw statistical inference. Therefore, bootstrapping is an option for standard error estimation.

Example 4.1. *The Schizophrenia Trial*

In this clinical trial for the treatment of schizophrenia, data were available on 523 patients allocated into three treatment groups: placebo (N = 88), haloperidol (N = 87), and risperidone (N = 348), where haloperidol was the standard treatment and risperidone a "novel chemical compound with useful pharmacological characteristics" (Henderson, Diggle, and Dobson, 2000[93]). Longitudinal measurements were available at baseline, 1, 2, 4, 6, and 8 weeks for the Positive and Negative Symptom Scale (PANSS), a quantitative score of psychiatric disorder. Two hundred and seventy patients dropped out of the study prior to completion, of which 183 were due to inadequate response and regarded as informative events. The remaining dropouts were treated as non-informatively censored times. Because the exact dropout time was not observed, it was imputed from a uniform distribution over the interval defined by the last observed and first missed measurement occasions. Figure 4.1(a) shows the within-group mean score of PANSS as a function of time. At each particular occasion, the average was taken on the patients who had not yet dropped out. Both haloperidol and risperidone groups show a greater amount of decrease in PANSS than the placebo group. The risperidone group has the lowest dropout rate, and the placebo group the highest (Figure 4.1(b)). The disparities in dropout rate across treatment groups may potentially bias the mean PANSS scores shown in Figure 4.1(a).

A saturated model was considered to characterize the change in PANSS over time; that is, a distinct regression coefficient was used for each treatment and occasion combination. The survival model for dropout had two binary covariates to indicate the treatment of risperidone or placebo, respectively, with the haloperidol group being the reference. Results from joint models with different $W_1(t)$ and $W_2(t)$ structures are summarized in Table 4.1. In the simplest setting, a random intercept U_1 was considered for PANSS (Models I and II), but introducing a stationary Gaussian process $V(t)$ into the PANSS trajectory improved the model fit (measured by the likelihood value) substantially (Models III–V). Almost equally sufficient fit was achieved when the Gaussian process $V(t)$ was replaced by a random slope $U_2 t$ (Models VI–X). Model X, which included the random slope U_2 and the current value of $W_1(t)$ as two separate factors for $W_2(t)$, was considered parsimonious without dramatic reduction in fit compared to Model IX. Thus, it was chosen as the final model and the results are given in Table 4.2. Results from a separate analysis assuming no latent association (Model VI) are reported as well for comparison purposes. In the joint model, the estimated γ_2 and γ_3 are both positive with p-values < 0.05, suggesting that patients with either high values of PANSS or less decline in

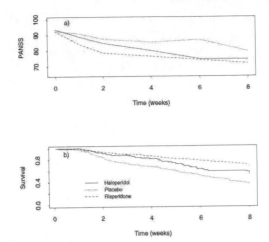

Figure 4.1 *Longitudinal and event time summaries for schizophrenia trial: (a) mean PANSS score and (b) survival curves for time to dropout due to inadequate response.*

the trajectory of PANSS show increased risk of dropout due to inadequate response. The impact of treatment on the dropout process is attenuated in the separate analysis (β_{21} and β_{22}), and the variance of the random slope (σ_2^2) is smaller than its counterpart in the joint model.

Figure 4.2 shows the estimated mean PANSS curves, which are compared to the observed profiles under various models. Under Model X (Figure 4.2(a)), the risperidone group has the lowest mean PANSS scores (and thus the best), and the placebo group is the highest, with the haloperidol group in the middle. The joint-model estimated mean curves are higher than the observed profiles. This

Table 4.1 *Log maximized likelihoods for schizophrenia data.*

	$W_1(t)$	$W_2(t)$	$\log L_Y$	$\log L_{N|Y}$	$\log L$
Intercept only					
I	U_1	0	-10251.85	-1228.55	-11480.40
II	U_1	$\gamma W_1(t)$	-10252.58	-1181.13	-11433.72
Intercept +SGP					
III	$U_1+V(t)$	0	-10126.66	-1228.55	-11355.21
IV	$U_1 + V(t)$	$\gamma W_1(t)$	-10132.55	-1146.14	-11278.69
V	$U_1 +V(t)$	$\gamma_1 U_1 + \gamma_2 V(t)$	-10139.79	-1107.61	-11247.40
Intercept +slope					
VI	$U_1 + U_2(t)$	0	-10127.31	-1228.55	-11355.86
VII	$U_1 + U_2(t)$	$\gamma W_1(t)$	-10133.76	-1137.41	-11271.17
VIII	$U_1 + U_2(t)$	$\gamma W_1(t) + U_3$	-10135.99	-1132.90	-11268.88
IX	$U_1 + U_2(t)$	$\gamma_1 U_1 + \gamma_2 U_2 + \gamma_3 W_1(t)$	-10147.75	-1096.05	-11243.80
X	$U_1 + U_2(t)$	$\gamma_2 U_2 + \gamma_3 W_1(t)$	-10148.42	-1095.60	-11244.03

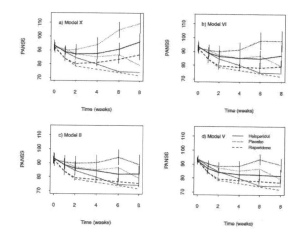

Figure 4.2 *Observed PANSS scores (fine lines) and hypothetical dropout-free estimates (thick lines) under various models, with ± two standard errors.*

can be explained by the fact that patients with high scores tend to drop out of the study because of inadequate response. Similar patterns are seen in Models II and V (Figure 4.2(c) and (d)) in which random intercept and random intercept plus stochastic Gaussian process were assumed in the longitudinal model for PANSS, respectively. This pattern is less pronounced in Model VI (Figure 4.2(b)) which assumed no latent association between PANSS and dropout. □

Table 4.2 *Parameter estimates and standard errors for final joint model with and without latent association.*

	Var(U_1) σ_1^2	Var(U_2) σ_2^2	Corr(U_1, U_2) ρ	Var(Z) σ_z^2	Placebo β_{21}	Resp. β_{22}	U_2 γ_2	$W_1(t)$ γ_3
Joint	283.37	12.59	0.06	100.24	0.779	−0.884	0.349	0.042
(X)	(18.17)	(1.31)	(0.02)	(3.95)	(0.344)	(0.322)	(0.051)	(0.007)
Separate	275.92	7.12	0.01	106.10	0.480	−0.508	0	0
(VI)	(21.42)	(0.81)	(0.08)	(4.18)	(0.218)	(0.196)	−	−

4.1.2 Mixture Models

In mixture models, the joint distribution $f(Y,T)$ is characterized as $f(Y|T)f(T)$, in which $f(T)$ is the marginal distribution of event times and $f(Y|T)$ is the conditional distribution of longitudinal data given event times. Such a model formulation is often applied to longitudinal studies with dropouts, where the primary interest focuses on statistical inference about longitudinal data after adjusting for informative dropout. The term *mixture* reflects the fact that the marginal distribution of Y is a mixture of its conditional distributions across all dropout patterns. That is,

$$f(Y) = \int f(Y|T)f(T)dT.$$

In the above density functions we omit parameters for simplicity. The marginal distribution of T may be associated with baseline characteristics, and the time T can be a covariate in the conditional model of Y. Discussions of mixture models can be found in Little (1995)[152], Hogan and Laird (1997)[95], and Ibrahim (2009)[107]. In what follows we review commonly used mixture models.

Pattern-Mixture Models

Pattern-mixture models are applied to longitudinal studies with prespecified observation times that are common to all study participants. Assume the maximum number of observations is K. In the presence of dropout, the data consists of up to K observations on Y, denoted as $Y_1, \ldots, Y_K$, and for subject i, $i = 1, \ldots, n$, this corresponds to $Y_i = (Y_{i1}, \ldots, Y_{iK})$ if dropout does not occur. The dropout time $T_i = k$ if a subject drops out between the $(k-1)$th and kth observation time; that is, $Y_{i1}, \ldots, Y_{i,k-1}$ are observed but $Y_{ik}, \ldots, Y_{iK}$ are missing. Note that $T_i = K + 1$ indicates a completer.

The conditional distribution of Y_i given T_i usually involves within-subject random effects (denoted as b_i). Let X_i collect between-subject covariates associated Y_i and T_i. The joint model generally can be written as

$$f(Y_i, T_i, b_i|X_i) = f(Y_i|b_i, T_i, X_i)f(b_i|T_i, X_i)f(T_i|X_i), \qquad (4.11)$$

where $f(Y_i|b_i, T_i, X_i)$ is the longitudinal data distribution stratified by missing data patterns, $f(b_i|T_i, X_i)$ models subject-specific random effects as a function of covariates X_i and missing data patterns, and $f(T_i|X_i)$ is the marginal distribution of missing data patterns as a function of covariates X_i.

Missing-Data Mechanisms in Pattern-Mixture Models

In a general setting, we assume that Y_i follows a multivariate normal distribution given dropout time T_i. Suppose there are M distinct dropout patterns with probabilities $\pi_1, \ldots, \pi_M$. The model can be written as $[Y_i|T_i] \sim N(\mu^{(m)}, \Sigma^{(m)})$, where $m = 1, \ldots, M$, and marginally T_i follows a multinomial distribution. Non-informative dropout can be tested by the null hypothesis $H_0 : (\mu^{(1)}, \Sigma^{(1)}) = \cdots = (\mu^{(M)}, \Sigma^{(M)})$.

The following sub-types of pattern-mixture models have been proposed. If the missing data mechanism depends on X_i only, then $f(Y_i|b_i, T_i, X_i) = f(Y_i|b_i, X_i)$ and $f(b_i|T_i, X_i) = f(b_i|X_i)$, and model (4.11) becomes

$$f(Y_i, T_i, b_i|X_i) = f(Y_i|b_i, X_i)f(b_i|X_i)f(T_i|X_i).$$

This is the so-called *covariate-dependent dropout*, a strong assumption which may be unrealistic in many applications.

If the random effects b_i have a same distribution across the dropout patterns, then model (4.11) becomes

$$f(Y_i, T_i, b_i | X_i) = f(Y_i | b_i, T_i, X_i) f(b_i | X_i) f(T_i | X_i),$$

which indicates *outcome-dependent dropout*. An example of such models is given by

$$\begin{aligned}
\{Y_i | b_i, T_i = k, X_i\} &= N_K(X_{1i}\alpha^{(k)} + X_{2i}b_i, \Sigma^{(k)}), \\
\{b_i | X_i\} &= N_q(0, \Gamma), \\
\{T_i | X_i\} &= Multinomial(\pi_{i0}, \pi_{i1}, \ldots, \pi_{iK}), \quad (4.12)
\end{aligned}$$

where Γ and $(\alpha^{(k)}, \Sigma^{(k)})$, $k = 1, \ldots, K$, are unknown fixed parameters and $\pi_{ik} = Pr(T_i = k)$, $k = 1, \ldots, K$, are functions of X_i (and possibly some unknown parameters). The assumption of pattern-specific fixed parameters $\alpha^{(k)}$ and $\Sigma^{(k)}$ creates identification problems because the parameters of complete-data distribution of Y_i are not estimable for incomplete patterns. The model can be identified by imposing supplemental restrictions on the missing data mechanism, which, unlike selection models, does not require explicit assumptions about the functional form of missing mechanisms. Illustration of this idea is given in Examples 4.2, 4.3, and 4.4.

A third type of pattern-mixture models is based on the assumption of *random effect-dependent dropout*, which indicates that b_i is a function of T_i. One example is given by

$$\begin{aligned}
\{Y_i | b_i, T_i = k, X_i\} &= \{Y_i | b_i, X_i\} = N_K(X_{1i}\alpha + X_{2i}b_i, \Sigma), \\
\{b_i | X_i, T_i = k\} &= N_q(X_{3i}\beta^{(k)}, \Gamma^{(k)}), \\
\{T_i | X_i\} &= Multinomial(\pi_{i0}, \pi_{i1}, \ldots, \pi_{iK}),
\end{aligned}$$

where α, Σ, and $(\beta^{(k)}, \Gamma^{(k)})$, $k = 1, \ldots, K$, are fixed unknown parameters, X_{1i}, X_{2i}, and X_{3i} are covariates, and π_{ik}, $k = 1, \ldots, K$, may be dependent on unknown parameters ρ. A special case of this model is provided in Example 4.5.

Random-Effects Mixture Models

In random-effects mixture models, the dropout time T_i is not treated as a discrete variable. Conditional on T_i, the distribution of Y_i is specified by a random effects model

$$\begin{aligned}
\{Y_i | b_i, T_i, X_i\} &= N_K(X_{1i}\alpha + X_{2i}b_i, \Sigma), \\
\{b_i | X_i, T_i\} &= N_q(X_{3i}\beta, \Gamma), \quad (4.13)
\end{aligned}$$

where X_{3i} includes T_i as a covariate. One example is that the mean of random slope b_{1i} is a linear function of T_i:

$$E(b_{1i}|T_i = t_i) = \beta_0 + \beta_1 t_i. \tag{4.14}$$

The marginal distribution of T_i can be left unspecified. An illustration of this model is given in Example 4.6.

Parameter estimation can be done via maximum likelihood. For example, for model (4.13), consider a general situation where there may be censored events with respect to efficacy-related dropout. This could happen when dropouts are due to administrative reasons or adverse events unrelated to treatment efficacy. The likelihood function is

$$L(\alpha, \beta, \Sigma, \Gamma) = \prod_{i=1}^{n} \int_{b_i} \{f(Y_i, b_i, \tilde{t}_i)^{\Delta_i} [\int_{\tilde{t}_i}^{\infty} f(Y_i, b_i, t) dt]^{1-\Delta_i}\} db_i,$$

where $\tilde{t}_i$ is the observed or censored time, Δ_i is an indicator such that $\Delta_i = 1$ if the dropout time is observed, and $f(Y_i, b_i, T_i) = f(Y_i|b_i, T_i)f(b_i|T_i)f(T_i)$. Maximum likelihood estimates can be obtained via an EM algorithm.

Example 4.2. *A Bivariate Normal Pattern-Mixture Model*
Consider the following pattern-mixture model for bivariate monotone data with two patterns $T_i = 0$ and $T_i = 2$:

$$\begin{aligned} \{Y_i|T_i = k\} &= N_2(\alpha^{(k)}, \Sigma^{(k)}), \\ \{T_i\} &= Multinomial(\pi_0, \pi_1, \pi_2), \end{aligned}$$

where $k = 0, 2$, $\pi_0 + \pi_2 = 1$, and $\pi_1 = 0$. Marginally, Y_i is a mixture of two normal distributions which are determined by 11 parameters, but only eight are identifiable. The 3 parameters in the conditional distribution $[Y_2|Y_1, T = 2]$ do not appear in the likelihood, so need to be identified by restrictions or prior information. Restrictions can be provided by the missing data mechanism. Assuming that for some known λ,

$$Pr(T_i = 2|Y_i) = g(Y_{i1} + \lambda Y_{i2}),$$

where $g(\cdot)$ is an arbitrary unspecified function, then the conditional distribution of Y_1 given $Y_1 + \lambda Y_2$ is identical for the two missing-data patterns, yielding restrictions that just identify the model. When $\lambda = 0$, the resulting maximum likelihood estimates reduce to the estimates from the MAR selection model. When $\lambda = \infty$, the dropout process depends entirely on Y_2, and maximum likelihood estimates reduce to the so-called protective estimates. When $\lambda = -1$, it indicates the missing probability depends on the increment $Y_2 - Y_1$. Note that λ is not identifiable from the data and thus a sensitivity analysis needs to be conducted for a range of plausible values of λ. $\square$

Example 4.3. *Trivariate Data with Dropout at the Third Time Point*

Consider data measured at three occasions with dropouts occurring only at $k = 3$. *The model for longitudinal data is*

$$\{Y_i | T_i = k\} = N_3(\alpha^{(k)}, \Sigma^{(k)}),$$

and $P(T_i = k) = Multinomial(\pi_0, \pi_1, \pi_2, \pi_3)$ *with* $\pi_1 = \pi_2 = 0$ *and* $\pi_0 + \pi_3 = 1$. *Assume that the probability of dropout at time 3 is an arbitrary function of* Y_{i2} *and* Y_{i3}. *This mechanism implies that the conditional distribution of* Y_1 *given* Y_2 *and* Y_3 *is identical for complete and incomplete cases, the restrictions that just identify the model. The mean of* Y_3 *is estimated by*

$$\hat{\alpha}^{(3)} = \bar{Y}_3 + (\hat{\alpha}^{(1)} - \bar{Y}_1)/b_{13.23},$$

where $\bar{Y}_j$ *is the mean of* Y_j *from the complete cases,* $\hat{\alpha}^{(1)}$ *is the mean of* Y_1 *from all the cases, and* $b_{13.23}$ *is the coefficient of* Y_3 *in the regression of* Y_1 *on* Y_2 *and* Y_3 *using the completed cases only. This estimate could be very unstable because* $b_{13.23}$ *estimates a quantity close to zero if the correlation of* Y_1 *and* Y_3 *is small after* Y_2 *is partialed out. In order-1 autoregressive cases,* $b_{13.23}$ *is estimating the parameter* $\beta_{13.23}$ *whose true value is zero. This indicates that the estimates are not data driven, but rely heavily on model assumptions and the dropout mechanism.* □

Example 4.4. *A Dose-Comparison Study for Treatment of Schizophrenia*
This is a clinical trial on 65 schizophrenia patients to compare three alternative dosing regimens of haloperidol, 5, 10, or 20 mg/day, for 4 weeks. The outcome, Brief Psychiatric Rating Scale Schizophrenia (BPRSS) factor, was measured at baseline, week 1, and week 4. The main interest is to estimate the change in BPRSS from baseline to week 4 in each dose group. Twenty-nine patients (45%) dropped out at week 4, possibly due to a poor BPRSS score and/or side effects with high doses. The following model was proposed:

$$\begin{aligned}
\{Y_i | X_i, T_i = k\} &= N_3(B^{(k)} X_i, \Sigma^{(k)}), \\
\{T_i | X_i\} &= Multinomial(\pi_{0i}, \pi_1, \pi_2, \pi_{3i}), \\
logit\pi_{3i} &= \rho^T X_i,
\end{aligned}$$

where $k = 0, 3$, $\pi_1 = \pi_2 = 0$, $\pi_{0i} + \pi_{3i} = 1$, *and* X_i *represents the three dose groups. The parameter* ρ *is a (3 × 1) vector, estimated by dropout rates at week 4 for each group. The six parameters of the distribution of* Y_3 *given* Y_1, Y_2, X, *and* $T = 3$ *are not identifiable from the data. Therefore, it is assumed that*

$$Pr(T_i = 3 | Y_{i1}, Y_{i2}, Y_{i3}, X_i) = g(c_1 Y_{i1} + c_2 Y_{i2} + c_3 Y_{i3}, X_i), \qquad (4.15)$$

where $g(\cdot)$ *is an arbitrary unspecified function and* c_1, c_2, *and* c_3 *are prespecified coefficients. Equation (4.15) indicates that the distribution of* (Y_1, Y_2, Y_3) *given* X *and* $(c_1 Y_1 + c_2 Y_2 + c_3 Y_3)$ *is the same for complete and incomplete cases, yielding 11 parameter restrictions for the six unidentified parameters.*

The model is thus overidentified. Four alternative choices were examined:
$(c_1, c_2, c_3) = (0.4, 0.4, 0.2), (0.3, 0.4, 0.4), (0.1, 0.1, 0.8),$ *and* $(0, 0, 1),$ *which represent progressively more extreme departures from MAR. The estimate of treatment effect was found to be moderately sensitive to the choice of missing data mechanisms.*□

Example 4.5. *A Special Case of Random Effect-Dependent Dropout Models*
Assume the following model for repeated measurements on subjects in J treatment groups:

$$\{Y_i | b_i\} = N_K \left(\begin{bmatrix} 1 & t_{i1} \\ \cdots & \cdots \\ 1 & t_{iK} \end{bmatrix} \begin{bmatrix} b_{i0} \\ b_{i1} \end{bmatrix}, \sigma_e^2 I \right),$$

$$\{b_i | x_i = j, T_i = k\} = N_2(\beta_j^{(k)}, \Gamma), j = 1, \ldots, J,$$
$$\{T_i | x_i = j\} = Multinomial(\pi_{j0}, \ldots, \pi_{jK}),$$

where $b_i^T = (b_{i0}, b_{i1})$ *is a vector of random intercept and slope for subject* i, x_i *a treatment group indicator,* π_{jk} *the proportion of the population receiving treatment* j *for which* $T_i = k$, *and* $\beta_j^{(k)} = (\beta_{j0}^{(k)}, \beta_{j1}^{(k)})^T$ *the expected intercept and slope for subjects in treatment group* j *with dropout pattern* $T_i = k$. *The parameters of interest are the mean of intercept and slope for subjects in treatment group* j, *averaged over missing data patterns:*

$$E(b_i | x_i = j) = \sum_{k=1}^K \pi_{jk} \beta_j^{(k)}.$$

Note that in this model, $\beta_j^{(1)}$ *and* $\beta_j^{(2)}$ *are not identifiable because patterns* $T = 1$ *and* $T = 2$ *contain at most one observation and estimation of straight lines requires at least two observed time points. These cases can be omitted from the analysis.* □

Example 4.6. *A Conditional Linear Model*
A conditional linear model has been proposed to characterize random effects distributions given dropout time. Specifically, the model assumes that the mean slope is a linear (or polynomial) function of dropout time as specified in equation (4.14). The model further assumes that conditional on $T_i = t_i$, *longitudinal data follow the same distribution pre- and post- dropout. To estimate the unconditional mean of* b_{1i}, *ordinary least squares (OLS) estimates* $\hat{b}_{1i}^{ols}$ *are first obtained by fitting model (4.13), and then* (β_0, β_1) *are estimated via a weighted least squares (WLS) regression, in which* $\hat{b}_{1i}^{ols}$ *is the response and the weights are proportional to* $1/(var(\hat{b}_{1i}) + \omega_1)$ *with* ω_1 *being the estimated variance of the random slope in* Γ. *Note that this procedure assumes that all dropout times are observed. Denote* $(\hat{\beta}_0, \hat{\beta}_1)$ *the WLS estimates of* (β_0, β_1). *The unconditional mean slope is then estimated by*

$$\hat{b}_1 = \hat{\beta}_0 + \hat{\beta}_1 \left(\frac{1}{n} \sum_{i=1}^n t_i \right),$$

and its standard error can be obtained by bootstrap methods. □

Terminal Decline Models

Terminal decline models, as a type of mixture models, have been developed for palliative care studies on patients with life-threatening illness such as advanced cancer. The main interest of a terminal decline model is to estimate the trajectory of longitudinal data in a period shortly before death. One unique feature of the approach is that longitudinal measurements are modeled retrospectively from death. In the model developed by Li et al. (2013) [140], the longitudinal outcome $Y_i(t)$ is characterized by

$$Y_i(t) = X_i^T(t)\beta + b_i + W_i(t) + \epsilon_i(t), \tag{4.16}$$

where t is the time calculated retrospectively from death (so at the time of death $t = 0$), $X_i^T(t)$ a vector of covariates which may include non-stochastic functions of time t such as piecewise linear functions or polynomials, and β a vector of fixed unknown regression coefficients. The remaining three terms in the model, b_i, $W_i(t)$, and $\epsilon_i(t)$, introduce random variations into $Y_i(t)$ and are mutually independent. Specifically, $b_i \sim N(0, \sigma^2)$ is the random intercept, $W_i(t)$ is a zero-mean stationary Gaussian process with $Cov(W_i(t), W_i(s)) = \nu^2 \rho(|t - s|)$, and $\epsilon_i(t) \sim N(0, \tau^2)$ is measurement error and $\epsilon_i(t) \perp \epsilon_i(s)$ if $t \neq s$. The function $\rho(t)$ is assumed to be $exp(-\alpha t^c)$ with a prespecified c.

The death time T_i is calculated as the time elapsed between study initiation and the occurrence of death, and may be right censored by C_i. The censorship mechanism is assumed to be noninformative. Li et al. (2013) [140] in their terminal decline model posited that T_i followed a piecewise exponential distribution with a density function $p(T_i; \theta)$, where θ is a vector of parameters. An example of $p(T_i; \theta)$ is given in the ENABLE II study at the end of this section.

The connection between the above terminal decline model and a mixture model can be seen by rewriting equation (4.16) as

$$Y_i(t^*)|T_i = X_i^T(T_i - t^*)\beta + b_i + W_i(T_i - t^*) + \epsilon_i(T_i - t^*),$$

where t^* is the time in study from baseline. Moreover, with this formulation, it is straightforward to calculate the conditional distribution of $Y_i(t^*)$ given $T_i > t^*$:

$$f(Y_i(t^*)|T_i > t^*) = \frac{\int_{t^*}^{\infty} f(Y_i(t^*)|T_i)f(T_i)dT_i}{\int_{t^*}^{\infty} f(T_i)dT_i}.$$

The terminal decline model specified above is fully parametric if change points in the piecewise exponential distribution of T_i are pre-determined. Maximum

likelihood estimates of model parameters can be obtained, and standard errors
are computed from the Fisher information matrix. Note that for censored
subjects, the likelihood function is an integral of the joint distribution of Y_i
and T_i over (C_i, ∞) with respect to T_i.

Example 4.7. *The ENABLE II Study*

*More details of the study can be found in Section 1.1.3. The objective is to
estimate and compare trajectories of quality of life (QOL) in the palliative and
usual care groups over a period shortly before death. Li et al. (2013) [140] analyzed the data using the terminal decline model described above. Specifically,
a piecewise linear model with a change point at $t = 6$ months as suggested by
previous results was proposed to characterize the mean trajectory of QOL:*

$$
\begin{aligned}
Y_i(t) \quad = \quad & \beta_0 + \beta_1 A_i + 6(\beta_2 + \beta_4 A_i - \beta_3 - \beta_5 A_i)I(t > 6) + (\beta_2 + \beta_4 A_i)t \\
& \times I(t \le 6) + (\beta_3 + \beta_5 A_i)tI(t > 6) + b_i + W_i(t) + \epsilon_i(t),
\end{aligned}
$$

*where A_i is a binary variable to indicate if patient i received palliative care
$(A_i = 1)$ or usual care $(A_i = 0)$. Thus, for the usual care group, the response
function is then specified as*

$$
Y_i(t) = \beta_0 + 6(\beta_2 - \beta_3)I(t > 6) + \beta_2 tI(t \le 6) + \beta_3 tI(t > 6) + b_i + W_i(t) + \epsilon_i(t),
$$

*so β_0 is interpreted as mean of Y_i at the time of death $(t = 0)$, and β_2 and
β_3 are slopes before and after 6 months, respectively. For the palliative care
group,*

$$
\begin{aligned}
Y_i(t) \quad = \quad & (\beta_0 + \beta_1) + 6(\beta_2 + \beta_4 - \beta_3 - \beta_5)I(t > 6) + (\beta_2 + \beta_4)tI(t \le 6) \\
& + (\beta_3 + \beta_5)tI(t > 6) + b_i + W_i(t) + \epsilon_i(t),
\end{aligned}
$$

*where β_1 is the treatment effect on Y_i at the time of death, and β_4 and β_5
are the treatment effect on the slopes before and after 6 months. In this analysis, c in the correlation function of $W_i(t)$ was set to 2, which corresponds to
Gaussian correlation.*

*The cumulative hazard of death shown in Figure 4.3 suggests a change in the
hazard rate at 13 months. Therefore, a two-piece exponential distribution was
proposed for T_i:*

$$
p(T_i; \theta) = \left\{
\begin{array}{ll}
\theta_1 exp(-\theta_1 T_i) & T_i \le 13, A_i = 1 \\
\theta_2 exp(-\theta_2 T_i - 13(\theta_1 - \theta_2)) & T_i > 13, A_i = 1 \\
\theta_3 exp(-\theta_3 T_i) & T_i \le 13, A_i = 0 \\
\theta_4 exp(-\theta_4 T_i - 13(\theta_3 - \theta_4)) & T_i > 13, A_i = 0
\end{array}
\right\},
$$

*where θ_1 and θ_2 are hazard rates in the palliative care group before and after
13 months, respectively, and θ_3 and θ_4 are hazards in the usual care group.*

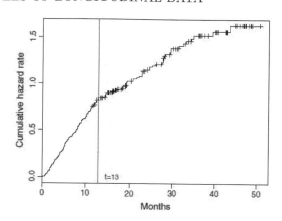

Figure 4.3 *Cumulative hazard rate of death.*

Table 4.3 *Estimates of model parameters (including baseline as outcome).*

	Terminal decline model		Survival model	
Sample used	Parameter	Estimate (SE)	Parameter	Estimate (SE)
Full sample	β_0	108.44(3.18)	θ_1	0.052(0.006)
	β_1	12.03(4.87)	θ_2	0.033(0.006)
	β_2	3.99(0.58)	θ_3	0.077(0.008)
	β_3	0.088(0.059)	θ_4	0.019(0.005)
	β_4	$-1.37(0.89)$		
	β_5	$-0.060(0.096)$		
	σ	18.22(1.18)		
	τ	11.36(0.44)		
	ν	9.95(1.03)		
	α	0.019(0.009)		

Table 4.3 shows the parameter estimates from this terminal decline model. At the time of death, the QOL scores in the palliative care group were on average 12.03 (SE = 4.87) higher than those in the usual care group, and this difference was statistically significant at an alpha level of 0.05. However, there was no significant treatment effect on the slopes of QOL before and after 6 months (β_4 = −1.37, SE = 0.89; β_5 = −0.06, SE = 0.096). The between-group difference in QOL was 12.03 − 1.37t for t < 6 months and 3.81 − 0.06t for t > 6 months, and this difference became significant when patients approached the last 4.4 months of life (6.02, 95% CI [0.03 − 12.01)]). The hazard rates were 0.052 (%95 CI [0.041 − 0.064]) and 0.033 (%95 CI [0.022 − 0.045]) before and after 13 months in the palliative care group, and were 0.077 (%95 CI [0.062 − 0.092]) and 0.019 (%95 CI [0.010 − 0.027]) in the usual care group. There

was a significant treatment effect in both time intervals, though usual care had a lower hazard after 13 months.

Model goodness of fit was assessed graphically by comparing fitted survival probabilities against Kaplan-Meier curves. The estimated trajectories of QOL were compared to the observed individual profiles. For censored patients, the profiles were estimated based on expected death times calculated from the survival model, conditional on $T_i > C_i$. Both suggest that the model fits observed data reasonably well. □

4.1.3 Remarks on Selection and Mixture Models

The two general classes of joint models for longitudinal and failure time data have distinct features. Selection models require the event time distribution be specified conditional on longitudinal data. If the event is dropout or death, it is straightforward to establish correspondence between model formulation and missing data mechanisms. The marginal distribution of longitudinal data, which is often the primary interest of analysis, is also readily obtained. Thus, selection models have conceptual advantages. On the other hand, pattern-mixture models do not require a specific functional form of the dropout process. Non-parametric and semiparametric models have been employed to specify $f(T)$ in the presence of censoring. The conditional distribution of Y can be estimated up to time T, but estimation of $f(Y|T)$ requires additional assumptions for post-event longitudinal measurements. One disadvantage of mixture models is that the marginal distribution of longitudinal data is not directly available, and thus the impact of covariates is unclear. This approach could be computationally intensive in the presence of many dropout patterns.

It should be noted that, in the presence of nonignorable missing data, joint models must make some unverifiable assumptions, or the model would be nonidentifiable. Thus, sensitivity analysis is needed to investigate the impact of modeling assumptions on parameter estimation. It is easier to carry out a sensitivity analysis in mixture models because there are explicit assumptions about the distribution of unobserved data. Sensitivity analysis in selection models will be discussed in Chapter 7. Other issues to consider for both selection and mixture models include parameter interpretation, estimation efficiency, and implementation. We refer readers to Little (1995)[152], Hogan and Laird (1997)[95], and Ibrahim (2009)[107] for a detailed discussion.

4.2 Joint Models with Discrete Event Times and Monotone Missingness

In this section, we pay closer attention to joint modeling approaches for longitudinal studies with discrete dropout times, in which data are recorded at pre-scheduled visits (or occasions) and all subjects follow the same measurement schedule. Following a similar set of notations in pattern-mixture models, we assume there are a total of K visits, so the complete data vector of outcome measurements on subject i can be written as $Y_i = (Y_{i1}, \ldots, Y_{iK})$, $i = 1, \ldots, n$. Further assume the distribution of Y is $f(Y|\psi)$, indexed by some unknown parameter ψ. Research interest often focuses on statistical inference for ψ, which, in the presence of ignorable missing data, can be easily obtained using the methods discussed in Chapter 2.

Dropout in such studies is often described by a vector of indicator variables $R_i = (R_{i1}, \ldots, R_{iK})$, $i = 1, \ldots, n$. Let $R_{i1} = \cdots = R_{ij} = 1$ and $R_{ij+1} = \cdots = R_{iK} = 0$ if a subject drops out in between visits j and $j + 1$, so that $Y_{i1}, \ldots, Y_{ij}$ are observed and $Y_{ij+1}, \ldots, Y_{iK}$ are missing. Let Y_{obs} and Y_{mis} denote the observed and missing components in Y, respectively. When dropout is *informative*, i.e., the dropout mechanism is non-ignorable, valid inference on ψ can be obtained from the joint distribution $f(Y_{obs}, R|\psi, \theta)$, where θ is a set of parameters to describe the distribution of R. Because $f(Y_{obs}, R|\psi, \theta) = \int f(Y_{obs}, Y_{mis}, R|\psi, \theta) dY_{mis}$, the joint distribution of observed data and dropout patterns relies on specification of $f(Y_{obs}, Y_{mis}, R|\psi, \theta)$.

As discussed in Section 4.1, there are two main approaches to characterize the dependence between Y and R, namely, *selection* models and *pattern-mixture* models. In selection models, the joint distribution is factorized into marginal distribution of Y, $f(Y|\psi)$, and conditional distribution of R given Y, $f(R|Y, \theta)$; in pattern-mixture models, the joint distribution is expressed as the product of $f(R|\theta)$ and $f(Y|R, \psi)$, so that marginal distribution of Y is a mixture of distributions classified by dropout patterns. Here we focus on two general approaches in selection models in which dropout is explicitly modeled as an event or process.

4.2.1 Outcome-Dependent Dropout Models

An outcome-dependent dropout model characterizes the probability of observing longitudinal data at occasion j for subjects who have not dropped out at occasion $j - 1$. Longitudinal measurements are incorporated as a covariate in the model for missing data probabilities. Diggle and Kenward (1994)[54] were among the first to develop outcome-dependent dropout models for normally distributed longitudinal data, which were later extended to generalized linear mixed models by Ibrahim, Chen, and Lipsitz (2001)[106], and non-monotone missing data patterns by Troxel, Lipsitz, and Harrington (1998)[209] and Parzen et al. (2006)[171]. Yang and Kang (2010)[242] proposed joint analysis of mixed Poisson and continuous longitudinal data with dropouts. Roy and Lin (2005)[192] studied estimation bias and statistical inference in the presence of missing covariates. Overview of methods for outcome-dependent dropout models can be found in Little (1995)[152], Hogan and Laird (1997)[95], Kenward and Molenberghs (1999)[115], Daniels and Hogan (2008)[49], and Ibrahim and Molenberghs (2009)[107].

Model Formulation

Outcome-dependent dropout models characterize the marginal distribution of Y through a mixed (conditional) or marginal model. In the first case, the distribution can be generally expressed using generalized linear mixed effects models. As introduced previously, conditional on random effects b_i and covariates X_{ij} and $\tilde{X}_{ij}$, we have that

$$g(E(Y_{ij}|b_i, \beta)) = X_{ij}^T \beta + \tilde{X}_{ij}^T b_i, \tag{4.17}$$

where g is a link function to characterize the association between the conditional mean of Y and linear predictor $X_{ij}^T\beta + \tilde{X}_{ij}^T b_i$. Normally distributed longitudinal data are included as a special case with g as an identity link. Assume random effects b_i are i.i.d. $N(0, \Sigma_b)$ and independent of covariates $X_i = (X_{i1}, \ldots, X_{in_i}, \tilde{X}_{i1}, \ldots, \tilde{X}_{in_i})^T$. Therefore, ψ contains β and parameters that specify variance-covariance matrix Σ_b. Note that ψ also includes a dispersion parameter that pertains to the variance of Y_{ij}.

In the case of a marginal model, the expectation of Y_{ij} is parameterized via β only; that is, $g(E(Y_{ij}|\beta)) = X_{ij}^T\beta$. Regression coefficients β then have a population-level interpretation. In addition, a marginal variance-covariance matrix V for $Y_i = (Y_{i1}, \ldots, Y_{in_i})$ needs to be specified. Again, let ψ denote the parameters in β and V.

Outcome-dependent models assume that the probability of observing Y_{ij} given the subject has not yet dropped out at occasion $j-1$ is related to responses up to occasion j, conditional on all observations of Y_i. That indicates the hazard of dropout at occasion j depends on the history (or path) of Y up to occasion j. The dropout process is often modeled through a logistic regression, such that for subject i,

$$logit\{P(R_{ij} = 1|R_{ij-1} = 1, Y_i, \theta)\} = H(\bar{Y}_{ij}; \theta), \tag{4.18}$$

where $\bar{Y}_{ij} = (Y_{i1}, \ldots, Y_{ij})$. Various formulations for $H(\bar{Y}_{ij}; \theta)$ have been proposed to characterize the relationship between longitudinal data and dropouts. One appealing feature of such models lies in the fact that there is a direct correspondence between the functional form of $H(\bar{Y}_{ij}; \theta)$ and missing data mechanisms: (1) when $H(\bar{Y}_{ij}; \theta) \neq H(\bar{Y}_{ij-1}; \theta)$, which indicates that the dropout probability is related to the current (possibly missing) response, data are missing not at random (MNAR); (2) when $H(\bar{Y}_{ij}; \theta) = H(\bar{Y}_{ij-1}; \theta)$, data are missing at random (MAR) because the dropout probability is a function of observed values, not missing components in Y_{ij}; (3) $H(\bar{Y}_{ij}; \theta) = H(\theta)$ (note that $H(\theta)$ could still depend on some covariates which contain no missing data) corresponds to the missing completely at random (MCAR) mechanism.

One typical example of $H(\bar{Y}_{ij}; \theta)$ is given by

$$logit\{P(R_{ij} = 1 | R_{ij-1} = 1, Y_i, \theta)\} = \theta_0 + \theta_1^T \bar{Y}_{ij-1} + \theta_2 Y_{ij} + \theta_3^T W_i, \quad (4.19)$$

where W_i is baseline covariates. This formulation provides insight into the missing data mechanism through θ_1 and θ_2. The missing data are MNAR if $\theta_2 \neq 0$ and are MAR if $\theta_2 = 0$, $\theta_1 \neq 0$; $\theta_1 = \theta_2 = 0$ indicates that the data are MCAR.

Parameter Estimation and Inference

Estimation of ψ and θ in the joint model (4.17)–(4.18) may proceed using either likelihood or Bayesian approaches. Here we focus on likelihood methods. We refer the reader to the literature in Section 4.1.1 for Bayesian models.

In likelihood approaches, estimation and inference methods discussed in Section 4.1.1 for selection models can be readily applied here. Specifically, because the model for longitudinal measurements involves unobserved random effects, estimation of ψ and θ often relies on an Expectation-Maximization (EM) algorithm or its analog, the so-called Monte Carlo EM (MCEM) algorithm if b_i has a high dimension. The EM algorithm is based on the complete-data log-likelihood function, assuming that random effects b_i are known:

$$
\begin{aligned}
\ell(\psi, \theta; Y, R, b) &= log\{\prod_{i=1}^{n} f(Y_i, b_i, R_i | \beta, D, \theta)\} \\
&= \sum_{i=1}^{n} \ell(\psi, \theta; Y_i, b_i, R_i) \\
&= \sum_{i=1}^{n} log\{f(Y_i | \psi, b_i)\} + \sum_{i=1}^{n} log\{f(b_i | D)\} \\
&\quad + \sum_{i=1}^{n} log\{f(R_i | \theta, Y_i)\}, \quad (4.20)
\end{aligned}
$$

in which the density function $f(R_i | \theta, Y_i)$ for $R_i = (R_{i1}, \ldots, R_{iK})$ is the product of a sequence of one-dimensional conditional distributions specified by model (4.18):

$$
\begin{aligned}
f(R_i | \theta, Y_i) &= f(R_{i1}, \ldots, R_{iK} | \theta, Y_i) \\
&= \prod_{j=1}^{d_i} f(R_{ij} | R_{ij-1}, \theta, Y_i),
\end{aligned}
$$

where $d_i = max(n_i + 1, K)$ with n_i being the number of observations on subject i. Define $R_{i0} = 1$. Note that there is no need to include R_{ij} for $j > d_i$. This is a feature of the likelihood for monotone missing data patterns, which is not applicable for non-monotone missing data.

The expectation step (E-step) calculates expected value of the complete data log-likelihood (4.20) given observed data and current parameter estimates $\psi^{(t)}$ and $\theta^{(t)}$:

$$Q_i(\psi, \theta | \psi^{(t)}, \theta^{(t)})$$
$$= E\{\ell(\psi, \theta; Y_i, b_i, R_i) | Y_{obs,i}, R_i, \psi^{(t)}, \theta^{(t)}\}$$
$$\int \int log\{f(Y_i | \psi, b_i)\} f(Y_{mis,i}, b_i | Y_{obs,i}, R_i, \psi^{(t)}) dY_{mis,i} db_i$$
$$+ \int \int log\{f(b_i | D)\} f(Y_{mis,i}, b_i | Y_{obs,i}, R_i, \psi^{(t)}) dY_{mis,i} db_i$$
$$+ \int \int log\{f(R_i | \theta, Y_i)\} f(Y_{mis,i}, b_i | Y_{obs,i}, R_i, \psi^{(t)}) dY_{mis,i} db_i. \quad (4.21)$$

The maximization step (M-step) maximizes $Q(\psi, \theta | \psi^{(t)}, \theta^{(t)}) = \sum_{i=1}^{n} Q_i(\psi, \theta | \psi^{(t)}, \theta^{(t)})$ to obtain updated parameter estimates $\psi^{(t+1)}$ and $\theta^{(t+1)}$. The algorithm iterates between the E-step and M-step until convergence is achieved.

In general the integrals in (4.21) do not have a closed-form, so numerical integration techniques, such as Gaussian quadrature, can be used. When the dimension of integrals is high, a MCEM algorithm may be used as an alternative. It works by sampling $Y_{mis,i}$ and b_i from $f(Y_{mis,i}, b_i | Y_{obs,i}, R_i, \psi^{(t)}, \theta^{(t)})$ for each subject i. This can be done by a Gibbs sampler in conjunction of an adaptive rejection algorithm as long as the densities are log-concave. Let $(Y_{mis,i}^{(1)}, b_i^{(1)}), \ldots, (Y_{mis,i}^{(m_i)}, b_i^{(m_i)})$ be a sample of m_i observations drawn from the the distribution $f(Y_{mis,i}, b_i | Y_{obs,i}, R_i, \psi^{(t)}, \theta^{(t)})$. In the $(t+1)$-th iteration the E-step evaluates

$$Q_i(\psi, \theta | \psi^{(t)}, \theta^{(t)})$$
$$= \frac{1}{m_i} \sum_{k=1}^{m_i} \ell(\psi, \theta; Y_{obs,i}, Y_{mis,i}^{(k)}, b_i^{(k)}, R_i)$$
$$= \frac{1}{m_i} \sum_{k=1}^{m_i} log f(Y_{obs,i}, Y_{mis,i}^{(k)} | \psi^{(t)}, b_i^{(k)}) + \frac{1}{m_i} \sum_{k=1}^{m_i} log f(b_i^{(k)} | D)$$
$$+ \frac{1}{m_i} \sum_{k=1}^{m_i} log f(R_i | \theta^{(t)}, Y_{obs,i}, Y_{mis,i}^{(k)}). \quad (4.22)$$

Estimates of ψ and θ are then updated by maximizing $Q(\psi, \theta | \psi^{(t)}, \theta^{(t)}) = \sum_{i=1}^{n} Q_i(\psi, \theta | \psi^{(t)}, \theta^{(t)})$. A closed-form solution exists for ψ if Y follows a (multivariate) normal distribution, but not for θ in general. When there are no closed-form solutions, estimates can be used using a one-step Newton–Raphson algorithm in each M-step.

Standard errors of $\hat{\psi}$ and $\hat{\theta}$ are estimated at the convergence of the EM or

MCEM algorithm. Define $\gamma = (\psi, \theta)$. The observed information matrix of γ is

$$I(\hat{\gamma}) = -\ddot{Q}(\hat{\gamma}|\hat{\gamma}) - \sum_{i=1}^{n} E\{S_i(\hat{\gamma}; Y_i, b_i, R_i)S_i(\hat{\gamma}; Y_i, b_i, R_i)^T\}$$

$$+ \sum_{i=1}^{n} \dot{Q}_i(\hat{\gamma}|\hat{\gamma})\dot{Q}_i(\hat{\gamma}|\hat{\gamma})^T, \tag{4.23}$$

where $\dot{Q}(\hat{\gamma}|\hat{\gamma})$ and $\ddot{Q}(\hat{\gamma}|\hat{\gamma})$ are the first and second derivatives of Q with respect to γ, evaluated at $\hat{\gamma}$,

$$S_i(\hat{\gamma}; Y_i, b_i, R_i) = [\frac{\partial\ell(\gamma; Y_i, b_i, R_i)}{\partial\gamma}]_{\gamma=\hat{\gamma}},$$

and the expectation E is taken with respect to $Y_{mis,i}$ and b_i conditional on $Y_{obs,i}$, R_i, and $\hat{\gamma}$. When a MCEM algorithm is used,

$$E\{S_i(\hat{\gamma}; Y_i, b_i, R_i)S_i(\hat{\gamma}; Y_i, \tag{4.24}$$

$$b_i, R_i)^T\} = \sum_{k=1}^{m_i} \frac{1}{m_i} S_i(\hat{\gamma}; Y_i, b_i, R_i)S_i(\hat{\gamma}; Y_i, b_i, R_i)^T.$$

Parameter estimation in a marginal model can be done via EM and MCEM algorithms outlined above, but with a minor modification. Under a marginal model, the complete data log-likelihood function (4.20) becomes

$$\ell(\psi, \theta; Y, R) = log\{\prod_{i=1}^{n} f(Y_i, R_i|\psi, \theta)\}$$

$$= \sum_{i=1}^{n} \ell(\psi, \theta; Y_i, R_i)$$

$$= \sum_{i=1}^{n} log\{f(Y_i|\psi)\} + \sum_{i=1}^{n} log\{f(R_i|\theta, Y_i)\}, \tag{4.25}$$

and in the E-step, the expectation is taken with respect to $Y_{mis,i}$:

$$Q_i(\psi, \theta|\psi^{(t)}, \theta^{(t)})$$

$$= E\{\ell(\psi, \theta; Y_i, R_i)|Y_{obs,i}, R_i, \psi^{(t)}, \theta^{(t)}\}$$

$$\int log\{f(Y_i|\psi)\}f(Y_{mis,i}|Y_{obs,i}, R_i, \psi^{(t)})dY_{mis,i}$$

$$+ \int log\{f(R_i|\theta, Y_i)\}f(Y_{mis,i}|Y_{obs,i}, R_i, \psi^{(t)})dY_{mis,i}. \tag{4.26}$$

Example 4.8. *Milk Protein Trial*

The milk protein trial studied effects of three diets, barley, mixed barley-lupins,

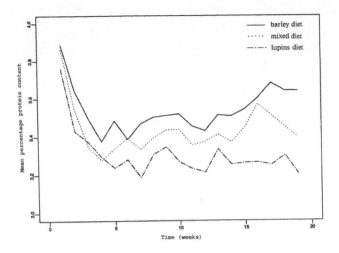

Figure 4.4 *Observed mean of the milk protein data.*

and lupins, on milk protein content from cows [54]. A total of 79 cows were randomized into three groups, with 25, 27, and 27 cows in each of the barley, mixed barley-lupins, and lupins diets, respectively. Protein content of milk samples was recorded on each cow up to 19 weeks. Dropout occurred when the cows stopped producing milk prior to study completion. There were 38 (48%) dropouts, all of which happened from week 15 onward. The mean protein content calculated using observed data is shown in Figure 4.4.

The objective of data analysis is to evaluate the impact of missing data on estimation of diet effect. The mean response is modeled by

$$\mu_{ij} = \begin{cases} \gamma_i - j\alpha & j < 3, \\ \gamma_i - 3\alpha + \eta(j-3) + \xi(j-3)^2 & j \geq 3, \end{cases}$$

in which i = 1, 2, and 3 denotes diet group and j is the index for time (in weeks). The quadratic term for j ≥ 3 reflects the fact that milk protein tended to rise at study completion. Data correlation is characterized by the following covariance structure:

$$Cov[Y_{ij}, Y_{ik}] = \begin{cases} \sigma^2 + \tau^2 & j = k, \\ \sigma^2 exp\{-\rho(j-k)^2\} & j \neq k. \end{cases}$$

Dropout at occasion j is modeled as

$$logit\{P(R_{ij} = 0 | R_{ij-1} = 1, Y_i, \beta)\} = \beta_{0,k-14} + \beta_1 Y_{ik} + \beta_2 Y_{ik-1}, \quad (4.27)$$

Table 4.4 *Milk protein trial: maximum likelihood estimates†.*

Parameter	Maximum likelihood estimates for the following models:		
	ID(int)	ID(app)	RD
γ_1	4.15	4.15	4.15
γ_2	4.05	4.05	4.05
γ_3	3.93	3.93	3.93
α	-0.23	-0.23	-0.23
$\eta \times 100$	0.51	0.05	0.72
$\xi \times 100$	-0.02	-0.02	-0.05
β_{01}	18.98	19.64	19.36
β_{02}	17.65	18.32	18.60
β_{03}	16.59	17.20	17.80
β_{04}	‡	‡	‡
β_{05}	18.28	18.89	18.54
β_1	5.65	5.53	
β_2	-12.01	-12.08	-6.29
σ^2	0.066	0.066	0.070
γ^2	0.027	0.027	0.026
ρ	0.86	0.86	0.86
2 log-likelihood	2402.7	2402.7	2388.8

†ID(int), ID using numercial integration; ID(app), ID using the approximation to the integral. ‡Extrinsically aliased.

for $k = 15, 16, 17$, and 19, since there were no dropouts at week 18. In addition, the dropout probability is set to 0 for $j \leq 14$. In the above model, parameters β_1 and β_2 are interpreted as effects of current and previous measurements on dropout.

Maximum likelihood estimates are shown in Table 4.4 for a joint model assuming random dropout (RD; i.e., $\beta_1 = 0$) and a model assuming nonignorable missing data due to informative dropout (ID; i.e., $\beta_1 \neq 0$). The likelihood ratio test statistic for $\beta_1 = 0$ is $2402.7 - 2388.8 = 14.2$ with 1 degree of freedom (p-value $= 0.0002$), which indicates that dropout was likely informative. Note that this conclusion is based upon the assumption that the joint model has correctly specified the longitudinal and dropout processes.

Since it seems difficult to interpret the opposite signs of estimated β_1 and β_2, the following reparametrization is examined:

$$logit\{P(R_{ij} = 0 | R_{ij-1} = 1, Y_i, \beta)\} = \beta_{0,k-14} + \theta_1(Y_{ik} + Y_{ik-1}) + \theta_2(Y_{ik} - Y_{ik-1}).$$

In this model, $\hat{\theta}_1 = (\hat{\beta}_1 + \hat{\beta}_2)/2 = -3.18$ and $\hat{\theta}_2 = (\hat{\beta}_1 - \hat{\beta}_2)/2 = 8.83$, which indicates that lower protein content or a large increase from the previous observation was associated with a higher probability of dropout.

The likelihood ratio test produces non-significant results for the null hypothesis $\eta = \xi = 0$, suggesting that there was no significant change in milk protein in week 15–19. The observed increase in mean responses (Figure 4.4) could be an

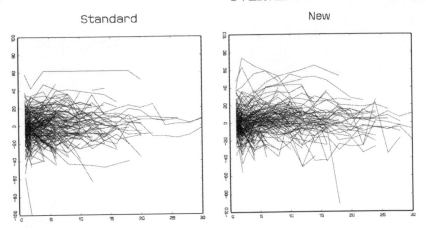

Figure 4.5 *Vorozole study: patient profiles of change in FLIC from baseline.*

artifact caused by informative dropouts, which were more likely to occur when the protein content was low. □

Example 4.9. *Vorozole Study*

The vorozole study is an open-label, randomized trial comparing vorozole (new) with megestrol acetate (standard) in post-menopausal patients with histologically confirmed estrogen-receptor positive metastatic breast carcinoma [115]. Four hundred and fifty-two patients were accrued at 67 centers and measurements were taken at baseline, month 1, month 2, and every two months onward until month 44. This analysis focuses on overall quality of life measured by the total Functional Living Index for Cancer (FLIC), with a higher value indicating a better condition. The longitudinal profiles of FLIC are displayed in Figure 4.5.

Table 4.5 *Vorozole study: selection models.*

Effect	Parameter	Estimate (standard error)
Fixed-effect parameters:		
Time	α_0	7.78(1.05)
Time × baseline	α_1	−0.065(0.009)
Time × treatment	α_2	0.086(0.157)
Time^2	α_3	−0.30(0.06)
Time^2× baseline	α_4	0.0024(0.0005)
Variance parameters:		
Random intercept	d	105.42
Serical variance	γ_2	77.96
Serical association	λ	7.22
Measurement error	σ_2	77.83

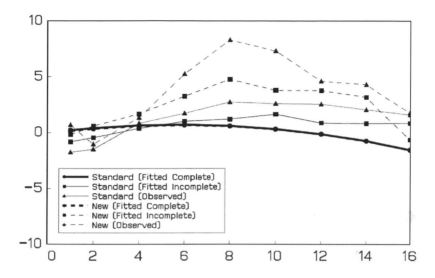

Figure 4.6 *Fitted profiles, based on averaging the predicted means for the incomplete and complete measurement sequences.*

Covariates considered for the longitudinal outcome included baseline FLIC, treatment, and time. A quadratic effect was shown to provide adequate fit because of a nonlinear time trend. Data correlation was captured by a random intercept and a spatial Gaussian process. Estimates of the longitudinal model are shown in Table 4.5. The following two dropout models were fit to the data, one with Y_{ij-1} and Y_{ij}, and the other with Y_{ij-2}, Y_{ij-1}, and Y_{ij} as predictors:

$$
\begin{aligned}
logit\{P(R_{ij} = 0 | R_{ij-1} = 1, Y_i)\} &= 0.53 - 0.015base_i - 0.076Y_{ij-1} \\
&\quad +0.057Y_{ij}, \\
logit\{P(R_{ij} = 0 | R_{ij-1} = 1, Y_i)\} &= 1.38 - 0.021base_i - 0.0027Y_{ij-2} \\
&\quad -0.064Y_{ij-1} + 0.035Y_{ij},
\end{aligned}
$$

where $base_i$ stands for baseline FLIC measured on subject i. Statistical tests could be conducted for the coefficients of Y_{ij}, but should be interpreted with caution because the estimated effects are, in principle, driven by unverifiable modeling assumptions, not observed data.

Figure 4.6 displays three estimated longitudinal profiles for each treatment group: (1) the mean of model-based predicted values, assuming all subjects completed the study; (2) the mean of predicted values for occasions with actual observations; and (3) the mean based on observed data only. For both groups, curve (3) is the highest, followed by the fitted incomplete, and complete profiles. This pattern suggests that subjects with low FLIC values tended to drop out of the study, so the observed data overestimated true trajectories. □

4.2.2 Random-Effects Dependent Dropout Models

Random-effects dependent dropout models are developed upon the belief that the association between longitudinal and dropout processes is induced by underlying smooth trends or characteristics, usually expressed as a function of random effects, in longitudinal trajectories. Such an assumption is appealing in many applications, specially when Y is prone to measurement errors and/or high biological variability. Methods for random-effects dependent dropout models are discussed in Wu and Carroll (1988)[240], Roy and Lin (2002)[191], Gao (2004)[74], and Yuan and Yin (2010)[246] for dropout as well as intermittent missing data. This topic is also covered by the review articles provided in Section 4.2.1. Tsonaka, Verbeke, and Lesaffre (2009)[219] extended existing methods by allowing random effects distributions completely unspecified.

In random-effects dependent dropout models, longitudinal data are characterize by a mixed model of form (4.17), and dropout is dependent on random effects b_i via a logistic regression:

$$logit\{P(R_{ij} = 1 | R_{ij-1} = 1, b_i, \theta)\} = H(b_i, \theta). \tag{4.28}$$

The above model can be adapted to intermittent or arbitrary missingness patterns, so that the response indicator R_{ij} is not necessarily dependent on R_{ij-1}:

$$logit\{P(R_{ij} = 1 | b_i, \theta)\} = H(b_i, \theta). \tag{4.29}$$

We assume conditional independence of Y and R given random effects and covariates. If the trajectory of Y is described by a random intercept b_{0i} and slope b_{1i}, then function $H(b_i, \theta)$ could take the form

$$H(b_i, \theta) = \theta_0 + \theta_1 b_{0i} + \theta_2 b_{1i}.$$

If $\theta_1 \neq 0$ or $\theta_2 \neq 0$, the dropout process (or missing data mechanism) is informative, i.e., missing data in Y are nonignorable.

Note that the underlying dropout process is continuous in nature, but usually we do not know exact dropout times because longitudinal data are measured intermittently at pre-scheduled occasions. Strictly speaking, the dropout time is interval-censored if we know that a subject is observed at time t_j, but has dropped out of the study by time t_{j+1}. The above logistic regression does not capture the continuous nature of actual dropout times. In light of this issue, a probit model has been proposed to characterize the probability of dropout:

$$\Phi^{-1}\{P(R_j = 0 | b_i, \theta)\} = \theta_{0j} + \theta_1 b_{0i} + \theta_2 b_{1i}, \tag{4.30}$$

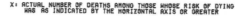
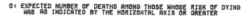
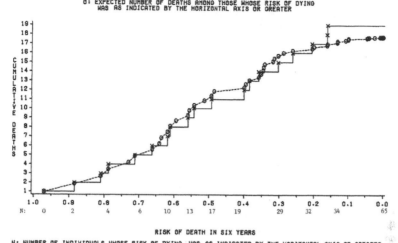

Figure 4.7 *Actual versus expected number of deaths in 6 years.*

where $\Phi^{-1}(\cdot)$ is inverse of the cumulative density function for a standard normal distribution. Note that the intercept θ_{0j} is dependent on j.

Under either (4.28) or (4.30), the joint distribution of Y_i and R_i conditional on b_i can then be written as

$$f(Y_i, R_i|b_i, \beta, D, \theta) = f(Y_i|b_i, \beta, D)f(R_i|b_i, \theta),$$

and the likelihood function is thus

$$
\begin{aligned}
L(\psi, \theta; Y, R) &= \prod_{i=1}^{n} \int_{b_i} f(Y_i, R_i|b_i, \beta, D, \theta)dF(b_i) \qquad (4.31) \\
&= \prod_{i=1}^{n} \int_{b_i} f(Y_i|b_i, \beta, D)f(R_i|b_i, \theta)dF(b_i).
\end{aligned}
$$

Likelihood and Bayesian methods described in Section 4.2.1 can be applied here for parameter estimation and inference.

Random-effects dependent dropout models are a type of shared parameter models. As discussed in Section (4.1.1), shared parameter models characterize the dependence between longitudinal and missing data mechanisms using random effects instead of actual but possibly censored longitudinal observations. This assumption seems restrictive because a common set of random effects are used to link together the two endpoints, but provide a good approximation to situations where random effects at the longitudinal endpoint capture most of uncertainty in dropouts.

Table 4.6 *Estimation for the expected FEV_1 slope, the missing-value coefficients, and likelihood-ratio test statistics for the coefficients.*

	Three-year mortality	Six-year mortality
Estimates and test statistics	Three-year FEV_1 follow-up	Six-year FEV_1 follow-up
Estimated FEV_1 change/year		
Unweighted	$-.093(.0164)^a$	$-.078(.0138)^b$
Weighted	$-.090(.0151)$	$-.076(.0136)$
Probit information missing	$-.095(.0152)$	$-.085(.0133)$
Estimated missing-value coefficients		
FEV_1 Initial value	$-3.80(2.01)$	$-4.61(1.70)$
FEV_1 slope	$-11.30(7.46)$	$-13.80(6.76)$
Likelihood-ratio test statistics		
Initial value $(H_1 vs H_0)^b : \chi_1^2$	11.02	26.97
Slope $(H_2 vs H_1)^b : \chi_1^2$	2.81	7.13
No. at risk at baseline	81	65
No. of deaths	8	19

^{a} Numbers in parentheses are estimated standard errors.
$^b H_0 : \theta_1 = \theta_2 = 0; H_1 : \theta_1 \neq 0, \theta_2 = 0; H_2 : \theta_1 \neq 0, \theta_2 \neq 0.$

Example 4.10. *PiZ Emphysema Study*

This is a feasibility study among subjects with PiZ phenotype who tended to develop pulmonary emphysema and hence rapid decline in lung function [240]. Retrospective data on PiZ subjects from ten US institutions were collected to estimate rates of decline in a 1-second forced expiratory volume (FEV1) and the estimates were then used in sample size calculations for a prospective study comparing a therapeutic group and control. Both 3-year and 6-year analyses of FEV1 were conducted; the former included 81 subjects (8 deaths) and the latter included 65 subjects (19 deaths). The average number of FEV1 measurements was 2.9 and 3.6 (median = 3 for both) and average (median) duration between baseline and last observed FEV1s was 28 (33) and 48 (55) months for the 3- and 6-year follow-ups, respectively. The analyses excluded individuals with only one FEV1 measurement.

In the joint model, FEV1 trajectories were specified by a linear mixed model with a random intercept b_{0i} and random slope b_{1i}. A probit model of form (4.30) was used to characterize time to death. Therefore, missing data caused by death were associated with baseline and slope of FEV1. Change in FEV1 per year was estimated using an unweighted average of individual simple least-squares estimates, a weighted average of simple least-squares estimates, and the joint model (Table 4.6). The weighted (or unweighted) estimates corresponded to maximum likelihood estimates of regression coefficients when individuals have different (or identical) time points. These quantities were derived under the assumption of ignorable missingness in FEV1. Likelihood ratio tests indicate statistical significance for θ_1 in both analyses and θ_2 in the 6-year analysis. Estimates of θ_1 and θ_2 were -3.8 and -11.3, and -4.6 and -13.8 in the 3- and 6-year analyses, respectively, which suggests that low baseline FEV1 and fast decline in follow-up were associated with a higher risk of death.

A graphical approach to check model fit was used to compare observed versus estimated cumulative counts of death for the 6-year follow-up data (Figure 4.7), suggesting that the probit model provides a reasonable fit. □

4.3 Longitudinal Data with Both Monotone and Intermittent Missing Values

Joint models we have discussed in Sections 4.1 and 4.2 are applied to studies in which missing data are caused by terminating events such as death or dropout so that missing data patterns are monotone. However, it is common to encounter both monotone and non-monotone (or intermittent) missing data in longitudinal studies. The term *intermittent* refers to a situation where a subject misses one or more occasions but returns to the study at later visits.

One way of handling monotone and intermittent missing data simultaneously is to augment joint models of longitudinal and survival data with a third component to characterize intermittent missingness. In what follows, we introduce a joint analysis developed by Tseng et al. (2012)[211] in which random effects are used to model the inter-dependence between longitudinal data, monotone, and intermittent missing patterns. As will be discussed in more detail, adaptive Gaussian–Hermite quadrature and Taylor series expansion are used to reduce computational burden due to high dimensional integration in the EM algorithm.

4.3.1 Model Formulation for Monotone and Intermittent Missing Data

Following the notation in previous sections, let Y_{ij} denote outcome Y measured on subject i at occasion j, T_i the survival time (death or dropout) that leads to monotone missing data, R_{ij} the intermittent missingness indicator such that $R_{ij} = 1$ if Y_{ij} is observed and $R_{ij} = 0$ if Y_{ij} is missing, $i = 1, \ldots, n$ and $j = 1, \ldots, K$. Note that T_i could be censored by C_i, and $\Delta_i = 1$ indicates that T_i is observed. Note that both Y_{ij} and R_{ij} are truncated by the survival/censoring time.

A linear mixed effects model for Y_{ij} is specified as:

$$Y_{ij} = X_{1ij}^T \beta_1 + Z_{1ij}^T b_{1i} + \sigma \epsilon_{ij}, \tag{4.32}$$

where β_1 and b_{1i} are fixed and random effects, respectively, X_{1ij} and Z_{1ij} are corresponding covariates, and σ is a dispersion parameter. When measurement errors ϵ_{ij} are standard normal random variables, σ^2 is the variance. To reduce the impact of outlying observations and achieve robust inference, a t-distribution can be posited for ϵ_{ij}. There are various ways to incorporate a t-distribution for robust inference. For example, given sufficient data, one can estimate the degree of freedom based on likelihood methods. As recommended in the literature, to simplify the model and computational effort, a fixed $\nu = 3$ degrees of freedom can be used here. Other robust joint models via t-distributed measurement errors are introduced in Chapter 5.

Intermittent missingness, i.e., $\pi_{ij} = Prob(R_{ij} = 0)$, for subject i at occasion j is modeled by a mixed effects logistic regression:

$$logit(\frac{\pi_{ij}}{1 - \pi_{ij}}) = X_{2ij}\beta_2 + Z_{2ij}b_{2i}, \tag{4.33}$$

where X_{2ij} and Z_{2ij} are covariates and β_2 and b_{2i} are associated fixed and random effects, respectively. The covariates X_{1ij}, X_{2ij}, Z_{1ij}, and Z_{2ij} can be disjoint or overlapped.

Survival time (monotone missingness) is characterized by a proportional hazards frailty model

$$\begin{aligned} \lambda(t|X_{3i}, Z_{3i}, b_{3i}) &= \lim_{h \to 0} \frac{Prob(t \le T_i < t + h | T \ge t, X_{3i}, Z_{3i}, b_{3i})}{h} \\ &= \lambda_0(t) exp(X_{3i}\beta_3 + Z_{3i}b_{3i}), \end{aligned} \tag{4.34}$$

where $\lambda_0(t)$ is the baseline hazard function, X_{3i} and Z_{3i} are vectors of covariates, and β_3 and b_{3i} are fixed and random effects (frailty), respectively.

Suppose the dimension of random effects b_{1i}, b_{2i}, and b_{3i} in the above models is q_1, q_2, and q_3, respectively, then $b_i = (b_{1i}, b_{2i}, b_{3i})$ is a $q_1 + q_2 + q_3$ dimensional vector of random effects to capture dependence among all observations. A multivariate normal distribution can be assumed for b_i: $b_i \sim N(0, \Sigma)$, where

$$\Sigma = \begin{pmatrix} \Sigma_{11} & \Sigma_{12} & \Sigma_{13} \\ \Sigma_{21} & \Sigma_{22} & \Sigma_{23} \\ \Sigma_{31} & \Sigma_{32} & \Sigma_{33} \end{pmatrix}.$$

This joint model implies that missing data from missed visits and/or study dropouts are nonignorable when b_{1i} is not independent of either b_{2i} or b_{3i}. Note that all fixed effects covariates $(X_{1ij}, X_{2ij}, X_{3i})$ and random effects covariates $(Z_{1ij}, Z_{2ij}, Z_{3i})$ can be disjoint or overlapped.

4.3.2 Likelihood and Estimation

Let $Y_{obs,i}$ and $Y_{mis,i}$ be the observed and missing outcome measurements on subject i, and $R_{obs,i}$ and $R_{mis,i}$ the observed and missing indicators for intermittent missingness. Survival data $S_{obs,i} = (\tilde{T}_i, \Delta_i)$ is observed for all subjects, where $\tilde{T}_i = min(T_i, C_i)$. The likelihood function for subject i is

$$\begin{aligned} L_i &= \int f(Y_{obs,i}, Y_{mis,i}, R_{obs,i}, R_{mis,i}, S_{obs,i}|X_i, Z_i, b_i) f(b_i) dY_{mis,i} dR_{mis,i} db_i \\ &= \int f(Y_{obs,i}, Y_{mis,i}|X_i, Z_i, b_i) f(R_{obs,i}, R_{mis,i}|X_i, Z_i, b_i) f(S_{obs,i}|X_i, Z_i, b_i) \\ &\quad \times f(b_i) dY_{mis,i} dR_{mis,i} db_i, \end{aligned}$$

where X_i and Z_i collect all covariates in (4.32)–(4.34). Assume that the observed data $(Y_{obs,i}, R_{obs,i})$ and unobserved data $(Y_{mis,i}, R_{mis,i})$ are conditionally independent given random effects b_i. Furthermore, because $\int f(Y_{mis,i}|b_i)dY_{mis,i} = 1$ and $\int f(R_{mis,i}|b_i)dR_{mis,i} = 1$ for each given value of b_i, the likelihood function reduces to:

$$L_i = \int f(Y_{obs,i}|X_i, Z_i, b_i)f(R_{obs,i}|X_i, Z_i, b_i)f(S_{obs,i}|X_i, Z_i, b_i)f(b_i)db_i.$$

Let $\psi = (\beta_1, \beta_2, \beta_3, \sigma^2, \theta)$ and $\Lambda_0(t) = \int_0^t \lambda_0(u)du$, where θ is a vector of parameters in Σ.

The goal is to calculate the maximum likelihood estimate for (ψ, Λ_0) over a space in which ψ belongs to a bounded set and Λ_0 is in a space consisting of all increasing functions in t with $\Lambda_0(0) = 0$. As discussed previously, in likelihood-based estimation methods, the EM algorithm is a natural choice to estimate (ψ, Λ_0). At the $(m+1)$th iteration, the E-step evaluates the expected value of functions of b_i that appear in the complete-data log-likelihood with respect to its conditional distribution given parameters estimated in the mth iteration. For example, the conditional expectation for function $h(b_i)$ is evaluated by

$$
\begin{aligned}
E(h(b_i)|D_i, \Lambda^{(m)}, \psi^{(m)}) &= \int h(b_i)f(b_i|D_i, \Lambda^{(m)}, \psi^{(m)})db_i \\
&= \frac{\int h(b_i)f(D_i, b_i|\Lambda^{(m)}, \psi^{(m)})db_i}{\int f(D_i, b_i|\Lambda^{(m)}, \psi^{(m)})db_i}, \quad (4.35)
\end{aligned}
$$

where $D_i = (Y_{obs,i}, R_{obs,i}, S_{obs,i})$ denotes the observed data for subject i, and $\Lambda^{(m)}$ and $\psi^{(m)}$ are estimates from the mth iteration.

Integrals in the E-step are computationally intensive if the dimension of b_i is 3 or higher. This joint model has motivated exploration of several techniques to reduce computational burden and to achieve better accuracy in numerical approximation of integration. The numerator and denominator in equation (4.35) can be approximated separately by Gauss–Hermite quadrature. It has been suggested that the two integrands in the numerator and denominator are similar in shape. By taking the ratio of them, the leading error term may cancel out and result in better approximation accuracy. However, computation could be heavy even with a moderate number of random effects b_i.

To reduce computational burden, $E(h(b_i))$ can be approximated by Taylor series expansion, which is augmented by adaptive quadrature to increase computation efficiency. Specifically, the expectation for all functions $h(b_i)$ is approximated by the first two moments of b_i:

$$E(h(b_i)) \approx h(Eb_i) + \frac{1}{2}h^{(2)}(Eb_i)Vb_i,$$

where $Eb_i = E(b_i)$ is the expectation of b_i, $Vb_i = E[(b_i - Eb_i)(b_i - Eb_i)^T]$

is the variance of b_i, and $h^{(2)}(b) = \frac{\partial^2 h(b)}{\partial b^2}$ is the second partial derivative of $h(b)$. Under this Taylor series approximation, the only integrals that need to be evaluated in the E-step are the first two moments of b_i.

Adaptive Gaussian–Hermite quadrature can be used to calculate the first two moments of b_i. The quadrature method approximates integrals of functions with respect to a given kernel by evaluating the integrand at predetermined abscissas and taking a weighted average of these values. For a multidimensional integral, the number of abscissas required to achieve the same accuracy rises exponentially as the number of dimensions increases. It works for integrals of the form

$$\int h(b_i)db_i = \int g(b_i)\phi(b_i, \hat{\mu}, \hat{\sigma})db_i \approx \sum_{k=1}^{l} \frac{w_k}{\sqrt{\pi}} g(\hat{\mu} + \sqrt{2}\hat{\sigma}x_k),$$

where $g(b_i) = \frac{h(b_i)}{\phi(b_i, \hat{\mu}, \hat{\sigma})}$, l is the number of nodes, x_k and w_k are the kth node and weight. A critical step for the success of adaptive quadrature is the choice of importance distribution ϕ and its parameters $\hat{\mu}$ and $\hat{\sigma}$. It is suggested to use the Laplace method to estimate the mode and dispersion of $h(b_i)$ for $\hat{\mu}$ and $\hat{\sigma}$. This choice of importance distribution is near optimal. As described above, with Taylor series approximation, one only needs to compute the first two moments of b_i to approximate $E(h(b_i))$. Thus, a single importance distribution can be used for all functions $h(\cdot)$ of b_i. Specifically, one can recycle the mean and variance calculated in the previous E-step as the importance distribution parameters ($\hat{\mu}$ and $\hat{\sigma}$) for the current E-step. This choice of importance distribution parameters allows us to sample the integrand $h(b_i)$ in a suitable range with minimal cost in computation. It is shown using simulated data that the estimated first two moments converge faster to their true values using the proposed adaptive Gaussian–Hermite quadrature compared to Gaussian–Hermite quadrature.

The M-step needs to solve conditional score equations derived from complete-data log-likelihood given observed data. If longitudinal data are characterized by a linear mixed effects model with normal random effects and residuals, regression coefficients in the longitudinal model have a closed form solution. However, there is no closed form solution for parameters in the mixed effects logistic model, proportional hazard frailty model, and longitudinal model with t-distributed measurement errors, for which one-step of Newton–Raphson can be carried out in the M-step.

Example 4.11. *The Scleroderma Lung Study*

The Scleroderma Lung Study is a multi-center placebo-control double bind randomized study to evaluate the effects of oral cyclophosphamide (CYC) on lung function and other health-related symptoms in patients with evidence of active alveolitis and scleroderma-related interstitial lung disease. One hundred and fifty-eight eligible patients underwent randomization, and about 15% of them

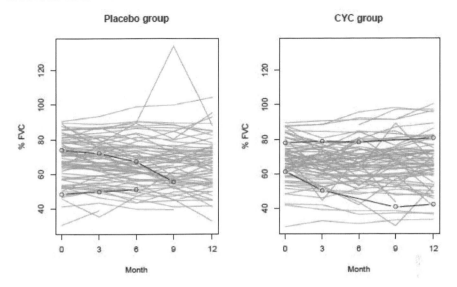

Figure 4.8 *Longitudinal %FVC in the placebo and CYC groups during the first 12 months. %FVC was measured at baseline and at three-month intervals throughout the study. Two subjects (01-ALS-013 and 04-JWW-010) in the placebo group are highlighted as examples of study dropouts at 6 and 9 months, and two subjects (08-S-L-018 and 09-NEP-005) in the CYC group are examples of missed visits at 6 and 9 months.*

dropped out of the study before 12 months. About 30% of dropouts were due to death and treatment failures. Intermittent missed visits also occurred during the course of the study. It is likely that the missing data were due to ineffectiveness of treatment and thus related to %FVC, the outcome of interest. A detailed description of the study is provided in Chapter 1, and %FVC is analyzed in Chapter 2 using methods assuming ignorable missing data.

Figure 4.8 shows profiles of %FVC during the first year, stratified by treatment group. Two subjects (01-ALS-013 and 04-JWW-010) in the placebo group are highlighted as examples of study dropouts at 6 and 9 months, and two subjects (08-S-L-018 and 09-NEP-005) in the CYC group are examples of missed visits at 6 and 9 months. Most patients showed a small variation in %FVC over time, but a few of them had outlying observations.

The longitudinal model assumed a linear time trend for %FVC:

$$\begin{aligned} FVC \quad = \quad & \beta_0^{(1)} + \beta_1^{(1)} Time + \beta_2^{(1)} FVC_0 + \beta_3^{(1)} MAXFIB_0 + \beta_4^{(1)} CYC \\ & + \beta_5^{(1)} CYC \times FVC_0 + \beta_6^{(1)} CYC \times MAXFIB_0 + \beta_7^{(1)} CYC \\ & \times Time + b_1 + \sigma\epsilon, \end{aligned}$$

where FVC_0 and $MAXFIB_0$ are baseline %FVC and maximum lung fibro-

sis, CYC a treatment indicator, b_1 a random intercept, and ϵ a t-distributed variable with 3 degrees of freedom.

Intermittent missing data were modeled by

$$logit(p) = \beta_0^{(2)} + \beta_1^{(2)} Time + b_2,$$

where p is the probability of missing a visit and b_2 is a random intercept. The event that led to monotone missing data in %FVC was death or treatment failure, which was characterized by a proportional hazards frailty model

$$\lambda(t) = \lambda_0(t) \exp(\beta_1^{(3)} FVC + \beta_2^{(3)} MAXFIB_0 + \beta_3^{(3)} CYC) + b_3,$$

where b_3 is a frailty.

Random effects (b_1, b_2, b_3) in the above three models were assumed to follow a three-dimensional multivariate normal distribution to capture the dependence among %FVC, missed visits, and time to death or treatment failure. Thus, the E-step involved three-dimensional integration. With 3 nodes for each dimension, adaptive Gauss–Hermite quadrature with 27 nodes was used for integrals in the E-step.

As this is a randomized trial, the assignment of CYC is independent of baseline characteristics. The overall treatment effect on %FVC at time t can be defined as:

$$E(FVC|CYC = 1, Time = t) - E(FVC|CYC = 0, Time = t)$$

$$= \int \{E(FVC|CYC = 1, Time = t, FVC_0, MAXFIB_0, b_1)$$

$$-E(FVC|CYC = 0, Time = t, FVC_0, MAXFIB_0, b_1)\}$$

$$\times f(FVC_0, MAXFIB_0, b_1)dFVC_0 dMAXFIB_0 db_1$$

$$\approx 1/n \sum_{i=1}^{n} eff_i,$$

where eff_i is the treatment(CYC) effect for the ith subject at time t:

$$eff_i = \quad E(FVC_i|CYC = 1, Time = t, FVC_{0i}, MAXFIB_{0i}, b_{1i})$$

$$-E(FVC_i|CYC = 0, Time = t, FVC_{0i}, MAXFIB_{0i}, b_{1i}).$$

Table 4.7 reports parameter estimates in the longitudinal model for %FVC, based on 6 to 18 months' data. %FVC is associated with its baseline measurement and maximum fibrosis score. In addition, the CYC effect appears to be modified by baseline %FVC measurement and maximum fibrosis. The second part of Table 4.7 shows estimated overall treatment effects at various time points, which indicates that the CYC effect rises to the maximum at month 18. □

Table 4.7 *Analysis of %FVC in the Scleroderma study, using data from 6 to 18 months.*

β	Estimate	Standard Error	p-value
β_1(Time)	−0.07	0.06	0.297
β_2(FVC$_0$)	0.92	0.013	<0.001
β_3(MAXFIB$_0$)	−1.62	0.16	<0.001
β_4(CYC)	−1.08	1.15	0.416
β_5(CYC×FVC$_0$)	0.081	0.019	<0.001
β_6(CYC×MAXFIB$_0$)	1.50	0.25	<0.001
β_7(CYC×Time)	0.24	0.09	0.009
overall effect at			
6 months	0.36	0.71	0.609
9 months	1.08	0.51	0.036
12 months	1.79	0.41	<0.001
15 months	2.50	0.47	<0.001
18 months	3.21	0.69	<0.001
$\beta_4 = \beta_5 = \beta_6 = \beta_7 = 0$			<0.001

4.4 Event Time Models with Intermittently Measured Time-Dependent Covariates

In this section we discuss a class of joint models to deal with practical issues with time-dependent covariates in event time models. Although it belongs to the broader realm of selection models, this topic deserves a separate treatment not only because it has a prominent position in the joint model literature, but development in this area has been one of the main forces driving prosperity of joint models. The initial interest of such models stemmed from research investigating predictiveness of repeatedly measured biomarkers for clinical meaningful events. Examples include AIDS studies to evaluate the relationship between CD4 counts (repeatedly measured) and time to progression or death, and prostate cancer studies using longitudinal prostate specific antigen (PSA) measurements to predict cancer recurrence. There is also interest in these studies to determine surrogacy of the biomarker; that is, treatment effect manifests through the biomarker so that the event is independent of treatment given biomarker trajectories.

In an ideal situation, the above research questions can be routinely addressed by an event time model in which the biomarker is included as a time-dependent covariate. For example, it is straightforward to incorporate the time-dependent biomarker into a Cox proportional hazards model and study its effect on the event. Treatment can be included as a time-fixed covariate, and its effect with and without adjustment for the biomarker is then examined to assess surrogacy. However, application of such models in practice is often problematic. First of all, the biomarker is not observed in a continuum interval of time; instead, measurements are available only at a set of specific time points. Thus, the biomarker may be missing at some observed event times, and partial likelihood discussed in Section 3.4 cannot be defined at these time points. Naive imputation methods, such as last observation carried forward, are likely to introduce bias into model estimation. Secondly, the biomarker is often subject to measurement error and high biological variation, so that the observed values may not accurately reflect true underlying trajectories. Thus, using observed values to predict the event could lead to further bias. The third issue is regarding possible nonignorable missing data in longitudinal measurements. Statistical analysis to characterize intra-subject changes and between-subject heterogeneity in the biomarker should take into account the missing data mechanism. This issue has been elaborated and discussed previously.

Joint modeling of time-dependent biomarkers and event times has been developed to address the above issues. In joint analysis, a longitudinal model is used to characterize the biomarker underlying (unobservable) trajectory, which is incorporated as a latent, time-dependent covariate in the survival model to predict failure times. In what follows, we discuss extensions of two standard approaches, Cox proportional hazards models and accelerated failure time models, to this area of joint analysis.

4.4.1 Cox Models with Intermittently Measured Time-Dependent Covariates

For subject i, let $Y_i(t)$ denote the underlying, smooth trajectory of biomarker, T_i the event time, and $Z_i(t)$ a set of possibly time-varying covariates. Because the biomarker is intermittently measured at time points t_{ij} and there are intra-subject measurement errors, $Y_i(t)$ is not directly observable; instead, measurements of $W_i(t_{ij})$ are available such that

$$W_i(t_{ij}) = Y_i(t_{ij}) + \epsilon_i(t_{ij}), \tag{4.36}$$

where $\epsilon_i(t_{ij})$ are measurement errors. In reality the event time T_i may be subject to right censoring so we observe $\tilde{T}_i = min(T_i, C_i)$ and $\Delta_i = I(T_i \leq C_i)$, where C_i is the censoring time. Measurements of $W_i(t_{ij})$ will then be available at time points $t_{ij} \leq \tilde{T}_i$, $j = 1, \ldots, n_i$.

The longitudinal model focuses on characterizing change in $Y_i(t)$ over time. If the change can be described by a polynomial function or splines of time t, then $Y_i(t)$ is specified as

$$Y_i(t) = \rho(t)^T b_i, \tag{4.37}$$

where b_i is a vector of subject-specific random effects. A simple example is

$Y_i(t) = \rho_{0i} + \rho_{1i}t$, or more flexibly, $Y_i(t) = \rho_{0i} + \rho_{1i}t + \cdots + \rho_{pi}t^p$, $b_i = (b_{0i}, \ldots, b_{pi})^T$. Model (4.37) assumes the trajectory of $Y_i(t)$ is determined by a relatively small set of time-fixed random effects, which may not fully account for within-subject variation over time. A mean-zero stochastic process $U_i(t)$ is thus added to the model such that

$$Y_i(t) = \rho(t)^T b_i + U_i(t). \tag{4.38}$$

The process $U_i(t)$ is usually assumed to be independent of b_i and covariates $Z_i(t)$. Examples of $U_i(t)$ include integrated Ornstein–Uhlenbeck (IOU) process and stationary Gaussian process. In fact, $U_i(t)$ captures biological fluctuations around the smooth trend $\rho(t)^T b_i$ and induces an additional within-subject autocorrelation structure on top of that by b_i. Choosing in between (4.37) and (4.38) reflects the belief whether the "inherent," dominant time trend in the biomarker is associated with T or the biological fluctuations are important features we should capture as well when characterizing the survival model.

In (4.37) and (4.38), random effects b_i are usually assumed to be normally distributed and the mean and covariance matrix may depend on $Z_i(t)$. Measurement errors $\epsilon_i(t_{ij}) \sim N(0, \sigma^2)$ are independent of b_i and $U_i(t)$ for all $t \geq 0$. Under (4.38), $\epsilon_i(t_{ij})$ takes into account measurement error as well as local, transient biological variation that is unlikely to carry over across j, so the independence assumption for $\epsilon_i(t_{ij})$ at different t_{ij} is reasonable. Model (4.38) reduces to (4.37) when the stochastic process $U_i(t)$ is absorbed into $\epsilon_i(t_{ij})$ so that $\epsilon_i(t_{ij})$ contains both measurement error and local biological fluctuations. In this case, a covariance structure may be necessary for $\epsilon_i(t_{ij})$ to characterize within-subject correlation over time. If time separation is sufficiently long so within-subject correlation due to biological variation is negligible, or if measurement error is in a much larger scale than biological variation, the independence assumption would still hold approximately.

A Cox proportional hazards model is used to specify the interrelationship between $Y_i(t)$, T_i, and $Z_i(t)$:

$$\lambda_i(t) = \lim_{dt \to 0} \frac{P\{t \leq T_i < t + dt | T_i \geq t, \bar{Y}_i(t), Z_i(t)\}}{dt}$$
$$= \lambda_0(t) exp\{\gamma Y_i(t) + \eta^T Z_i(t)\}, \tag{4.39}$$

where $\bar{Y}_i(t) = \{Y_i(u), 0 \leq u \leq t\}$ is the history of the biomarker up to time t. This specification implies that given covariates and past history $\bar{Y}_i(t)$, the biomarker is associated with the event risk through its current value $Y_i(t)$. Alternative specifications are possible, for example, $\lambda_i(t) = \lambda_0(t) exp\{\gamma b_{1i} + \eta^T Z_i(t)\}$, where b_{1i} is the random slope if $Y_i(t)$. This formulation is applied to circumstances where we believe that, given $\bar{Y}_i(t)$ and covariates, the main force that drives the event process is the underlying constant rate of change in $Y_i(t)$.

Parameter estimation and statistical inference for the joint model specified in

(4.36), (4.37), and (4.39), or (4.36), (4.38), and (4.39) have been studied using
likelihood-based or Bayesian approaches. The EM algorithm outlined in Section 4.1.1 is commonly used in likelihood approaches for parameter estimation.
However, as discussed previously, such an approach suffers from computational
burden when random effects b_i have a high dimension. In addition, parametric assumptions usually posited for b_i, such as normal distribution, raise the
concern about model robustness. In view of these potential issues, an estimating equation approach based on conditional score has been developed, which
relaxes parametric distributional assumptions for b_i and is relatively easy to
implement. In what follows we review the conditional score, likelihood-based,
and Bayesian approaches.

Conditional Score Approach

The conditional score approach, developed by Tsiatis and Davidian (2001,
2004)[217, 216], is an estimating-equation based method that conditions on a
"sufficient statistic" for b_i. Consider a random intercept and slope model for
$Y_i(t)$:

$$Y_i(t) = b_{0i} + b_{1i}t. \qquad (4.40)$$

Assume measurement errors $\epsilon_i(t_{ij})$ in (4.36) are i.i.d. normal variables
$N(0, \sigma^2)$ given random effects b_i, covariates $Z_i(t)$, $\bar{Y}_i(t_{ij})$ and that the
biomarker is measured at t_{ij} and subject i is at risk at t_{ij}. Let $\hat{Y}_i(t)$ be the ordinary least squares estimator for $Y_i(t)$ based on measurements up to t. In the
case of (4.40), $\hat{Y}_i(t) = (1, t)\hat{b}_i$, where $\hat{b}_i$ is the ordinary least squares estimates
of intercept and slope for subject i. Note that $\hat{b}_i$ is defined for subjects with at
least two measurements by time t. Let $J_i(t)$ be the at-risk indicator for subjects
with at least two measurements at time t, such that $J_i(t) = I(\tilde{T}_i \geq t, t_{i2} \leq t)$.
Under the assumption that censoring or seeing a measurement at time t given
b_i and biomarker data prior to t are not dependent on measurement errors
prior to t, it can be shown that

$$\hat{Y}_i(t)|J_i(t) = 1, \mathcal{T}_i(t), b_i, Z_i(t) \sim N(Y_i(t), \sigma^2\theta_i(t)),$$

where $\mathcal{T}_i(t) = \{t_{ij}, t_{ij} < t\}$ and $\sigma^2\theta_i(t)$ is the variance of predicted value $\hat{Y}_i(t)$.
In the case of (4.40),

$$\theta_i(t) = 1/n_{i,t} + (t - \bar{t}_{i,t})^2 / \sum_{j=1}^{n_{i,t}} (t_{ij} - \bar{t}_{i,t})^2,$$

where $n_{i,t}$ is the number of time points in $\mathcal{T}_i(t)$ and $\bar{t}_{i,t}$ is the mean of the $n_{i,t}$
time points.

The following derivation of conditional score estimating equations assumes σ^2
is known. Extension to the case of unknown σ^2 will be discussed in a moment.

Define the counting process $dN_i(t) = I(t \le \tilde{T}_i < t + dt, \Delta_i = 1, t_{i2} \le t)$. The conditional density for the joint distribution of $\{dN_i(t) = r, \hat{Y}_i(t) = y\}$ is

$$
\begin{aligned}
&Pr\{dN_i(t) = r, \hat{Y}_i(t) = y | J_i(t) = 1, \mathcal{T}_i(t), b_i, Z_i(t)\} \\
= \ &Pr\{dN_i(t) = r | \hat{Y}_i(t) = y, J_i(t) = 1, \mathcal{T}_i(t), b_i, Z_i(t)\} \\
&\times Pr\{\hat{Y}_i(t) = y | J_i(t) = 1, \mathcal{T}_i(t), b_i, Z_i(t)\}.
\end{aligned}
\tag{4.41}
$$

The first component of (4.41) is a Bernoulli variable with probability $\lambda_0(t)dt \exp\{\gamma Y_i(t) + \eta^T Z_i(t)\}$, and the second is a normal variable $N(Y_i(t), \sigma^2\theta_i(t))$. After simplifications it can be shown that to order dt, (4.41) is equal to

$$
\begin{aligned}
&\exp[Y_i(t)\{\frac{\gamma\sigma^2\theta_i(t)dN_i(t) + \hat{Y}_i(t)}{\sigma^2\theta_i(t)}\}] \\
&\times \frac{\{\lambda_0(t)\exp(\eta^T Z_i(t))dt\}^{dN_i(t)}}{\{2\pi\sigma^2\theta_i(t)\}^{1/2}} \exp\{-\frac{\hat{Y}_i^2(t) + Y_i^2(t)}{2\sigma^2\theta_i(t)}\},
\end{aligned}
$$

which indicates that a "sufficient statistic" for b_i is $S_i(t, \gamma, \sigma^2) = \gamma\sigma^2\theta_i(t)dN_i(t) + \hat{Y}_i(t)$. Conditional on $S_i(t, \gamma, \sigma^2)$, it can be shown that

$$
\begin{aligned}
&\lim_{dt\to 0} Pr\{dN_i(t) = 1 | S_i(t, \gamma, \sigma^2), Z_i(t), \mathcal{T}_i(t), J_i(t)\}/dt \\
= \ &\lambda_0(t)\exp\{\gamma S_i(t, \gamma, \sigma^2) - \gamma^2\sigma^2\theta_i(t)/2 + \eta^T Z_i(t)\}J_i(t) \\
= \ &\lambda_0(t)E_{0i}^*(t, \gamma, \eta, \sigma^2).
\end{aligned}
$$

This suggests that the conditional density of $dN(t) = \sum_{i=1}^{n} dN_i(t)$ given $S_i(t, \gamma, \sigma^2), Z_i(t), \mathcal{T}_i(t), J_i(t)$, $i = 1, \ldots, n$, is $\lambda_0(t)E_0^*(t, \gamma, \eta, \sigma^2)$, where $E_0^*(t, \gamma, \eta, \sigma^2) = \sum_{i=1}^{n} E_{0i}^*(t, \gamma, \eta, \sigma^2)$. Therefore, a natural estimator for $\lambda_0(t)dt$ is given by

$$
\hat{\lambda}_0(t)dt = dN(t)/E_0^*(t, \gamma, \eta, \sigma^2).
\tag{4.42}
$$

The parameters γ and η can be estimated by solving the following estimating equation which is an analogue to score equations of partial likelihood:

$$
\sum_{i=1}^{n} \int \{S_i(t, \gamma, \sigma^2), Z_i(t)\}^T \{dN_i(t) - E_{0i}^*(t, \gamma, \eta, \sigma^2)\lambda_0(t)dt\} = 0.
$$

Substitution of $\hat{\lambda}_0(t)$ in (4.42) for $\lambda_0(t)$ yields the conditional score estimating equation

$$
\sum_{i=1}^{n} \int [\{S_i(t, \gamma, \sigma^2), Z_i(t)\}^T - \frac{E_1^*(t, \gamma, \eta, \sigma^2)}{E_0^*(t, \gamma, \eta, \sigma^2)}]dN_i(t) = 0,
\tag{4.43}
$$

where

$$
E_1^*(t, \gamma, \eta, \sigma^2) = \sum_{i=1}^{n}\{S_i(t, \gamma, \sigma^2), Z_i(t)\}^T E_{0i}^*(t, \gamma, \eta, \sigma^2).
$$

When $\sigma^2 = 0$, the estimating equation (4.43) reduces to the partial likelihood score equations.

The above derivation assumes that σ^2 is known. However, in most cases σ^2 needs to be estimated from the data. A natural estimator of σ^2 is the pooled residual sum of squares from the least squares fit over subjects with at least three measurements:

$$\hat{\sigma}^2 = \frac{\sum_{i=1}^n I(n_i > 2)SS_i}{\sum_{i=1}^n I(n_i > 2)(n_i - 2)},$$

where SS_i is the residual sum of squares for the n_i measurements on subject i. It can be shown that $\hat{\sigma}^2$ is a consistent estimator of σ^2 under the assumption that the measurement errors $\epsilon_i(t_{ij})$ are i.i.d. $N(0, \sigma^2)$ random variables given random effects b_i, covariates $Z_i(t)$, the biomarker history prior to t_{ij}, and $J_i(t_{ij}) = 1$.

When $\hat{\sigma}^2$ is substituted for σ^2, solving the conditional score equation (4.43) yields $(\hat{\gamma}, \hat{\eta})$. It can be shown that $(\hat{\gamma}, \hat{\eta})$ are consistent and asymptotically normal. The usual sandwich approach may be used to derive their standard errors. Compared to likelihood approaches, the conditional score method is relatively easier to implement. Although the derivation is discussed in a simple situation where a linear time trend is assumed for each subject, the method can be extended to general polynomial and spline trajectories.

In a set of simulation studies, this method is compared to four other ways of fitting Cox models with time-dependent covariates. Altogether, the following five approaches are examined:

Method I: the "ideal" situation in which the true value of $Y_i(t)$ is known for all subjects at each observed event time;

Method CS: the conditional score approach discussed above;

Method RC: a regression calibration approach, using empirical Bayesian predictors of $Y_i(t)$ in the partial likelihood;

Method NR: "naive regression," using predicted values of $Y_i(t)$ by least squares fit for subjects with $n_i \geq 2$;

Method LV: at each observed event time carrying forward the last observation available for subjects at risk.

In Method RC, the missing biomarker measurements at each observed event time are imputed using predicted values from mixed effects models fitted to available data up to the 25th, 50th, 75th, and 100th percentiles of the observed event times. To avoid multiple roots that could exist for the conditional score equation, the starting value of γ in Method CS is set to the naive estimator when the observed biomarker is treated as a time-dependent covariate in the Cox model.

In each scenario, 500 data sets with $n = 200$ are generated from models (4.36), (4.39), and (4.40) with $\gamma = -1.0$ and $\eta = 0$. The biomarker is measured at 0, 2, 4, 8 weeks and every 8 weeks afterwards up to 80 weeks, with a missing

Table 4.8 *Simulation results for three random effect distributions.*

Method	Normal				Mixture				Skewed			
	Mean	SD	SE	Cov	Mean	SD	SE	Cov	Mean	SD	SE	Cov
I	−1.01	0.08	0.09	0.96	−1.02	0.10	0.12	0.95	−1.01	0.09	0.08	0.97
CS	−1.01	0.11	0.12	0.95	−1.03	0.24	0.25	0.95	−1.01	0.12	0.12	0.95
RC	−0.93	0.08	0.09	0.87	−0.88	0.07	0.09	0.75	−0.92	0.07	0.09	0.85
NR	−0.88	0.07	0.08	0.65	−0.83	0.06	0.08	0.44	−0.88	0.07	0.08	0.68
LV	−0.87	0.07	0.08	0.67	−0.87	0.06	0.08	0.65	−0.86	0.07	0.08	0.61

SD, Monte Carlo standard deviation; SE, average of estimated standard errors; Cov, Wald coverage probabilities. Methods: I, "ideal"; CS, conditional score; RC, regression calibration; NR, naive regression; LV, last value carried forward.

rate of 10% at each occasion except baseline. Event hazard is set to zero for $t < 16$ to exclude events that occur early after enrollment. C_i, the censoring time, is generated from an exponential distribution with mean equal to 110 weeks. All events and longitudinal measurements are censored at 80 weeks. The random effects b_i are generated from three distinct distributions, all of which have the same marginal mean $(4.173, -0.0103)^T$: (1) a normal distribution with $\text{cov}(b_i) = \Sigma$ and $\Sigma = (\Sigma_{11}, \Sigma_{12}, \Sigma_{22}) = (1.24, -0.0114, 0.003)$; (2) a bimodal mixture of normal variables with the same variances as in (1), but the covariance $\Sigma_{12} = 0.039$; (3) a bivariate skew-normal distribution with the same variance-covariance matrix as in (1) and coefficients of skewness -0.07 and 0.85 for b_{0i} and b_{1i}, respectively. The measurement error variance σ^2 is set to 0.30.

Table 4.8 presents results of the five approaches when the random effects b_i follow the above normal, mixture of normals, and skew-normal distributions. In all three scenarios, considerable bias is seen in the estimated γ for Methods RC, NR, and LV, which leads to marked lower than nominal-level confidence interval coverage probabilities, especially for Methods NR and LV. In contrast, the CS method produces results comparable to the "ideal" estimator for all three random effect distributions, with negligible bias and proper confidence interval coverage probabilities. Similar patterns are seen under other specifications of n and σ^2, and when σ^2 increases, Methods RC, NR, and LV tend to have larger bias in γ.

Song and Wang (2008)[200] developed an extended conditional score approach in which a time-varying regression coefficient was posited in the proportional hazards model to characterize non-constant CD4 effect on AIDS development. An estimator of the regression coefficient was obtained from the local conditional score estimating equation that involves local kernel smoothing.

Likelihood-Based Methods

Different from the conditional score method which relaxes parametric distributional assumptions for the random effects, likelihood-based approaches generally involve specification of the full distribution of $Y_i(t)$, including the distribution of random effects. For illustrative purposes, we look at an AIDS study in which the research interest is to characterize change in CD4 counts and its relationship with survival. The methods are discussed in Wulfsoh and Tsiatis (1997)[241] and Song, Davidian, and Tsiatis (2002)[199].

Consider a joint model consisting of (4.36), (4.37), and (4.39) as specified previously. The biomarker of interest is CD4 counts, whose measurement times are assumed to be non-informative; that is, occasions at which CD4 measurements are made do not predict the measurement itself or survival. Otherwise, their inter-dependence should be modeled as well to obtain unbiased estimates. This topic is discussed in Section 4.5. A growth curve model in the form of (4.37) can be used to specify the trajectory of CD4 counts. For simplicity, consider the mixed effects model

$$Y_i(t) = a_{0i} + a_{1i}t, \qquad (4.44)$$

where a_{0i} and a_{1i} are subject-specific intercept and slope, respectively. This model reflects the belief that the underlying trajectory of CD4 counts measured on each patient is linear in time. Due to skewness in the raw CD4 counts, $Y_i(t)$ is usually the log- or fourth-root transformed data. Fluctuations of CD4 counts commonly seen in the profile plot of observed data are a result of biological variation and measurement error. These features are considered "local," not predictive of survival under the perspective of (4.44). To fully specify the distribution of $Y_i(t)$, parametric distributional assumptions are needed for a_i. A natural choice is multivariate normal (or bivariate normal in the case of (4.44)). Write $a_i \sim N(\mu_a, \Sigma)$. As stated previously, the measurement errors in (4.36) are i.i.d. $N(0, \sigma^2)$, independent of a_i and covariates $Z_i(t)$ in (4.39).

Under the key assumption that the longitudinal biomarker and event times are independent given random effects a_i, the likelihood of joint model (4.36), (4.39), and (4.44) can be written out similar to (4.9). Parameter estimation and statistical inference may proceed using the methods discussed in Section 4.1.1. The EM algorithm is generally recommended for estimation of model parameters. As stated previously, under likelihood formulation, the baseline hazard $\lambda_0(t)$ in (4.39) is usually left unspecified. Denote $\Lambda_0(t) = \int_0^t \lambda_0(u)du$. The maximum likelihood estimator of Λ_0 is searched over a space consisting of all increasing functions in t with $\Lambda_0(0) = 0$. It can been shown that $\hat{\lambda}_0(t)$, the non-parametric maximum likelihood estimator of $\lambda_0(t)$, has a closed-form solution conditional on a_i, with point masses at non-censored event times and is zero everywhere else. Specifically, in the M-step, $\lambda_0(t)$ is updated by

$$\hat{\lambda}_0(t) = \sum_{i=1}^{n} \frac{\Delta_i I(\tilde{T}_i = t)}{\sum_{j=1}^{n} E_j[\exp\{\gamma(a_{0j} + a_{1j}t) + \eta^T Z_i(t)\}]I(\tilde{T}_j \geq t)},$$

where E_j stands for expectation with respect to a_i conditional on the observed longitudinal and survival data on subject j as well as most updated estimates of model parameters.

In the above discussions, the random effects a_i are assumed to follow a multivariate normal distribution, which may seem restrictive in some circumstances. Next, we introduce a likelihood approach that does not posit any specific parametric assumptions for a_i, but only requires the distribution of a_i be in a general class of smooth densities $\mathcal{H}$ that may be skewed, multi-modal, fat- or thin-tailed. In this approach, the normal density is included in $\mathcal{H}$ as a special case. For ease of discussion, express the random effects a_i as

$$a_i = f(\mu_a, Z_i) + R\xi_i,$$

where $f(\cdot)$ is a function of μ_a and time-fixed covariates Z_i, R is a lower triangular matrix, and the random variable ξ_i (vector valued) is independent of Z_i with density in $\mathcal{H}$. For example, if Z_i is a group indicator taking values in $\{0, 1\}$, a_i can be specified as

$$a_i = \mu_0(1 - Z_i) + \mu_1 Z_i + R\xi_i,$$

so that $\mu_a = (\mu_0^T, \mu_1^T)^T$. In the case of (4.44), R is a 2×2 lower triangular matrix with elements (R_{00}, R_{01}, R_{11}). The density of ξ_i can be approximated by

$$
\begin{aligned}
h_K(z) &= P_K^2(z)\varphi(z) \\
&= (\sum_{0 \le i_1 + i_2 \le K} c_{i_1 i_2} z_1^{i_1} z_2^{i_2})^2 \varphi(z),
\end{aligned}
\tag{4.45}
$$

where $K \ge 0$ is a given tuning parameter, $z = (z_1, z_2)^T$, $\varphi(z)$ is the bivariate standard normal density, and $P_K(z)$ is a Kth order polynomial with coefficients $c_{i_1 i_2}$, $i_1, i_2 = 0, 1, \ldots, K$ subject to $0 \le i_1 + i_2 \le K$. For example, when $K = 2$, $P_K(z) = c_{00} + c_{10} z_1 + c_{01} z_2 + c_{20} z_1^2 + c_{02} z_2^2 + c_{11} z_1 z_2$. The coefficients $c_{i_1 i_2}$ must be chosen such that $\int h_K(z) dz = 1$. When $K = 0$, ξ_i is standard normal and $a_i \sim N(\mu_0(1 - Z_i) + \mu_1 Z_i, RR^T)$. When $K > 0$, conditional on Z_i, the mean of a_i is $\mu_0(1 - Z_i) + \mu_1 Z_i + RE(\xi_i)$, and $var(a_i) = Rvar(\xi_i)R^T$, where $var(\cdot)$ stands for the variance-covariance matrix.

It has been shown that any density in $\mathcal{H}$ can be approximated and estimated by a density of form (4.45) with a fixed set of parameters given K; thus this approach is called "seminonparametric" (SNP) . In practice, K may be chosen by Akaike information criterion or other model selection measures. For fixed K, estimation can be done via the EM algorithm, but implementation is more complex compared to the model with normally distributed random effects a_i.

Example 4.12. *The ACTG study*

The SNP joint model is illustrated by the AIDS Clinical Trials Group (ACTG) Protocol 175 conducted on 2467 HIV-infected patients. It is a randomized trial to compare four therapies: zidovudine alone, zidovudine + didanosine, zidovudine + zalcitabine, or didanosine alone. This illustration focuses on comparisons of zidovudine alone versus the remaining three treatments (i.e., $Z_i \ne$

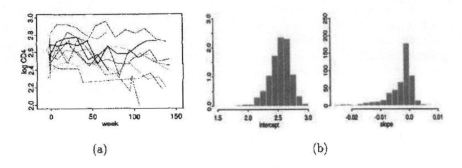

Figure 4.9 *(a) Trajectories of $\log_{10}$ CD4 for 10 randomly selected subjects. (b) Histograms of subject-specific intercept and slope estimates from simple least-squares fits.*

zidovudine) combined because previous analyses suggest that treatment with zidovudine alone is worse than the other three groups. The event of interest is progression to AIDS or death, and its relationship with CD4 counts, which were measured approximately every 12 weeks after randomization, is evaluated using the joint model (4.36), (4.39), and (4.44).

Prior to fitting the model, logarithm transformation was applied to CD4 counts to correct data skewness. Figure 4.9 (a) shows trajectories for 10 randomly selected patients. Subject-specific intercept and slope were empirically estimated by least-squares fit of a straight line to each individual. The histograms given in Figure 4.9 (b) indicate left skewness in estimated subject-specific slopes, which motivates the SNP approach discussed above to approximate the non-normal distribution.

Table 4.9 summarizes results of the SNP joint model applied to this data set with $K = 0, 2, 3, 4$. As a comparison, the estimates of γ and η from the conditional score approach (CS) are also presented. Similar results are obtained for γ, η, and random effects parameters across the SNP models with different K. There is a statistically significant negative association between CD4 counts and AIDS progression or death, i.e., an increase in CD4 counts correlates to a decreased risk of AIDS progression or death. The treatment effect, η, is close to zero, indicating that CD4 may be a surrogate marker because there was a significant marginal association between treatment and AIDS progression or death when CD4 was not included as a predictor. Similar conclusions are drawn from the CS method, but the standard errors inflate by a factor of 2 compared to their counterparts in the SNP models. Assuming the random effect distribution is correctly specified in the likelihood approach, the CS method, which is based on estimating equations, is less efficient.

Model fit is compared across K using AIC, BIC, and Hannan–Quinn criterion (HQ). All three measures suggest the best fit is achieved for a K of 3 or 4. Figure 4.10 (a) and (c) show the estimated density of a_i for each K, suggesting *that a_i has a bimodal distribution. However, this violation of the normality assumption does not seem to affect model estimation and statistical inference as shown in Table 4.9; similar results are obtained for $K = 0$ (the normal case) versus $K > 0$. This property of robust inference of normal distributions is interesting and deserves further investigation.* $\square$

Table 4.9 *Fit of the joint models to the ACTG 175 data using CS(conditional score) and SNP with K=0,2,3,4. Values in parentheses are estimated standard errors. The second entry of estimates of $E(a|Z_i = z)^T$ and its standard error are multiplied by 10^2 in each case. Estimates of $cov(a_{i0}, a_{i1})$ and $var(a_{i1})$ are multiplied by 10^3.*

	CS	K=0	K=2	K=3	K=4
γ	-2.214	-2.487	-2.487	-2.490	-2.498
	(0.207)	(0.091)	(0.092)	(0.092)	(0.092)
η	0.145	0.003	0.002	0.001	-0.007
	(0.264)	(0.132)	(0.132)	(0.132)	(0.131)
$E(a_i\|Z_i = 0)^T$	—	(2.523, -0.295)	(2.525, -0.223)	(2.525, -0.238)	(2.527, -0.234)
	—	(0.007, 0.017)	(0.007, 0.017)	(0.007, 0.014)	(0.008, 0.019)
$E(a_i\|Z_i = 1)^T$	—	(2.579, -0.207)	(2.572, -0.195)	(2.575, -0.214)	(2.578, -0.229)
	—	(0.004, 0.010)	(0.005, 0.014)	(0.004, 0.012)	(0.006, 0.017)
$var(a_{i0})$	—	0.024	0.024	0.023	0.023
$cov(a_{i0}, a_{i1})$	—	0.093	0.094	0.094	0.126
$var(a_{i1})$	—	0.014	0.013	0.013	0.012
Log likelihood	—	8558.465	9018.782	9310.945	9347.163
AIC	—	-0.412	-0.435	-0.449	-0.450
HQ	—	-0.397	-0.418	-0.432	-0.433
BIC	—	-0.364	-0.385	-0.397	-0.396

Bayesian Methods

Likelihood approaches for parameter estimation are computationally prohibitive when the dimension of latent variables b_i is high. Bayesian methods for joint modeling have developed as an appealing alternative to overcome computation difficulty involved in likelihood inference. Moreover, a complex form of biomarker trajectories, e.g., a stochastic process as in (4.38), can be easily introduced into Bayesian joint model framework. In addition, it is natural to incorporate prior information if available for parameters of interest.

Several Bayesian methods have been proposed to evaluate the association between time-dependent biomarkers and hazards of clinically meaningful events. The earliest work is dated back to Faucett and Thomas (1996)[65] who considered a model of the form (4.37) and (4.39). Faucett, Schenker, and Elashoff (1998)[64] posited a Markov model for an intermittently measured binary outcome which was used to predict survival times. Wang and Taylor (2001)[230] extended the model by incorporating a stochastic process into the biomaker trajectory. Brown and Ibrahim (2003)[28] used Dirichlet process priors for parameters at the longitudinal endpoint to relax their distributional assumptions.

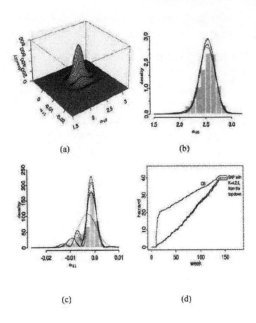

Figure 4.10 *Fit to the ACTG data using the SNP estimator for $Z_i = 0$. (a) Estimated density of a_i for $K = 4$. (b), (c) Estimated marginal densities for $K = 0$ (dotted line), $K = 2$ (solid line), $K = 3$ (dash-dotted line), $K = 4$ (long dashed line) with the histogram of ordinary least-squares estimates of the intercept and slope superimposed, respectively. (d) Estimated baseline cumulative hazard function.*

In this section we look at the approach developed by Wang and Taylor (2001)[230] with application to an AIDS study. An interesting feature of the model is that biological variation in CD4 counts is characterized by an integrated Ornstein–Uhlenbeck (IOU) process (i.e., $U_i(t)$ in (4.38)), which is believed to capture changes in CD4 that cannot be accounted for by a strong derivative tracking model (4.37). The IOU stochastic process assumes that $U_i(t)$ is Gaussian whose covariance function between times s and t is given by

$$cov(U_i(s), U_i(t)) = \frac{\tilde{\sigma}^2}{2\tilde{\alpha}^3}[2\tilde{\alpha}\min(s,t) + e^{-\tilde{\alpha}t} + e^{-\tilde{\alpha}s} - 1 - e^{-\tilde{\alpha}|t-s|}], \quad (4.46)$$

where the fixed but unknown parameters $\tilde{\alpha}$ and $\tilde{\sigma}^2$ characterize the degree of smoothness of the process. It is easy to show that $var(U_i(t)) = (\tilde{\sigma}^2/\tilde{\alpha}^3)[\tilde{\alpha}t + e^{-\tilde{\alpha}t} - 1]$. This model is motivated by the belief that CD4 does not have a constant change in unit time. The rate of change at time t for subject i is characterized by $\mathcal{B}_{t,i}$ as described in an Ornstein–Uhlenbeck process, i.e., an AR(1) process on the continuous time scale with correlation $e^{-\tilde{\alpha}\Delta t}$ between $\mathcal{B}_{t+\Delta t,i}$ and $\mathcal{B}_{t,i}$. When $\tilde{\alpha} \to 0$ while holding $\tilde{\sigma}^2/\tilde{\alpha}$ constant, it reduces to a random effects model with uncorrelated subject-specific intercept and linear time trend, whereas when $\tilde{\alpha} \to \infty$ and $\tilde{\sigma}/\tilde{\alpha}$ is constant, it corresponds to the scaled Brownian motion.

For ease of estimation, the time interval on which subject i is measured can be split into sufficiently small sub-intervals by K_i grid points, such that over the interval $(t^*_{i(k-1)}, t^*_{ik}]$ the IOU process $U_i(t)$ is approximated by a constant U_{ik}. Set $t^*_{i0} = 0$. Jointly the U_{ik}'s over the K_i intervals have a multivariate normal distribution with covariance matrix specified by (4.46). In the Bayesian framework, the baseline hazard $\lambda_0(t)$ in (4.39) is usually taken to be a piecewise constant function with pre-determined change points. Therefore, the joint model is fully parametric. The joint posterior distribution of model parameters is the product of likelihood and priors, and the posterior mean and standard deviation of each parameter can obtained by Markov chain Monte Carlo (MCMC) via the Gibbs sampler or Metropolis–Hastings sampling scheme.

Example 4.13. *The Multicenter AIDS Cohort Study*

The data set used in this analysis consisted of 115 homosexual men in the Los Angeles center of Multicenter AIDS Cohort Study. The trajectory of fourth-root power transformed CD4 measurements after 6 months of HIV infection was analyzed using model

$$Y_i(t) = b_i + \beta^{(1)}t + Z_i(t)^T\beta^{(2)} + U_i(t), \tag{4.47}$$

where $U_i(t)$ was an IOU process and $Z_i(t)$ consisted of two time-fixed factors: pcd4, the average of $CD4^{1/4}$ prior to HIV infection, and age at HIV infection; both were centered at their sample averages. The piecewise constant U_{ij} was 4 months apart. One to 32 (median = 11) CD4 measurements were available per patient. Fourth-root power transformation was applied to CD4 measurements to maintain homogeneity of within-subject variation. Impact of CD4 on the time to AIDS diagnosis was evaluated by (4.39). Among the 115 patients, 51 developed AIDS, and the median time to AIDS was 5.5 years. The baseline hazard in (4.39) was assumed to have eight constant pieces with 1.32 years apart.

A mixture of weakly informative and standard distributions were used as priors for model parameters, which, except $\tilde{\alpha}$, were not very sensitive to the choice of priors as suggested by additional analyses with other proper, improper, and "flat" priors. In model implementation, $(\tilde{\alpha}, \tilde{\sigma})$ was reparameterized as $(\tilde{\alpha}, \tilde{\theta})$ where $\tilde{\theta} = \tilde{\sigma}^2/\tilde{\alpha}^2$. Posterior mean and standard deviation of each parameter were estimated by MCMC sampling with 200,000 iterations after 200,000 burn-in. The joint model was compared to separate analysis of CD4 counts and time to AIDS. In particular, time to AIDS was analyzed by both Bayesian and partial likelihood methods, in which observed CD4 measurements were used to replace $Y_i(t)$ in (4.39).

In Table 4.10, results of joint model (column "Joint (MCMC)") indicate that $CD4^{1/4}$ declined post-HIV infection ($\beta^{(1)} = -0.191$, SD = 0.015) and lower CD4 measurements were associated with a increased risk of AIDS (γ

Table 4.10 *Joint and separate analyses of MACS data. Results are summarized by posterior means with standard deviations given in parentheses. (Note: μ_b and σ_b^2 are the mean and variance of b_i; σ_e^2 is the variance of measurement errors.)*

Parameter	IOU Joint(MCMC)	IOU Separate (MCMC)	IOU Separate (Partial likelihood)	Brownian motion Joint (MCMC)	Random effects Joint(MCMC)
$\beta^{(1)}$ (slope)	$-.191^a$ $(.015)^b$	$-.187$ $(.015)$		$-.191$ $(.015)$	$-.212$ $(.018)$
$\beta_1^{(2)}$ (pcd4)	.441 $(.074)$	.439 $(.073)$		.433 $(.074)$	.429 $(.080)$
$\beta_2^{(2)}$ (age)	$-.031$ $(.047)$	$-.031$ $(.047)$		$-.021$ $(.047)$	$-.078$ $(.051)$
μ_b (Intercept)	5.099 $(.036)$	5.096 $(.036)$		5.098 $(.036)$	5.141 $(.038)$
σ_b^2	.075 $(.018)$	.073 $(.018)$		.066 $(.018)$	.125 $(.021)$
σ_e^2	.049 $(.004)$	.048 $(.005)$		.039 $(.003)$	.087 $(.004)$
$\tilde{\theta}$	.127 $(.016)$	.122 $(.015)$		.116 $(.011)$	
$\tilde{\alpha}$	5.28 (4.80)	8.90 (11.11)		∞	0
median of $\tilde{\alpha}$ (95%probability limits)	3.68 $(1.70,13.14)$	4.32 $(1.78,33.41)$			
γ (cd4)	-1.486 $(.201)$	-1.322 $(.168)$	-1.383 $(.168)$	-1.485 $(.196)$	-1.409 $(.216)$
η_1 (pcd4)	.359 $(.348)$	.249 $(.332)$	.309 $(.339)$	.361 $(.347)$	.318 $(.341)$
η_2 (age)	$-.011$ $(.247)$	$-.016$ $(.231)$	$-.065$ $(.238)$	$-.008$ $(.248)$	$-.062$ $(.242)$
λ_{01}^c	.019 $(.014)$	.018 $(.013)$		.019 $(.014)$	.020 $(.014)$
λ_{02}^c	.025 $(.012)$	.026 $(.013)$		.025 $(.012)$	.026 $(.013)$
λ_{03}^c	.030 $(.012)$	.035 $(.014)$		.030 $(.012)$	.035 $(.014)$
λ_{04}^c	.052 $(.019)$	.063 $(.021)$		.051 $(.018)$	.058 $(.021)$
λ_{05}^c	.046 $(.019)$	.059 $(.023)$		.046 $(.019)$	.057 $(.022)$
λ_{06}^c	.052 $(.022)$	.086 $(.032)$		.053 $(.022)$	.060 $(.025)$
λ_{07}^c	.052 $(.029)$	.083 $(.043)$		.052 $(.029)$	.058 $(.033)$
λ_{08}^c	.034 $(.036)$	.045 $(.044)$		.034 $(.035)$	.040 $(.041)$

[a] Estimate = sample mean of the MCMC sequence.
[b] SD = sample standard deviation of the MCMC sequence.

$= -1.486$, $SD = 0.201$). *Surprisingly, age at HIV infection did not seem to affect CD4 postinfection or risk of AIDS. CD4 levels prior to HIV infection were positively correlated with CD4 measured postinfection ($\beta_1^{(2)} = 0.441$, SD $= 0.074$), but not related to AIDS development ($\eta_1 = 0.359$, SD $= 0.348$) after adjusting for post-infection CD4. Estimated λ_{0k}^c, $k = 1, \dots, 8$, indicate that the baseline hazard for AIDS increased over time. The separate analysis using MCMC method produced similar estimates for parameters in the*

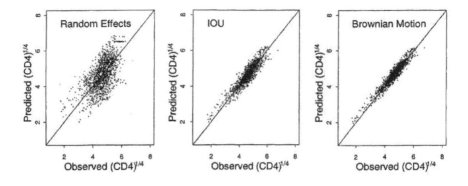

Figure 4.11 *Plot of observed CD4$^{1/4}$ data versus their predicted values.*

CD4 trajectory model, except that $\tilde{\alpha}$ is larger than its joint model counterpart. Both MCMC and partial likelihood methods in the separate analysis generated smaller estimates of γ, suggesting that noise caused by measurement error and "local" biological fluctuations in CD4 counts could attenuate the association with time to AIDS.

The posterior density of $\tilde{\alpha}$ estimated from the joint MCMC approach is right-skewed, with a posterior mean of 5.28. Moreover, results from the joint model assuming Brownian motion (which corresponds to $\tilde{\alpha} \to \infty$) are similar to those from the joint model with an IOU process, except that estimated σ_b^2, σ_e^2, and $\tilde{\theta}$ tended to be smaller. However, the opposite was observed for σ_b^2 and σ_e^2 when $\tilde{\alpha}$ was assumed to be zero (column "Random Effects Joint (MCMC)"). Figure 4.11 suggests that the joint model assuming Brownian motion provides the best fit since predicted values of CD4$^{1/4}$ are closest to the observed, suggesting that change in CD4 counts cannot be fully described by a pre-determined linear track model. □

Corrected Score Approach

Wang (2006)[228] proposed a corrected score approach to estimate time-dependent covariate effects in Cox proportional hazards models when there are measurement errors in the covariate. The method is based upon partial-score estimating equations. Similar to the conditional score approach, corrected score methods do not assume any parametric distributions for the random effects that describe covariate trajectories. Song and Wang (2008)[200] considered a varying-coefficient proportional hazards model and developed a local conditional score approach and a local corrected score approach, both allowing covariate effects to change over time. The estimators are shown to be consistent and asymptotically normal. Simulation studies indicate that the corrected score estimator performs less well than the conditional score counterpart in some circumstances, especially when measurement errors have a large variation.

4.4.2   Accelerated Failure Time Models with Intermittently Measured Time-Dependent Covariates

In some applications, the proportional hazards assumption in Cox models does not satisfactorily approximate the association between time-dependent covariates and risk of event times. Tseng, Hsieh, and Wang (2005)[212] proposed a joint analysis that considered an accelerated failure time (AFT) model when evaluating the effect of a time-dependent covariate. Let T be the event time, X time-fixed covariates, and ϵ the random error. In general, AFT models can be written as

$$logT = -X^T\gamma + e. \tag{4.48}$$

Let U be the survival time when $X = 0$, so $U = exp(e)$. Its associated survival function is denoted as S_0, which is also called baseline survival function. An extended AFT model for a time-dependent covariate $Y(t)$ is $U \sim S_0$, where

$$U = \Phi\{\bar{Y}(T); \gamma\} = \int_0^T exp\{\gamma Y(s)\}ds,$$

with $\bar{Y}(T)$ being the covariate history up to T. Thus, the survival function at time t is $S\{t|\bar{Y}(t)\} = S_0[\Phi\{\bar{Y}(t); \gamma\}]$ for a subject with covariate history $\bar{Y}(t)$. When S_0 is absolute continuous, the hazard function is

$$\begin{aligned} \lambda\{t|\bar{Y}(t)\} &= \lambda_0[\int_0^t exp\{\gamma Y(s)\}ds]exp\{\gamma Y(t)\} \\ &= \lambda_0[\Phi\{\bar{Y}(t); \gamma\}]\dot{\Phi}\{\bar{Y}(t); \gamma\}, \end{aligned} \tag{4.49}$$

where $\lambda_0(\cdot)$ is the hazard function for S_0 and $\dot{\Phi}$ is the first derivative of Φ. Equation (4.49) indicates that the event risk at time t depends on the whole covariate history up to t. This assumption is scientifically attractive, but requires that the entire covariate trajectory is observable and free of measurement error.

However, as pointed out previously, in reality the time-dependent covariate $Y(t)$ is intermittently measured and could be subject to measurement error and/or high biological variation, such as CD4 counts in AIDS studies. Similar to what has been discussed in Section 4.4.1, a linear mixed effects model can be used to describe the trajectory of $Y(t)$. For example,

$$Y(t) = \rho(t)^T b_i, \tag{4.50}$$

where $\rho(t) = \{\rho_1(t), \ldots, \rho_p(t)\}^T$ with each $\rho_j(t)$ being a known function and possibly time-varying, and the p-dimensional random effects $b_i \sim N_p(\mu, \Sigma)$. Choice of basis functions in $\rho(t)$ is driven by the feature of covariate time trend. For instance, $\rho(t) = \{\rho_1(t), \rho_2(t)\} = (logt, t - 1)$ is used to characterize the egg-laying trajectories of medfly data discussed in Example 4.14. Suppose the covariate is measured at t_{ij}, $j = 1, \ldots, n_i$, and we do not observe $Y_i(t_{ij})$; instead, measurements of W_{ij} are available such that

$$W_{ij} = Y_i(t_{ij}) + \epsilon_{ij}. \tag{4.51}$$

As usual the measurement errors ϵ_{ij} are i.i.d. $N(0, \sigma_\epsilon^2)$ and independent of b_i.

Incorporating (4.50) into the AFT hazard function (4.49) yields

$$\begin{aligned} \lambda\{t|\bar{Y}(t)\} &= \lambda_0\{\Phi(t; \gamma, b_i)\}\dot{\Phi}(t; \gamma, b_i) \\ &= \lambda_0[\int_0^t exp\{\gamma\rho(s)^T b_i\}ds]exp\{\gamma\rho(t)^T b_i\}. \end{aligned} \tag{4.52}$$

Under the assumption of noninformative censorship and measurement schedule, the likelihood function of the joint model (4.50)–(4.52) is expressed as

$$\begin{aligned} L(\theta) &= L(\gamma, \mu, \Sigma, \sigma_\epsilon^2, \lambda_0) \\ &= \prod_{i=1}^n [\int_{b_i} \{\prod_{j=1}^{n_i} f(W_{ij}|b_i, \sigma_\epsilon^2)\}f(\tilde{T}_i, \Delta_i|b_i, \lambda_0, \gamma) \\ &\quad \times f(b_i|\mu, \Sigma)db_i], \end{aligned} \tag{4.53}$$

where $f(W_{ij}|b_i, \sigma_\epsilon^2)$ and $f(b_i|\mu, \Sigma)$ are normal densities, $\tilde{T}_i = min(T_i, C_i)$ with C_i being the censoring time, and $\Delta_i = I(T_i \leq C_i)$. The density function of survival data is given by

$$\begin{aligned} f(\tilde{T}_i, \Delta_i|b_i, \lambda_0, \gamma) &= [\lambda_0\{\Phi(\tilde{T}_i; \gamma, b_i)\}\dot{\Phi}(\tilde{T}_i; \gamma, b_i)]^{\Delta_i} \\ &\quad \times exp\{-\int_0^{\Phi(\tilde{T}_i; \gamma, b_i)} \lambda_0(t)dt\}. \end{aligned} \tag{4.54}$$

Treating the random effects b_i as missing data, parameter estimation based on likelihood (4.53) can proceed using the EM algorithm. However, there is a computational challenge in the accelerated failure time model (4.54). Maximum likelihood estimation of $\lambda_0(\cdot)$ is not readily available because of unobserved baseline failure times $U_i = \Phi(\tilde{T}_i; \gamma, b_i)$ which involve random effects and unknown parameter γ. Thus, in a likelihood setting, it is difficult to employ the point-mass approach as for baseline functions in Cox models in which the masses are assigned at uncensored event times.

To make the EM algorithm feasible under the AFT setting, the baseline hazard $\lambda_0(\cdot)$ could be assumed constant between two adjacent estimated baseline failure times. Define $\hat{u}_k = \int_0^{\tilde{T}_k} exp\{\hat{\gamma}\rho(s)^T\hat{b}_k\}ds$, for $k = 1, \ldots, d$, with d being the number of distinct uncensored event times, $\hat{\gamma}$ the current estimate of γ in the EM algorithm, and $\hat{b}_k$ the current empirical Bayes estimate of b_k. Next, order $\hat{u}_k$ such that $0 = \hat{u}_{(0)} \leq \hat{u}_{(1)} \leq \ldots \leq \hat{u}_{(d)}$. The baseline hazard $\lambda_0(\cdot)$ is a step function taken to be constant between $\hat{u}_{(j-1)}$ and $\hat{u}_{(j)}$:

$$\lambda_0(u) = \sum_{j=1}^{d} C_j 1_{\{\hat{u}_{(j-1)} \leq u \leq \hat{u}_{(j)}\}}.$$

The cumulative baseline hazard Λ_0 is then given by

$$\int_0^{\Phi(\tilde{T}_i; \gamma, b_i)} \lambda_0(s)ds = \int_0^{u_i} \lambda_0(s)ds = \sum_{j=1}^{d} C_j(\hat{u}_{(j)} - \hat{u}_{(j-1)}) 1_{\{\hat{u}_{(j)} \leq u_i\}}.$$

In the EM algorithm, numerical integration or Monte Carlo integration can be used in the E-step to calculate expectation of functions of b_i that appear in the complete-date log-likelihood. Due to the fact that the baseline hazard function is nonparametric and the joint model (4.50)–(4.52) does not have a closed-form profile likelihood, standard errors of model parameters are estimated by the bootstrap technique.

Example 4.14. *The Medfly Fecundity Data*

The joint model (4.50)–(4.52) is applied to a data set of female Mediterranean fruit flies (medflies) on whom daily egg production was recorded until death. The relationship between egg production and medfly's life span is of particular interest. In a subset of most fertile medflies (N = 251), the data suggest that the proportional hazards assumption for survival times is questionable. Therefore, the AFT joint model outlined above is used here.

Figure 4.12 shows the number of eggs laid each day on four typical flies. The solid lines are fitted profile curves by the Gamma function, indicating that each fly had its own specific shape and scale parameters. Therefore, a suitable choice of the fecundity process could be:

$$Y_i^*(t) = t^{b_{1i}} exp(b_{2i}t), \tag{4.55}$$

where b_{1i} and b_{2i} are random effects. The observed number of eggs laid on day t is given by $W_i(t) = Y_i^*(t) + \epsilon_i(t)$. However, equation (4.55) is a nonlinear random effects model, which brings extra computational difficulty to the EM algorithm. To linearize it in terms of b_{1i} and b_{2i}, logarithmic transformation is applied to $W_i(t) + 1$ and $Y_i(t) + 1$. The value 1 is included here to avoid taking a logarithm of zeros. The final model proposed for fecundity is

$$log(W_{ij} + 1) = Y_{ij} + \epsilon_{ij},$$
$$Y_{ij} = b_{1i} log(t_{ij}) + b_{2i}(t - 1),$$

where the random effects $b_i = (b_{1i}, b_{2i})^T \sim N(\mu_{2 \times 1}, \Sigma_{2 \times 2})$, for $i = 1, \ldots, 251$,

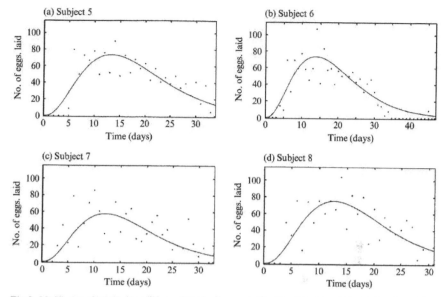

Fig. 2: Medfly data. Individual profiles are fitted by the gamma function. Number of eggs laid by (a) subject 5 is fitted by $t^{2 \cdot 710}e^{-0 \cdot 204t}$, (b) subject 6 by $t^{2 \cdot 652}e^{-0 \cdot 193t}$, (c) subject 7 by $t^{2 \cdot 725}e^{-0 \cdot 226t}$, and (d) subject 8 by $t^{2 \cdot 803}e^{-0 \cdot 221t}$. The shape and scale parameters are obtained by least squares.

Figure 4.12 *Medfly data. Individual profiles are fitted by the Gamma function.*

Table 4.11 *Medfly data. Parameter estimation based on (a) complete data and (b) incomplete data, together with results from 100 bootstrap samples under the joint accelerated failure time model.*

a. Complete data

	γ	μ_1	μ_2	σ_{11}	σ_{12}	σ_{22}	σ_ϵ^2
Fitted value	−0.4340	2.1227	−0.1442	0.3701	−0.0482	0.0068	0.8944
Boostrap mean	−0.4313	2.1112	−0.1429	0.3651	−0.0483	0.0066	0.8958
Boostrap SD	0.0115	0.0375	0.0051	0.0353	0.0002	0.0005	0.0223

b. Incomplete data

	γ	μ_1	μ_2	σ_{11}	σ_{12}	σ_{22}	σ_ϵ^2
Fitted value	−0.3890	2.2011	−0.1665	0.2833	−0.0382	0.0051	0.9775
Boostrap mean	−0.3526	2.1986	−0.1575	0.2862	−0.0398	0.0057	0.9712
Boostrap mean	0.0323	0.0461	0.0074	0.0351	0.0046	0.0006	0.0570

SD, standard deviation of 100 bootstrap estimates.

and ϵ_{ij} are i.i.d. $N(0, \sigma_\epsilon^2)$. The number of observation days per medfly ranged from 22 to 99, which are also the survival times since there were no censored events.

Table 4.11 part (a) summarizes parameter estimates in which the standard errors (bootstrap SD) were estimated using 100 bootstrap samples. The estimated β is −0.434 with a standard deviation of 0.012, indicating a significant posi-

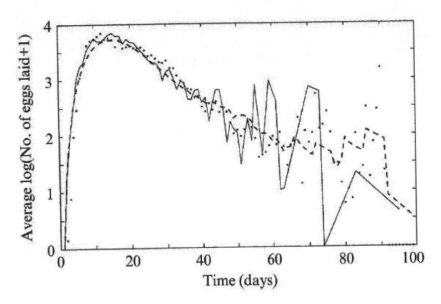

Figure 4.13 *Medfly data. Fitted cross-sectional mean curves for complete, dashed line, and incomplete, solid line, data. The dots represent the daily observed cross-sectional mean eggs of those medflies that are still alive.*

tive association between reproduction activity of the flies and their longevity. Note that the analytic sample of this illustration contains 251 medflies that laid more than 1150 eggs in their lifetime. In this group of highly fertile flies, reproduction reflects some sort of "good" genetic trait that may lead to a longer life span. The bootstrap procedure works reasonably well because its estimated parameters (the second row) are close to the model fitted values (the first row). In addition, the fitted cross-sectional mean curve fits well into the cross-sectional mean of log-transformed daily egg-laying data (Figure 4.13, dashed line). Substantial data variation is observed starting from day 60 because 90% of the flies had died by that time.

Model performance was also evaluated using artificially created incomplete data (from the same medfly cohort) with irregularly spaced, incomplete longitudinal measurements and censored survival times. First, a random number of egg-laying observations, ranging from 1 to 7, were drawn from each fly. The observation collected on the day of death was then added to the end of this sequence, resulting in 2 to 8 egg production measurements per fly. The egg-laying data generated this way were irregularly spaced with intermittent missing values. Second, the egg production data obtained in the first step were then censored (or truncated) by a random variable generated from an exponential distribution with mean 500. As a result, 20% of flies were censored and lost all longitudinal measurements after the censoring date. The joint model performs well on this artificially created incomplete data set since the results

(Table 4.11 part (b)) are close to those obtained from the complete data, and the fitted mean egg-laying trajectory shows a consistent trend with the observed data (Figure 4.13, solid line) up to day 50. Sparsity of the incomplete egg-laying data starting from day 50 results in an increased variability in the mean curve. □

4.5 Longitudinal Data with Informative Observation Times

This section introduces joint models that are applied to longitudinal studies with informative observation times, i.e., the observation time of longitudinal measurements is response dependent, or *informative*. One example is given by the bladder cancer study introduced in Chapter 1. Eighty-five patients with superficial bladder tumors were enrolled, and, at baseline, all tumors were removed transurethrally. The patients then received either placebo (N = 47) or thiotepa treatment (N = 38) and were followed to monitor tumor recurrence. One goal of the study was to compare recurrence rate between the two treatments. During follow-up, many patients had multiple recurrences and the recurrent tumors were removed at clinical visits. Some patients had significantly more clinical visits than others, with the smallest being 1 and the largest 38, suggesting that the observation time could be informative of recurrence rate.

In the literature of longitudinal data with informative observation times, most research focuses on conditional approaches, in which the observation time is characterized by event time models, such as Cox regression, and its association with the longitudinal endpoint is modeled via latent variables which are either discrete (latent class) or continuous (random effects). The former is called latent pattern mixture models, in which the data patterns are specified by latent classes that are shared by longitudinal measurements and observation times. In the second approach, the association between observation times and longitudinal data is characterized by random effects which are specified by either parametric or nonparametric distributions. The latent variable approaches and their extensions can be found in Huang, Wang, and Zhang (2006)[101], Sun, Sun, and Liu (2007)[205], Liu, Huang, and O'Quigley (2008)[154], Liang, Lu, and Ying (2009)[145], Sun et al. (2012)[206], and Han et al. (2014)[88]. Marginal approaches to tackle this problem include a class of inverse intensity-of-visit process-weighted estimators for marginal regression coefficients in the longitudinal model (Lin, Scharfstein, and Rosenheck, 2004[149]) and a marginal model for longitudinal data in which the counting process characterizing observation times was included as covariates (Sun et al., 2005[204]). In what follows, we look at the two conditional approaches, latent pattern mixture models and random effects models.

4.5.1   Latent Pattern Mixture Models

Different from pattern mixture models that stratify subjects based on observed missingness patterns, latent pattern mixture models classify subjects through joint patterns of longitudinal responses and observation times using latent classes and thus are more flexible in handling irregularly measured responses. Such models are also called latent class models. The number of latent classes K is prespecified, but model fit can be evaluated under various K. We illustrate latent pattern mixture models using the method developed by Lin, McCulloch, and Rosenheck (2004)[148] which assumes that there exists a small number of classes in the study population that affect trajectories and observation times of longitudinal responses.

Model Specification

The joint analysis is specified through three linked components: a class membership model, a longitudinal response model, and an intensity model for the visit process of longitudinal measurements. Assume there are K latent classes in the n study subjects. Let $c_i = (c_{i1}, \ldots, c_{iK})^T$ be a vector of binary indicators for subject i such that $c_{ik} = 1$ indicates that subject i is in class k and $c_{ik} = 0$ if not. The probability that subject i belongs to class k, π_{ik}, is modeled via a multinomial regression with logit link:

$$\pi_{ik} = P(c_{ik} = 1) = \frac{exp(v_i^T \eta_k)}{\sum_{j=1}^{K} exp(v_i^T \eta_j)}, \tag{4.56}$$

where $v_i = (v_{i1}, \ldots, v_{im})^T$ is a covariate vector and η_k the associated class-specific regression coefficients. Note that η_1 is set to zero for identifiability purposes.

The longitudinal measurements on subject i, $Y_i = (Y_{i1}, \ldots, Y_{in_i})$, are characterized by a linear mixed effects model with class-specific mean functions:

$$Y_i = X_i \beta + W_i(Mc_i) + Z_i b_i + \epsilon_i, \tag{4.57}$$

where X_i, W_i, and Z_i are observed covariate matrices which may contain time-varying covariates and/or deterministic functions of time, β a $p \times 1$ vector of fixed coefficients, and b_i a $r \times 1$ vector of random effects with a multivariate normal distribution that has mean zero and variance-covariance matrix D. The component $W_i(Mc_i)$ models class-specific mean functions. Specifically, the $q \times K$ matrix M, $M = (\mu_1, \ldots, \mu_K)$, contains class-specific parameters μ_i, such that when $c_{ik} = 1$, $Mc_i = \mu_i$. Note that vector μ_1 is taken to be zero to ensure model identifiability. The measurement error term $\epsilon_i = (\epsilon_{i1}, \ldots, \epsilon_{in_i})$, in which ϵ_{ij}, $j = 1, \ldots, n_i$, are i.i.d. $N(0, \sigma^2)$ and independent of b_i.

A multiplicative intensity model is used to characterize the visit process. Let

$N_i(t)$ be a counting process to denote the number of observations by time t, $0 \leq t \leq \tau$ with τ being the end of study follow-up, and $R_i(t)$ a left-continuous at-risk process with $R_i(t) = 1$ indicating that subject i has a non-zero probability of coming back for the next visit and 0 otherwise. The intensity of observing a measurement of Y at time t is specified as

$$\alpha_i(t|c_{ik} = 1, \omega_i) = \omega_i R_i(t) \lambda_k(t) exp(\gamma_k^T x_i(t)), \tag{4.58}$$

for all $0 \leq t \leq \tau$, where α_i is the intensity function of a visit process for subject i conditional on frailty ω_i, $\lambda_k(t)$ an unspecified baseline function for class k, $k = 1, \ldots, K$, and γ_k a vector of class-specific regression coefficients associated with covariates $x_i(t)$. The frailty ω_i captures dependence among observation times on the same subject and is assumed to follow a Gamma distribution with mean 1 and variance θ. Note that the choice of K is primarily driven by longitudinal trajectories of Y since the visit process model (4.58) itself is not identifiable.

Estimation and EM Algorithm

For a given number K of latent classes, the identifiability, existence, consistency, and weak convergence of maximum likelihood estimators for the above model can be established under regularity conditions. Similar to likelihood approaches to other joint models, maximum likelihood estimates can be obtained via the EM algorithm. The log-likelihood of observed data is given by

$$l(\Psi; Y, N, R, Q) = \sum_{i=1}^{n} log\{\sum_{k=1}^{K} f(c_{ik} = 1|Q_i; \Psi) f(Y_i|c_{ik} = 1, Q_i; \Psi)$$
$$f(N_i, R_i|c_{ik} = 1, Q_i; \Psi)\},$$

where $\Psi = (\eta_1, \ldots, \eta_K, \beta, M, D, \sigma, \gamma, \theta, \Lambda_1, \ldots, \Lambda_K)$ with Λ_k being the cumulative baseline intensity function for class k, and $Q_i = (v_i, X_i, Z_i, W_i, x_i)$ to denote all covariates.

The E-step of EM algorithm needs to calculate $\tilde{c}_{ik} = E(c_{ik}|Y_i, N_i, R_i, Q_i; \Psi)$, the condition expectation of class membership c_{ik} given observed data and current parameter estimates. Specifically, it is evaluated by

$$\tilde{c}_{ik} = E(c_{ik}|Y_i, N_i, R_i, Q_i; \Psi)$$
$$= \frac{\pi_{ik} f(Y_i|c_{ik} = 1, Q_i; \Psi) f(N_i, R_i|c_{ik} = 1, Q_i; \Psi)}{\sum_{j=1}^{K} \pi_{ij} f(Y_i|c_{ij} = 1, Q_i; \Psi) f(N_i, R_i|c_{ij} = 1, Q_i; \Psi)}.$$

The density $f(N_i, R_i|c_{ik} = 1, Q_i; \Psi)$ is obtained by integrating out frailty ω_i from $f(N_i, R_i|\omega_i, c_{ik} = 1, Q_i; \Psi)$.

In the M-step, closed-form solutions are available for β, M, D, σ, and $\lambda_k(t)$,

$k = 1, \ldots, K$, but not for η, γ, and θ, which can be updated using a Newton-type algorithm. Since the EM algorithm may converge to a stationary point, various starting values should be examined to ensure convergence to a global maximum. Standard errors are estimated by the inverse of empirical Fisher information of the log profile likelihood with nonparametric baseline intensity functions profiled out. Note that the model assumes conditional independence of longitudinal measurements and visit process given class membership. We refer the interested reader to Lin, McCulloch, and Rosenheck (2004)[148] for methods to check this assumption.

Example 4.15. *The HUD-VASH Homeless Study*

This is a randomized controlled trial comparing three housing interventions for homeless people with mental illness [148]. The study took place at four of 35 sites that implemented a joint program linking services of the US Department of Housing and Urban Development (HUD) and the US Department of Veterans Affairs (VA)—the HUD-VA Supported Housing (HUD-VASH) program. Four hundred and sixty (460) veterans, recruited between 1992 and 1995, were randomized to receive: (1) both vouchers for rent subsidies and intensive case management; (2) case management but no vouchers; or (3) standard VA care consisting of short-term broker case management. The randomization was weighted so that half of the veterans were assigned to case management alone to assure that the vouchers would be used in a timely fashion. Although the follow-up interviews were scheduled at every three months, study subjects often missed visits or showed up in between scheduled visits, so that the observations were irregularly spaced. The average number of visits (standard deviations) for groups (1)–(3) is 8.5 (3.2), 7.1 (3.6), and 6.0 (3.5). Out of the total 2837 visits made over 4 years, 686 visits were separated in time by more than 6 months, and 126 by more than one year.

The longitudinal outcome is log-transformed homeless days in the past 3 months. Covariates are selected from available variables that predict either longitudinal homeless measurements and/or visit process. Covariate vector v includes service received (service), receiving any social security or VA benefit (benefit), total number of visits made, baseline measure and changes of the last available measurements from baseline in days homeless in the past 90 days, income, and Lehman measure of quality of living (Qliv). Time trend is modeled by a restricted natural cubic spline with four knots evenly spaced at yearly intervals, which is included in X and W and is service-specific (coded as interaction between the service group and time trend vector). The final model considers a random intercept (in Z) since the class-specific time trends adequately characterize between individual heterogeneity in changes of homeless days over time. Covariates x in model (4.58) include income, Qliv, benefit, and service.

The choice of K depends on interpretability of the joint pattern of longitudinal data and visit process within each class. Also, the classification should provide adequate fit and not violate the conditional independence assumption.

The latent pattern mixture model specified previously was fit with K = 1–5 to the HUD-VASH data. For each K, the EM algorithm was run with different starting values, of which the one that produced the highest likelihood at convergence was chosen. Bayesian information criterion (BIC) was calculated for K = 1–5, and the smallest value was obtained when K = 4. Visual inspection of fitted homeless measurements and smoothed intensity of visit of the four-class model identifies distinct homeless profiles. The four classes are named as "Flat," "Low," "Down," and "Wavy." Estimated proportions of subjects in these classes are 0.18, 0.46, 0.21, and 0.15, respectively.

The results show that, being in the service group (1), higher baseline income and increased quality of living situation are significant predictors for being in the "Low" class. Those with more frequent visits are less likely to be in the "Low" class; this agrees with the consistently low visit intensity shown in Figure 4.14 (four-class visit intensity). A higher baseline homeless level is a significant predictor for being in class "Down" and "Wavy." The class "Down" has a significant decrease in homelessness over time. Table 4.12 shows the estimated fixed effects of longitudinal submodel (4.57). Better quality of living situation (Qliv) is significantly associated with a lower level of homelessness (the third row in the "Flat" column). Time trend in homelessness for service group (3) is not significant in the class "Flat." This is consistent with the flat profile trajectory in Figure 4.14. Changes in homelessness over time in classes "Low," "Down," and "Wavy" are statistically significant as assessed by a likelihood ratio test. The estimated γ indicates that better quality of living situation (Qliv) and being in service group (1) or (2) versus the standard care group (3) are associated with increased visit frequencies. □

Table 4.12 *Estimates of parameters in the model (4.57)–(4.58).*

		β(Flat)	M[a]			γ
	Intercept	2.16(0.26)	0.84(0.37)	2.08(0.44)	1.24(0.56)	
	Income[b]	0.01(0.03)				0.01(0.02)
	Qliv[b]	−0.35(0.02)				0.05(0.01)
	Benefit[b]	0.08(0.05)				−0.03(0.02)
Service(i)						0.20(0.02)
	First sp bs[c]	−0.00(0.21)	-0.42(0.34)	−1.80(0.49)	−0.77(0.40)	
	Second sp bs	−0.03(0.11)	0.13(0.21)	0.63(0.28)	0.44(0.21)	
	Third sp bs	0.02(0.45)	−0.18(0.85)	−1.74(1.06)	−1.22(0.79)	
Service(ii)						0.08(0.02)
	First sp bs	0.04(0.34)	-0.85(0.52)	−1.32(0.56)	0.11(0.61)	
	Second sp bs	-0.09(0.12)	0.75(0.25)	0.37(0.22)	−0.07(0.27)	
	Third sp bs	0.39(0.53)	−2.94(1.07)	−1.05(0.99)	0.54(1.04)	
Service(iii)						
	First sp bs	0.48(0.18)	-0.99(0.29)	−1.60(0.33)	−0.52(0.47)	
	Second sp bs	-0.33(0.10)	0.40(0.20)	0.61(0.18)	0.87(0.22)	
	Third sp bs	1.03(0.35)	−0.96(0.83)	−1.69(0.66)	−3.11(0.77)	

[a]Estimated coefficients for classes "Low," "Down," and "Wavy" are signed differences from those of class "Flat" which is the baseline class.
[b]Income is in thousands of dollars in the past three months, Qliv represents Lehman Measures of quality of living situation, Benefit is the indicator of whether social security or VA benefit was received during past three months.
[c]sp bs is shorthand for spline basis.

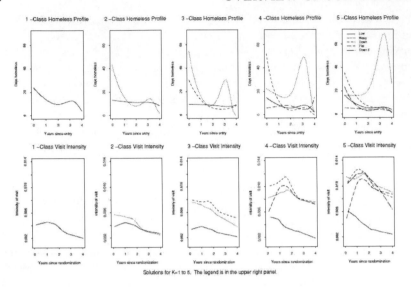

Figure 4.14 *Fitted homeless measurement and smoothed intensity of visit.*

4.5.2 Latent Random Effects Models

Latent random effects models assume that the visit process is linked to longitudinal measurements through continuous, but unobservable, random effects. Selection models using random effects to link together longitudinal and event time data discussed previously can be easily extended to this area of application. Different distributional assumptions, parametric or non-parametric, have been made for the random effects. Models with parametric assumptions for random effects are generally easy to interpret and computationally efficient, but may bear the criticism of non-robustness when the assumption is violated. As an illustration, we review the method proposed by Sun, Sun, and Liu (2007)[205], in which the distribution of random effects is left completely unspecified and parameter estimation is done via estimating equations.

Model and Inference

Similar to Section 4.5.1, denote $Y_i(t)$ the longitudinal response and $N_i(t)$ the counting process of observation number up to time t for subject i, $i = 1, \ldots, n$. Further, let Z_i be a vector of covariates and C_i the follow-up or censoring time. Note that $Y_i(t)$ is observed only at the time points where $N_i(t)$ jumps for $t \leq C_i$. Consider a situation where the counting process and censoring time are informative to the longitudinal response, in the sense that $Y_i(t)$, $N_i(t)$, and C_i depend on each other through a subject-specific latent variable (frailty) V_i. Note that the model does not require parametric assumptions for the distributions of V_i and C_i.

Assume V_i is non-negative with $E(V_i|Z_i) = 1$. Given Z_i and V_i, $Y_i(t)$ is posited to follow the marginal model

$$E\{Y_i(t)|Z_i, V_i\} = \mu_0(t) + Z_i^T\beta + V_i, \qquad (4.59)$$

where $\mu_0(t)$ is an unspecified smooth function of t and β a vector of regression parameters. Conditional on Z_i and V_i, assume $N_i(t)$ is a nonstationary Poisson process with intensity function

$$\lambda(t|Z_i, V_i) = V_i\lambda_0(t)exp(Z_i^T\gamma), \qquad (4.60)$$

where γ is a vector of regression parameters and $\lambda_0(t)$ a continuous baseline intensity function. The censoring time C_i is assumed to be dependent on Z_i and V_i in an arbitrary way, but conditional on Z_i and V_i, $Y_i(\cdot)$, $N_i(\cdot)$, and C_i are mutually independent. Note that the joint model (4.59)–(4.60) assumes a positive correlation between $Y_i(t)$ and $N_i(t)$, which is appropriate for the bladder cancer study discussed in Example 4.16.

Note that V_i, C_i, $\mu_0(t)$, and $\lambda_0(t)$ are nonparametric components of the joint model. An estimating equation approach is proposed with the focus towards estimating β, which is the main interest of statistical inference. For a random sample of n subjects, data on subject i include $Y_i(t_{i1}), \ldots, Y_i(t_{i,n_i})$, Z_i, V_i, C_i, and $N_i(t)$, $i = 1, \ldots, n$, $t \leq \tau$, where $t_{i1}, \ldots, t_{i,n_i}$ are the observation times with n_i being the total number of observations for subject i and τ is the longest follow-up time. If V_i and γ are known, β can be estimated using the estimating equation

$$U(\beta;\gamma) = n^{-1}\sum_{i=1}^{n}\int_0^\tau Q(t)\{Z_i - \tilde{Z}^\star(t;\gamma)\}\{Y_i(t) - V_i - Z_i^T\beta\}$$

$$\times R_i(t)dN_i(t) = 0, \qquad (4.61)$$

where $Q(t)$ is a weight function (possibly data-dependent), $R_i(t) = I(C_i \geq t)$, and

$$\tilde{Z}^\star(t;\gamma) = \frac{\sum_{i=1}^{n} R_i(t)V_i \exp(Z_i^T\gamma)Z_i}{\sum_{i=1}^{n} R_i(t)V_i \exp(Z_i^T\gamma)}.$$

The parameter β cannot be estimated directly using (4.61) since γ and V_i are unknown. To solve this issue, estimates of γ and V_i can be obtained first and then plugged into equation (4.61).

To this end, let $\Lambda_0(t) = \int_0^t \lambda_0(u)du$ and $F(t) = \Lambda_0(t)/\Lambda_0(\tau)$, for $0 \leq t \leq \tau$. The nonparametric maximum likelihood estimator of $F(t)$ is

$$\hat{F}(t) = \prod_{s_{(l)} > t}(1 - \frac{d_{(l)}}{N_{(l)}}),$$

where $\{s(l)\}$ denote the ordered and distinct observation times $\{T_{ij}, i = 1, \ldots, n, j = 1, \ldots, n_i\}$, $d_{(l)} = \sum_{i=1}^{n} dN_i(s_{(l)})$, the number of observations at $s_{(l)}$, and $N_{(l)} = \sum_{i=1}^{n} R_i(s_{(l)})N_i(s_{(l)})$, the total number of observations satisfying $T_{ij} \leq s_{(l)} \leq C_i$. Note that $\hat{F}(t)$ is taken to be 1 if there is no $s_{(l)} > t$. To estimate γ, let $X_i = (1, Z_i^T)^T$, $\alpha_1 = log\Lambda_0(\tau)$, and $\alpha = (\alpha_1, \gamma^T)^T$. Under model (4.60), the following estimation equation is used to estimate α:

$$n^{-1} \sum_{i=1}^{n} W_i X_i \{n_i \hat{F}^{-1}(C_i) - \exp(X_i^T \alpha)\} = 0, \qquad (4.62)$$

where W_i is a weight function that may depend on $(Z_i, \alpha, \hat{F})$. Let $\hat{\alpha} = (\hat{\alpha}_1, \hat{\gamma}^T)^T$ be the solution to equation (4.62), then V_i can be estimated by

$$\hat{V}_i = \frac{n_i}{\hat{\Lambda}_0(C_i) \exp(Z_i^T \hat{\gamma})},$$

based on the fact that $E(n_i | V_i, Z_i, C_i) = V_i \Lambda_0(C_i) \exp(Z_i^T \gamma)$, where $\hat{\Lambda}_0(t) = \hat{F}(t) \exp(\hat{\alpha}_1)$.

A closed-form solution for β exists by replacing V_i and γ with $\hat{V}_i$ and $\hat{\gamma}$, respectively, in equation (4.61). The estimate of β is given by

$$\begin{aligned} \hat{\beta} &= [\sum_{i=1}^{n} \int_0^{\tau} Q(t)\{Z_i - \bar{Z}(t; \hat{\gamma})\}Z_i^T R_i(t) dN_i(t)]^{-1} \\ &\quad \times \sum_{i=1}^{n} \int_0^{\tau} Q(t)\{Z_i - \bar{Z}(t; \hat{\gamma})\}\{Y_i(t) - \hat{V}_i\} R_i(t) dN_i(t), \end{aligned}$$

where

$$\bar{Z}(t; \gamma) = \frac{\sum_{i=1}^{n} R_i(t)\hat{V}_i \exp(Z_i^T \gamma) Z_i}{\sum_{i=1}^{n} R_i(t)\hat{V}_i \exp(Z_i^T \gamma)}.$$

There are graphical and numerical procedures available for model checking. We refer the reader to Sun, Sun, and Liu (2007)[205] for more information.

Example 4.16. *The Bladder Cancer Data*

The proposed methodology is illustrated by the longitudinal bladder cancer data introduced in Chapter 1. The observed data for each patient include clinical visits (or observation times, in months) and number of bladder tumors that patients developed between clinical visits. Note that recurrent tumors were removed at clinical visits. The analysis focuses on effects of thiotepa treatment and baseline number of tumors on recurrence of bladder cancer [205].

The outcome $Y_i(t)$ is the natural logarithm of the number of observed tumors (plus 1 to avoid 0) at time t, $i = 1, \ldots, 85$. Covariate Z_{i1} is equal to 0 for the placebo group and 1 for the thiotepa group, and Z_{i2} is the baseline number of *tumors. Setting the weight functions W_i and $Q(t)$ to 1, the proposed method produced estimates $\hat{\beta}_1 = -0.47$ (SE = 0.11) and $\hat{\beta}_2 = 0.01$ (SE = 0.03). After setting $Q(t) = n^{-1} \sum_{i=1}^{n} R_i(t)$, the estimates became $\hat{\beta}_1 = -0.52$ (SE = 0.11) and $\hat{\beta}_2 = 0.01$ (SE = 0.03). The results indicate that the thiotepa group had a reduced recurrence rate of bladder tumor, but the baseline number of tumors did not appear to be related to tumor recurrence. Goodness-of-fit tests indicate that model (4.59) provides reasonable overall fit to the observed data.*

The data were also analyzed by the joint model (4.59)–(4.60) but assuming $V_i = 1$ for all i, that is, the response and observation processes were assumed to be independent given covariates. This model yielded estimates $\hat{\beta}_1 = -0.19$ (SE = 0.05) and $\hat{\beta}_2 = 0.05$ (SE = 0.01); that is, the baseline number of tumors was a significant predictor in this analysis and there was a substantial reduction in the effect size of treatment. One explanation of the discrepancy between the two sets of results is that the observation process carried information about tumor recurrence, and the independence assumption could falsely transform the association between $Y(t)$ and $N(t)$ and between $Y(t)$ and the covariates.
□

4.6   Dynamic Prediction in Joint Models

When the research interest is to predict clinical meaningful events such as death or disease recurrence using a biomarker, the joint model that characterizes the association between these two endpoints can be used as a prognostic tool for dynamic prediction of the event probability. Such prediction is conditional on the biomarker trajectory for a specific patient up to a given time point at which the event is yet to occur. This will facilitate better understanding of disease progression to make early decisions. Dynamic prediction has been proposed in joint models that use latent classes to characterize the association between the biomarker and event times (Garre et al., 2008[75]; Proust-Lima and Taylor, 2009[179]) and that use shared random effects (Rizopoulos, 2011[184]). It has also been discussed in a joint analysis that considers cure-rate survival data (Yu, Taylor, and Sandler, 2008[245]). Below we describe in detail the dynamic prognostic tool developed by Proust–Lima and Taylor (2009)[179]. The idea is applicable to joint analysis using either latent classes or random effects to model the relationship of longitudinal data and event times.

Denote Y the longitudinally measured biomarker and T the event time. For a new patient i who has not experienced the event at time s, the objective is to predict the probability that $T_i \leq s + t$ conditional on covariates X_i and $Y_i^{(s)} = \{Y_i(t_{ij}), t_{ij} \leq s\}$ that contains all biomarker measurements up to time s. This probability is defined as

$$P_i(s+t, s; \theta) \quad = \quad P(T_i \leq s + t | T_i > s, Y_i^{(s)}, X_i; \theta), \qquad (4.63)$$

where θ denotes the joint model parameters. If the association between Y and T is modeled by random effects b_i and assumed that $Y \perp T$ conditional on b_i, the probability (4.63) can be calculated as

$$
\begin{aligned}
&P(T_i \leq s + t | T_i > s, Y_i^{(s)}, X_i; \theta) \\
&= \int P(T_i \leq s + t | T_i > s, Y_i^{(s)}, X_i, b_i; \theta) f(b_i | T_i > s, Y_i^{(s)}, X_i; \theta) db_i \\
&= \int P(T_i \leq s + t | T_i > s, X_i, b_i; \theta) f(b_i | T_i > s, Y_i^{(s)}, X_i; \theta) db_i \\
&= \int \frac{S(s | X_i, b_i; \theta) - S(s + t | X_i, b_i; \theta)}{S(s | X_i, b_i; \theta)} f(b_i | T_i > s, Y_i^{(s)}, X_i; \theta) db_i,
\end{aligned}
$$

$$(4.64)$$

where $S(\cdot | X_i, b_i; \theta)$ is the survival function of T_i conditional on the covariates and random effects. The posterior density of b_i, $f(b_i | T_i > s, Y_i^{(s)}, X_i; \theta)$, is given by

$$
\begin{aligned}
f(b_i | T_i > s, Y_i^{(s)}, X_i; \theta) &= \frac{f(T_i > s, Y_i^{(s)}, X_i, b_i; \theta)}{f(T_i > s, Y_i^{(s)}, X_i; \theta)} \\
&= \frac{S(s | X_i, b_i; \theta) f(Y_i^{(s)} | X_i, b_i; \theta) f(b_i | X_i; \theta)}{\int S(s | X_i, b_i; \theta) f(Y_i^{(s)} | X_i, b_i; \theta) f(b_i | X_i; \theta) db_i}.
\end{aligned}
$$

In latent-class joint models, the dependence between Y_i and T_i is captured by latent class $c_i \in \{1, \ldots, G\}$. The probability for the event to occur between s and $s + t$ is given by

$$
\begin{aligned}
&P(T_i \leq s + t | T_i > s, Y_i^{(s)}, X_i; \theta) \\
&= \sum_{g=1}^{G} P(T_i \leq s + t | T_i > s, Y_i^{(s)}, X_i, c_i = g; \theta) P(c_i = g | T_i > s, Y_i^{(s)}, X_i; \theta) \\
&= \sum_{g=1}^{G} P(T_i \leq s + t | T_i > s, X_i, c_i = g; \theta) P(c_i = g | T_i > s, Y_i^{(s)}, X_i; \theta) \\
&= \sum_{g=1}^{G} \frac{S(s | X_i, c_i = g; \theta) - S(s + t | X_i, c_i = g; \theta)}{S(s | X_i, c_i = g; \theta)} \\
&\quad P(c_i = g | T_i > s, Y_i^{(s)}, X_i; \theta).
\end{aligned}
$$

$$(4.65)$$

The posterior class membership $P(c_i = g | T_i > s, Y_i^{(s)}, X_i; \theta)$ is

$$
\begin{aligned}
&P(c_i = g | T_i > s, Y_i^{(s)}, X_i; \theta) \\
&= \frac{\pi_{ig} S(s | X_i, c_i = g; \theta) f(Y_i^{(s)} | X_i, c_i = g; \theta)}{\sum_{k=1}^{G} \pi_{ik} S(s | X_i, c_i = k; \theta) f(Y_i^{(s)} | X_i, c_i = k; \theta)},
\end{aligned}
$$

where $\pi_{ig} = P(c_i = g | X_i; \theta)$.

The dynamic prediction $P_i(s + t, s; \theta)$ based on either (4.64) or (4.65) is calculated using $\hat{\theta}$ that is estimated by the joint model. The standard error of predicted probability can be approximated by the Bayesian posterior distribution of $P_i(s + t, s; \hat{\theta})$. That is, a sample of $\theta^{(d)}$, $d = 1, \ldots, D$, is drawn from the approximated asymptotic distribution of θ, $N(\hat{\theta}, \hat{V}(\hat{\theta}))$. The standard error is then estimated by $\sqrt{D^{-1} \sum_{d=1}^{D} (P_i(s + t, s; \theta^{(d)}) - P_i(s + t, s; \hat{\theta}))^2}$. This method does not need extra efforts for estimation or bootstrap resampling, but requires the model to be fully parametric. For semiparametric joint models, the bootstrap resampling scheme would be an option.

A measure of predictive accuracy of this prognostic tool has been developed through contrasting the predicted values with observed data. The error of prediction (EP) is defined as $err_{L,Y}(t) = E_{Y,T}[L(\eta(t) - \hat{S}(t|Y))]$, where $L(\cdot)$ is a loss function, $\eta(t)$ a binary variable to indicate the event status at time t, and $\hat{S}(t|Y)$ the predicted survival probability. Note that the expectation $E_{Y,T}$ is with respect to the joint distribution of T and Y. Denote the dynamic prediction rule $\hat{S}(s + t | T_i > s, Y_i^{(s)}) = S(s + t | T_i > s, Y_i^{(s)}, X_i; \hat{\theta})$. An estimator of absolute EP proposed by Henderson et al. (2002)[93] looks at the prediction error at time $s + t$ conditional on the data history up to time s:

$$\hat{err}_{Y,s}(s + t)$$

$$= \frac{1}{N_s} \sum_{i=1}^{N_s} I(T_i > s + t) |1 - \hat{S}(s + t | T_i > s, Y_i^{(s)})|$$

$$+ \Delta_i I(T_i \leq s + t) |0 - \hat{S}(s + t | T_i > s, Y_i^{(s)})| + (1 - \Delta_i) I(T_i \leq s + t)$$

$$\times [|1 - \hat{S}(s + t | T_i > s, Y_i^{(s)})| \frac{\hat{S}(s + t | T_i > s, Y_i^{(s)})}{\hat{S}(T_i | T_i > s, Y_i^{(s)})}$$

$$+ |0 - \hat{S}(s + t | T_i > s, Y_i^{(s)})| (1 - \frac{\hat{S}(s + t | T_i > s, Y_i^{(s)})}{\hat{S}(T_i | T_i > s, Y_i^{(s)})})],$$

where N_s is the number of patients in the risk set at time s and Δ_i the event indicator such that $\Delta_i = 1$ if T_i is not censored for patient i.

Let τ denote the end of follow-up for a given study. The predictive accuracy measure varies with t, so a summary score that integrates $\hat{err}_{Y,s}(s + t)$ over the interval $[s, \tau]$ is useful:

$$D_Y(s, \tau) = \frac{\sum_{k=1}^{n_\tau^{(s)}} d_k^{(s)} (\hat{G}(s) / \hat{G}(t_k)) \hat{err}_{Y,s}(t_k)}{\sum_{k=1}^{n_\tau^{(s)}} d_k^{(s)} (\hat{G}(s) / \hat{G}(t_k))},$$

where $d_k^{(s)}$ is the number of events at time t_k among patients in the risk set for s, and $\hat{G}(s)$ and $\hat{G}(t_k)$ the Kaplan–Meier estimates of censoring distribution at times s and t_k. This summary measure can be interpreted as a weighted average of absolute EP in which the weights compensate for reduction in observed events towards the end of follow-up due to censoring.

Note that these prediction measures are attached to a specific biomarker Y. When comparing two models that contain the marker information (Y_1) and (Y_1, Y_2), the added predictive accuracy by including Y_2 can be calculated as $1 - D_{Y_1,Y_2}(s, \tau)/D_{Y_1}(s, \tau)$, an analogue of the coefficient of determination R^2 in linear regression.

Chapter 5

Joint Models for Longitudinal Data and Continuous Event Times from Competing Risks

The joint models discussed in Chapter 4 assume that the event times are generated from a single failure type, so are not applicable to studies with multiple failure types or competing risks. Use the scleroderma lung study we have introduced in Chapter 1 as an example. Recall that the primary outcome is forced vital capacity (FVC, as % predicted) determined at 3-month intervals from baseline. The event of interest is time to treatment failure or death. The longitudinal and survival data are possibly correlated, which could introduce nonignorable non-response missing values for %FVC after event times. Dependence between the two endpoints is further complicated by informatively censored events due to dropout during follow-up. Note that both death and dropout could lead to nonignorable missing data in %FVC measurements. The joint model developed by Elashoff, Li, and Li (2008)[61], as described in Section 5.1, has the capacity to handle multiple failure types, or competing risks at the survival endpoint. Parameter estimation and inference of this model via a Bayesian approach can be found in Hu, Li, and Li (2009)[100]. A robust joint model with t-distributed random errors (Li, Elashoff, and Li, 2009[137]) is described in Section 5.2. Li et al. (2010)[138] developed a model for studies with ordinal longitudinal measurements and competing risks, and this approach is discussed in Section 5.3. Section 5.4 extends joint models with competing risks to the scenario where there exists heterogeneity in the random effects covariance across study subjects (Huang, Li, and Elashoff, 2010[103]; Huang, Li, Elashoff, and Pan, 2011[104])

5.1   Joint Analysis of Longitudinal Data and Competing Risks

5.1.1   The Model Formulation

Let $Y_i(t)$ be the longitudinal outcome measured at time t for subject i, where $i = 1, 2, \ldots, n$, and n is the total number of subjects in study. Each subject may experience one of g distinct failure types or could be right censored during follow-up. Let $C_i = (T_i, D_i)$ denote the competing risks data on subject i, where T_i is the failure/censoring time, and D_i takes a value in $\{0, 1, \ldots, g\}$, with $D_i = 0$ indicating a censored event and $D_i = k$ showing that subject i fails from the kth type of failure, $k = 1, \ldots, g$. The censoring mechanism is assumed to be independent of event times.

Model settings for the longitudinal data are similar to those introduced in Chapter 4; that is, a linear mixed effects model (or a generalized linear mixed effects model in the case of discrete outcomes) can be used to specify the trajectory of $Y_i(t)$. To accommodate multiple failure types, a cause-specific hazards model is incorporated into the joint analysis framework to characterize the distribution of competing risks. Specifically, the model has the following two linked components:

$$Y_i(t) = X_i^{(1)}(t)^T \beta + \tilde{X}_i^{(1)}(t)^T b_i + \epsilon_i(t), \tag{5.1}$$

and

$$
\begin{aligned}
& \lambda_k(t; X_i^{(2)}(t), u_i, \gamma_k, \nu_k) \\
= & \lim_{h \to 0} \frac{P\{t \le T_i < t + h, D_i = k | T_i \ge t, X_i^{(2)}(t), u_i\}}{h} \\
= & \lambda_{0k}(t) exp\{X_i^{(2)}(t)^T \gamma_k + \nu_k u_i\},
\end{aligned} \tag{5.2}
$$

where in (5.1), $X_i^{(1)}(t)$ and $\tilde{X}_i^{(1)}(t)$ are vectors of covariates associated with $Y_i(t)$ and are allowed to change over time, β represents the fixed effects of $X_i^{(1)}(t)$, b_i is a vector of random effects for $\tilde{X}_i^{(1)}(t)$, and $\epsilon_i(t)$ is measurement error and assumed to be $\sim N(0, \sigma^2)$ for all $t \ge 0$. Further assume that b_i is independent of $\epsilon_i(t)$ and $\epsilon_i(t_1)$ is independent of $\epsilon_i(t_2)$ for any $t_1 \ne t_2$. In (5.2), $\lambda_k(t; X_i^{(2)}(t), u_i, \gamma_k, \nu_k)$ is the instantaneous rate for failures of type k at time t in the presence of all other failure types, conditional on covariates $X_i^{(2)}(t)$ and frailty u_i. In particular, $\lambda_{0k}(t)$ is a completely unspecified baseline hazard function for risk k, $k = 1, \ldots, g$. Denote $\gamma = (\gamma_1^T, \ldots, \gamma_g^T)^T$ and $\nu = (\nu_1, \ldots, \nu_g)^T$, in which ν_1 is set to 1 to ensure identifiability.

Assume that the longitudinal and survival data are independent conditional on the random effects and covariates. Thus, the association between $Y_i(t)$ and C_i is induced by the joint distribution of b_i and u_i. As one example, u_i can be a linear function of b_i, or, in a more general setting as discussed in Section

4.1.1, b_i and u_i are posited to have a joint multivariate normal distribution:

$$a_i = \begin{pmatrix} b_i \\ u_i \end{pmatrix} \sim N \left(\begin{pmatrix} 0 \\ 0 \end{pmatrix}, \begin{pmatrix} \Sigma_{bb} & \Sigma_{bu}^T \\ \Sigma_{bu} & \sigma_u^2 \end{pmatrix} \right).$$

There are three sources of data correlation in the above joint model. At the longitudinal endpoint, the correlation among repeated measurements within subject is modeled by the random effects b_i; at the survival endpoint, the association between multiple failure types is characterized by the frailty u_i; and lastly, the linkage between longitudinal and survival data is modeled through the joint distribution of b_i and u_i. When $\Sigma_{bu} = 0$, the joint model reduces to separate analyses of $Y_i(t)$ and C_i.

For competing risks failure data, it is well known that the distribution of $C = (T, D)$ is the identified minimum and that the joint distribution of underlying failure times is not identifiable from the observed data (Tsiatis, 1975[213]). Under the assumptions that the variation of observed regressors $\{exp(X_2(t)^T \gamma_d), d = 1, \dots, g\}$ contains a non-empty open set in R^g and that the expectation of frailty $exp(u)$ is finite, Abbring and Van den Berg (2003)[6] have shown that parameters of a mixed proportional cause-specific hazards model are identifiable for competing risks data. The arguments can be applied here to establish identifiability of model parameters in equation (5.2).

5.1.2 Estimation and Inference Procedure

Suppose the longitudinal outcome $Y_i(t)$ is observed at time points t_{ij} for $j = 1, \dots, n_i$, and denote $Y_i = (Y_{i1}, \dots, Y_{in_i})$. Note that $(t_{i1}, \dots, t_{in_i})$ can be different among subjects, due to different event times and the fact that some patients may miss one or more visits. The joint distribution of (Y, C) is completely determined by $f(Y|a, \Psi)$, $f(C|a, \Psi)$, and $f(a|\Psi)$, where $\Psi = (\beta, \sigma^2, \gamma, \nu, \Sigma, \lambda_{01}(t), \dots, \lambda_{0g}(t))$ containing all unknown parameters from (5.2)–(5.2). The likelihood function for Ψ, conditional on the observed data (Y_i, C_i), $i = 1, \dots, n$, and covariates, is thus

$$
\begin{aligned}
L(\Psi; Y, C) \quad &\propto \quad \prod_{i=1}^n f(Y_i, C_i | \Psi) \\
&= \quad \prod_{i=1}^n \int_a f(Y_i | C_i, a, \Psi) f(C_i | a, \Psi) f(a|\Psi) da \\
&= \quad \prod_{i=1}^n \int_a f(Y_i | a, \Psi) f(C_i | a, \Psi) f(a|\Psi) da \\
&= \quad \prod_{i=1}^n \int_a [\prod_{j=1}^{n_i} \frac{1}{\sqrt{2\pi\sigma^2}} exp\{-\frac{1}{2\sigma^2}(Y_{ij} - X_i^{(1)}(t_{ij})^T \beta -
\end{aligned}
$$

$$\tilde{X}_i^{(1)}(t_{ij})^T b)^2\}]\{\prod_{k=1}^{g} \lambda_k(T_i; X_i^{(2)}(T_i), u, \gamma_k, \nu_k)^{I(D_i=k)}\}$$

$$\times exp[-\int_0^{T_i}\{\sum_{k=1}^{g}\lambda_k(t; X_i^{(2)}(t), u, \gamma_k, \nu_k)\}dt]$$

$$\times \frac{1}{\sqrt{2\pi|\Sigma|}}exp(-\frac{1}{2}a^T\Sigma^{-1}a)da,$$

where the second equality follows from the assumption that Y and C are independent, conditional on the covariates and random effects.

Similar to likelihood approaches for selection models discussed in Chapter 4, the maximum likelihood estimate of Ψ can be obtained through the EM algorithm. Given a_i, the complete-data likelihood is

$$L(\Psi; Y, C, a)$$

$$\propto \prod_{i=1}^{n}[\prod_{j=1}^{n_i}\frac{1}{\sqrt{2\pi\sigma^2}}exp\{-\frac{1}{2\sigma^2}(Y_{ij} - X_i^{(1)}(t_{ij})^T\beta -$$

$$\tilde{X}_i^{(1)}(t_{ij})^T b_i)^2\}]\{\prod_{k=1}^{g}\lambda_k(T_i; X_i^{(2)}(T_i), u_i, \gamma_k, \nu_k)^{I(D_i=k)}\}$$

$$\times exp[-\int_0^{T_i}\{\sum_{k=1}^{g}\lambda_k(t; X_i^{(2)}(t), u_i, \gamma_k, \nu_k)\}dt]$$

$$\times \frac{1}{\sqrt{2\pi|\Sigma|}}exp(-\frac{1}{2}a_i^T\Sigma^{-1}a_i).$$

The E-step of the $(m+1)th$ iteration calculates expected values of all functions of a_i, say $h(a_i)$, that appear in $l(\Psi; a) = logL(\Psi; Y, C, a)$ conditional on (Y, C) and $\Psi^{(m)}$. The expectation can be derived by

$$E_{a_i|Y_i,C_i,\Psi^{(m)}}(h(a_i)) = \int h(a_i)f(a_i|Y_i, C_i, \Psi^{(m)})da_i.$$

In the M-step, Ψ is updated using

$$\Psi^{(m+1)} = argmax_\Psi\ Q(\Psi; \Psi^{(m)}),$$

where $Q(\Psi; \Psi^{(m)}) = E_{a|Y,C,\Psi^{(m)}}(l(\Psi; a))$. Integrals in the E-step can be evaluated using the methods discussed in Chapter 4. Parameters β, σ^2, Σ, and cumulative baseline hazard functions $\Lambda_{0k}(t)$, $k = 1, \ldots, g$, can be updated with closed forms; in particular, the nonparametric maximum likelihood estimate of $\Lambda_{0k}(t)$ is a step function with jumps at observed event times due to risk k. No closed-form solutions exist for γ and ν, which can be updated using a one-step Newton–Raphson algorithm in each M-step. Iterations stop when the convergence criterion is met. Standard errors can be estimated using methods outlined in Section 4.1.

Example 5.1. *The Scleroderma Lung Study*

Recall that the study was designed to evaluate the effectiveness and safety of oral cyclophosphamide (CYC) versus placebo in patients with active, symptomatic scleroderma-related interstitial lung disease. The primary outcome %FVC was repeatedly measured every 3 months up to 2 years postrandomization. Missing data in %FVC following death, dropout, and treatment failure could be missing not at random (MNAR) (or nonignorable) if these events were correlated with the unobserved %FVC values. In this analysis the CYC treatment effect on %FVC is evaluated using a joint model that consists of two sub-models (5.1) and (5.2). Results from this joint model that assume nonignorable missing data are compared to the analysis via a linear mixed effects model (Table 2.1) to examine the impact of assumed missing data assumptions on parameter estimation and inference. The longitudinal model for %FVC takes the form of equation (2.9); that is, the fixed effects include treatment (CYC), baseline %FVC (FVC_0), baseline fibrosis score (FIB_0), interaction between treatment and fibrosis, and a linear spline with one knot at 18 months. Three-dimensional random effects b_i are used to capture between-individual heterogeneity at baseline and in the two spline slopes. The study has 16 treatment failures or deaths and 47 dropouts, in which 37 of the dropouts are considered informative as they were related to patient disease condition. In this illustration, treatment failure or death is treated as risk 1 and informative dropout is treated as risk 2. Jointly, the frailty u_i and random effects b_i are assumed to follow a multivariate normal distribution.

The results of this joint model are presented in Table 5.1. It can be seen that the time trend estimates (β_5–β_8) are similar to their counterparts in the linear mixed effects model (Table 2.1). However, the joint analysis identifies a significant interaction effect between CYC and baseline fibrosis score ($\beta_4 = 1.699$, $p = 0.0040$), and the overall treatment effect becomes statistically significant ($H_0 : \beta_3 = \beta_4 = \beta_7 = \beta_8 = 0$, $p = 0.0090$). This difference in estimated β comparing the separate and joint analyses can be explained by the marginally significant negative association between u_i and b_{2i} ($Cov(u_i, b_{2i}) = -0.282$, $p = 0.0636$). For a positive ν, a more rapid decline in %FVC before 18 months is associated with a higher risk of treatment failure, death, or informative dropout. As a result, ignoring the missing data caused by these events potentially biases the results. In the competing risks sub-model (5.2), none of the covariates are associated with treatment failure, death, or informative dropout, so the results are not included here. □

5.2   A Robust Model with t-Distributed Random Errors

The joint model discussed in Section 5.1 assumes a normal random error in the longitudinal sub-model, which is not robust against outlying observations. Figure 5.1 shows individual profiles of %FVC in the scleroderma lung study,

Table 5.1 *Join analysis of %FVC, treatment failure or death (risk 1), and dropout (risk 2) in the Scleroderma Lung Study*

Parameter	Estimate	SE	p-value
Fixed Effects			
$Intercept$	66.668	1.106	<0.0001
FVC_0	0.943	0.029	<0.0001
FIB_0	−1.413	0.435	0.0012
CYC_i	−1.403	1.456	0.3352
$CYC_i \times FIB_0$	1.699	0.591	0.0040
t_{ij}	−0.090	0.082	0.2724
$(t_{ij} - 18)_+$	−0.067	0.253	0.7911
$CYC_i \times t_{ij}$	0.211	0.110	0.0551
$CYC_i \times (t_{ij} - 18)_+$	−0.460	0.310	0.1378
$H_0 : \beta_3 = \beta_4 = \beta_7 = \beta_8 = 0$			0.0090
Random Effects			
$Var(b_{1i})$	18.243		
$Var(b_{2i})$	0.339		
$Var(b_{3i})$	0.496		
$Cov(b_{1i}, b_{2i})$	−0.974	0.720	0.1761
$Cov(b_{1i}, b_{3i})$	0.166	1.325	0.9003
$Cov(b_{2i}, b_{3i})$	−0.273	0.131	0.0372
$Var(u_i)$	1.082		
$Cov(u_i, b_{1i})$	−2.307	1.470	0.1166
$Cov(u_i, b_{2i})$	−0.282	0.152	0.0636
$Cov(u_i, b_{3i})$	0.119	0.312	0.7029
ν_2	0.220	0.285	0.4402
σ^2	15.192		

which suggest existence of outlying observations in both treatment groups. Li, Elashoff, and Li (2009)[137] proposed a joint analysis that is robust against outlying longitudinal measurements by assuming a t-distributed measurement error in the longitudinal model. With a t-distributed random error, the model implicitly reweights observations according to their residuals when estimating fixed effects at the longitudinal endpoint, which effectively downweights outlying observations.

This robust joint model has the same functional form as (5.1)–(5.2), but the measurement errors $\epsilon_i(t)$ are assumed to have a $t(0, \sigma^2, \kappa)$ distribution, where κ denotes degrees of freedom. The normal distribution is included as a special

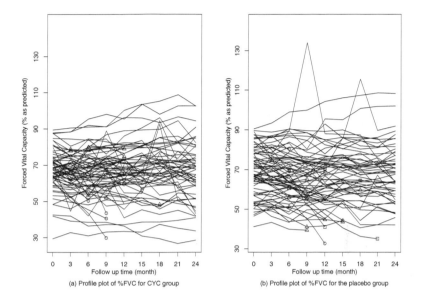

Figure 5.1 *Profile plot of %FVC in the scleroderma lung study*

case when $\kappa \to \infty$. This parameter can be prespecified or estimated from the data, but usually a value of 3 or 4 works well in practice.

Parameter estimation may proceed via the EM algorithm as outlined previously. However, under the t-distribution, estimation of β and σ^2 is intractable. This problem can be solved by making use of the fact that the t-distribution $t(0, \sigma^2, \kappa)$ is a mixture of ϵ_{ij} with a scaling variate w_{ij}, such that

$$\epsilon_{ij}|w_{ij} \sim N(0, \sigma^2/w_{ij}), \ w_{ij} \sim \chi_\kappa^2/\kappa,$$

where w_{ij} are i.i.d. *Gamma* random variables. Given w_{ij} and $a_i = (b_i, u_i)$, the complete-data likelihood function can be written as

$$
\begin{aligned}
& L(\Psi; Y, C, a, w) \\
& \propto \prod_{i=1}^{n}\{\prod_{j=1}^{n_i} \frac{\sqrt{w_{ij}}}{\sqrt{2\pi\sigma^2}} exp[-\frac{w_{ij}}{2\sigma^2}(Y_{ij} - X_i^{(1)}(t_{ij})^T\beta - \tilde{X}_i^{(1)}(t_{ij})^T b_i)^2] \\
& \quad [\prod_{k=1}^{g} \lambda_k(T_i; X_i^{(2)}(T_i), u_i, \gamma_k, \nu_k)^{I(D_i=k)}] \\
& \quad \times exp\{-\int_0^{T_i} [\sum_{k=1}^{g} \lambda_k(t; X_i^{(2)}(t), u_i, \gamma_k, \nu_k)]dt\}
\end{aligned}
$$

$$\times \prod_{j=1}^{n_i} \frac{(\frac{\kappa}{2})^{\frac{\kappa}{2}} w_{ij}^{\frac{\kappa}{2}-1}}{\Gamma(\frac{\kappa}{2})} \exp(-\frac{\kappa}{2}w_{ij}) \times \frac{1}{\sqrt{2\pi|\Sigma|}} exp(-\frac{1}{2}a_i^T \Sigma^{-1} a_i)\}.$$

It is fairly straightforward to derive an EM algorithm from the above likelihood. Because the expectation of the complete-data log-likelihood $l_i(\Psi; w_{ij}, a_i)$ for subject i is linear (up to a certain constant) in w_{ij}, we can write $E_{w_{ij},a_i|Y_i,C_i,\Psi^{(m)}}[l_i(\Psi; w_{ij}, a_i)] = E_{a_i|Y_i,C_i,\Psi^{(m)}}[l_i(\Psi; a_i, E_{w_{ij}|a_i,Y_i,C_i,\Psi^{(m)}}(w_{ij}))]$, where m indicates that the parameter estimates are from the mth iteration of the EM algorithm. In the E-step of the $(m+1)$th iteration, for subject i, calculate

$$E_{w_{ij}|a_i,Y_i,C_i,\Psi^{(m)}}(w_{ij}) = \frac{\kappa+1}{\kappa+\delta_{ij}^2(\Psi^{(m)})},$$

where

$$\delta_{ij}^2(\Psi^{(m)}) = (Y_{ij} - X_i^{(1)}(t_{ij})^T\beta - \tilde{X}_i^{(1)}(t_{ij})^T b_i))^2/\sigma^2.$$

Use E to stand for $E_{a_i|Y_i,C_i,\Psi^{(m)}}$. In the M-step, the regression coefficients β is updated by

$$\beta^{(m+1)} = [\sum_{i=1}^{n}\sum_{j=1}^{n_i} E(w_{ij})X_i^{(1)}(t_{ij})X_i^{(1)}(t_{ij})^T]^{-1}\{\sum_{i=1}^{n}\sum_{j=1}^{n_i}[E(w_{ij})Y_{ij} - E(w_{ij}\tilde{X}_i^{(1)}(t_{ij})^T b_i)]X_i^{(1)}(t_{ij})\}.$$

As can be seen from the above, w_{ij} implicitly weights the observations according to their residuals. Since outliers with large residuals have smaller weights, robust estimates are then obtained by downweighting the outliers.

The t-distribution in this robust joint model can be replaced by other distributions such as a slash distribution and contaminated normal distribution [126], but as Rosa, Padovani, and Gianola (2003)[190] pointed out, the t process is often a good alternative to a Gaussian distribution and is the most commonly used thick-tailed distribution to achieve robust inference.

Example 5.2. *The Scleroderma Lung Study (continued)*

The robust joint model with t-distributed random errors is applied to the Scleroderma Lung Study. There are a few outliers in %FVC, especially in the placebo group as indicated in Figure 5.1. In particular, the %FVC measurement for one patient in the placebo group is above 130 at month 9, which is most likely a measurement error as suggested by the study investigator. The joint analysis presented in Table 5.1 has eliminated this data point. In this illustration, the robust joint model is fit to all data points without eliminating any outliers and the results are shown in Table 5.2. Compared to the joint model with normally distributed random errors, the robust joint model tends to produce more efficient parameter estimates (i.e., smaller standard errors) *by reducing the impact of noises from outliers in %FVC. The results indicate that there was a significant increase in %FVC in the CYC group before 18 months compared to placebo, but after 18 months, %FVC in the CYC group dropped quickly. The Wald test of overall treatment effect on %FVC after adjusting for treatment failure, death, and dropout has a p-value of 0.0002. Interestingly, different from the results in Table 5.1, the frailty u_i is significantly associated with the random intercept b_{1i} and random slope b_{3i} in 18–24 months.* □

Table 5.2 *Application of the robust joint model to %FVC, treatment failure or death (risk 1), and dropout (risk 2) in the Scleroderma Lung Study*

Parameter	Estimate	SE	p-value
Fixed Effects			
$Intercept$	66.891	0.583	<0.0001
FVC_0	0.956	0.034	<0.0001
FIB_0	−2.315	0.519	<0.0001
CYC_i	0.780	0.887	0.3792
$CYC_i \times FIB_0$	3.268	0.786	<0.0001
t_{ij}	−0.091	0.052	0.0801
$(t_{ij} - 18)_+$	0.106	0.158	0.5023
$CYC_i \times t_{ij}$	0.140	0.071	0.0486
$CYC_i \times (t_{ij} - 18)_+$	−0.431	0.207	0.0373
$H_0 : \beta_3 = \beta_4 = \beta_7 = \beta_8 = 0$			0.0002
Random Effects			
$Var(b_{1i})$	12.480		
$Var(b_{2i})$	0.186		
$Var(b_{3i})$	0.196		
$Cov(b_{1i}, b_{2i})$	0.055	0.224	0.8060
$Cov(b_{1i}, b_{3i})$	−1.473	0.414	0.0004
$Cov(b_{2i}, b_{3i})$	−0.068	0.054	0.2079
$Var(u_i)$	3.714		
$Cov(u_i, b_{1i})$	−6.773	1.578	<0.0001
$Cov(u_i, b_{2i})$	−0.113	0.159	0.4773
$Cov(u_i, b_{3i})$	0.825	0.265	0.0019
ν_2	0.046	0.156	0.7681
σ^2	5.039		

5.3 Ordinal Longitudinal Outcomes with Missing Data Due to Multiple Failure Types

Longitudinal ordinal outcomes are commonly encountered in biomedical studies. For example, in the NINDS rt-PA stroke trial introduced in Chapter 1, patients treated with rt-PA were compared with those given a placebo on their Modified Rankin Scale, an ordinal measure of disability with categories ranging from no symptoms, no significant disability, and up to severe disability. During the follow-up, patients could dropout, die, or experience treatment failure. A treatment failure occurred if the patient remained in severe disability in two consecutive visits after treatment initiation. Both death and dropout could result in nonignorable missing values in the Modified Rankin Scale measurements because these events are highly related to patient disease condition. One objective of the study is to estimate treatment effects on both longitudinal measurements of Modified Rankin Scale and risk of treatment failure or death, but due to the previously stated reasons, the analysis needs to adjust for possible nonignorable missing data in Modified Rankin Scale and informative censoring of treatment failure or death caused by dropout. In this regard, dropout can be treated as a competing risk at the survival endpoint.

5.3.1 Model Formulation

Li et al. (2010)[138] developed a general joint model that can be applied to studies similar to the rt-PA stroke trial; that is, the longitudinal outcome is ordinal in nature and the survival endpoint contains competing risks failure time data. The formulation of this joint model is similar to (5.1)–(5.2), but with (5.1) replaced by a partial proportional odds model. Specifically, the partial proportional odds model is built upon popular proportional odds models for ordinal data, but allows non-proportional odds for a subset of covariates. It is a more flexible approach and also serves as a useful tool to test the proportional odds assumption.

Suppose there are n subjects in the study, each with n_i observations, $i = 1, \ldots, n$. Let Y_{ij} denote the jth response for subject i, where Y_{ij} takes values in $\{1, \ldots, K\}$ for some integer $K \geq 2$. The partial proportional odds model for Y_{ij} is specified as:

$$
\begin{aligned}
& P(Y_{ij} \leq k | X_{ij}, \tilde{X}_{ij}, W_{ij}, \theta, \beta, \alpha, b_i) \\
= {} & \frac{1}{1 + \exp(-\theta_k - X_{ij}^T \beta - \tilde{X}_{ij}^T \alpha_k - W_{ij}^T b_i)}
\end{aligned}
\tag{5.3}
$$

for $k = 1, \ldots, K-1$, where β is a vector of fixed effects associated with covariates X_{ij} that satisfy the proportional odds assumption, $\tilde{X}_{ij}$ contains a subset of covariates in X_{ij} for which the proportional odds assumption is violated,

α_k, $k = 1, \ldots, K - 1$, are regression coefficients with α_1 set to zero, so that $\tilde{X}_{ij}^T \alpha_k$ is the increment in the logit of probability $Y_{ij} \leq k$ comparing to that of $Y_{ij} \leq 1$, and b_i is a vector of random effects associated with covariates W_{ij} and assumed to be $N(0, \Sigma_b)$. The level-specific intercepts $\theta_1, \ldots, \theta_{K-1}$ satisfy $\theta_1 < \theta_2 < \ldots < \theta_{K-1}$. Denote $\theta = (\theta_1, \ldots, \theta_{K-1})^T$ and $\alpha = (\alpha_2^T, \ldots, \alpha_{K-1}^T)^T$.

The association between Y and C can be similarly modeled by the joint multivariate normal distribution of random effects u_i and b_i:

$$a_i = \begin{pmatrix} b_i \\ u_i \end{pmatrix} \sim N_{(q+1)} \left(\begin{pmatrix} 0 \\ 0 \end{pmatrix}, \begin{pmatrix} \Sigma_b & \Sigma_{bu}^T \\ \Sigma_{bu} & \sigma_u^2 \end{pmatrix} \right).$$

Again, ν_1 in (5.2) is set to 1 to ensure identifiability. A test of the null hypothesis $H_0 : \Sigma_{bu} = 0$ can be used to evaluate the association between Y and C, and it can be seen that the joint model reduces to separate analysis of the two endpoints if $\Sigma_{bu} = 0$. However, keep in mind that the conclusion from this test is valid based on the assumption that the joint model is correctly specified. Li et al. (2012)[139] developed an extended model to allow multiple longitudinal ordinal outcomes, in which the association between multiple longitudinal outcomes was modeled by shared random effects and the normality assumption for these random effects was relaxed by employing the nonparametric approach outlined in Section 4.1.1.

5.3.2 Estimation and Inference

For the notation, write $Y_i = (Y_{i1}, \ldots, Y_{in_i})^T$ and $C_i = (T_i, D_i)$. It is assumed that Y_i and C_i are independent conditional on the covariates and random effects, $i = 1, \ldots, n$. Let $\pi_{ij}(k)$ denote the probability that $Y_{ij} \leq k$ given the covariates and random effects, and thus $\pi_{ij}(K) = 1$ and $\pi_{ij}(0) = 0$ for all i and j. The observed-data likelihood function for $\Psi = (\theta, \beta, \alpha, \gamma, \nu, \Sigma, \lambda_{01}(t), \ldots, \lambda_{0g}(t))$ is therefore

$$\begin{aligned} L(\Psi; Y, C) &\propto \prod_{i=1}^{n} f(Y_i, C_i | \Psi) \\ &= \prod_{i=1}^{n} \int_a f(Y_i | C_i, a, \Psi) f(C_i | a, \Psi) f(a | \Psi) da \\ &= \prod_{i=1}^{n} \int_a f(Y_i | a, \Psi) f(C_i | a, \Psi) f(a | \Psi) da \\ &= \prod_{i=1}^{n} \int_a [\prod_{j=1}^{n_i} \prod_{k=1}^{K} \{\pi_{ij}(k) - \pi_{ij}(k-1)\}^{I(Y_{ij}=k)}] \\ &\qquad \{\prod_{d=1}^{g} \lambda_d(T_i; Z_i(T_i), u, \gamma_d, \nu_d)^{I(D_i=d)}\} \end{aligned}$$

$$\times exp[-\int_0^{T_i} \{\sum_{d=1}^{g} \lambda_d(t; Z_i(t), u, \gamma_k, \nu_k)\}dt]$$

$$\times \frac{1}{\sqrt{(2\pi)^{q+1}|\Sigma|}} exp(-\frac{1}{2}a^T \Sigma^{-1} a)da. \qquad (5.4)$$

The maximum likelihood estimate of Ψ can be obtained via the EM algorithm and statistical inference may proceed in a similar fashion as outlined in Section 5.1.

Example 5.3. *The rt-PA Stroke Trial*

A detailed description of the study is given in Chapter 1. The longitudinal outcome, modified Rankin scale, was recorded at baseline, 7–10 days, 3 months, 6 months, and 12 months poststroke onset. This variable is in an ordinal scale and defined as: 1 = no symptoms or no significant disability despite symptoms, 2 = slight disability, 3 = moderate disability or moderately severe disability, 4 = severe disability or dead. Note that some categories are collapsed to reduce the number of distinct levels, so this definition is slightly different from what is used in medical practice. Although death is one outcome at the longitudinal endpoint, in this analysis it is separated from modified Rankin scale and considered at the survival endpoint. There are around 30% missing data at 12 months due to death or dropout. The missing data could be non-ignorable since patients with a higher Rankin score were more likely to die or drop out of the study because of low treatment efficacy.

Baseline characteristics and changes in modified Rankin scale over time are summarized in Table 5.3. Subtypes of acute stroke (small vessel occlusive disease, large vessel atherosclerosis or cardioembolic stroke, and unknown reasons) and baseline modified Rankin scale were evenly distributed between treatment groups. Although for both groups the modified Rankin scale decreased over time, it was significantly lower in the rt-PA group after treatment initiation. The Kendall's tau correlation among modified Rankin scale measurements at 7–10 days, 3, 6, and 12 months is in between 0.65–0.87 (p-values < 0.0001).

The following covariates were considered when modeling modified Rankin scale poststroke onset: treatment group (rt-PA versus placebo), disease subtypes, modified Rankin scale prior to stroke onset, and time since randomization. An unstructured time trend was modeled using three dummy variables, time3, time6, time12, to represent 3, 6, and 12 months, respectively, so that the measure at 7–10 days served as reference. The likelihood ratio test was carried out to assess the proportional odds assumption and identified a violation by disease subtype. A random intercept was assumed in (5.3) since the time trend did not vary substantially between patients. Two competing risks, dropout (risk 1) and death or treatment failure (risk 2), were considered at the survival

Table 5.3 *Baseline characteristics of study subjects and changes in modified Rankin scale over time (mean (standard deviation) and frequency (%) are shown for modified Rankin scale and disease subtypes, respectively).*

	rt-PA group (n = 292)	Placebo group (n = 295)	p-value
Disease subtypes			
small vessel	31 (10.62%)	30 (10.17%)	
large vessel or cardioembolic stroke	181 (61.99%)	184 (62.37%)	0.9804
Modified Rankin scale			
modified Rankin scale prior onset	0.27 (0.73)	0.29 (0.80)	0.9872
modified Rankin scale (7-10 days)	2.55 (1.20)	2.90 (1.07)	0.0006
modified Rankin scale (3 months)	1.97 (1.07)	2.27 (1.02)	0.0017
modified Rankin scale (6 months)	1.91 (1.04)	2.18 (1.04)	0.0060
modified Rankin scale (12 months)	1.81 (1.01)	2.13 (1.04)	0.0015

endpoint. Death and treatment failure were combined into one risk because both events are strong evidence of low treatment efficacy.

Table 5.4 shows the joint model results. Note that at the longitudinal endpoint, $\tilde{X}$ = (small vessel, large vessel, or cardioembolic stroke)^T. The modified Rankin scale decreased over time. Conditional on the covariates and random effects, the cumulative odds ratio for $Y \leq k$, $k = 1, 2, 3$, is $exp(2.12) = 8.33$ at 3 months compared to 7–10 days post stroke onset (the 95% confidence interval is (5.63, 12.33)), and is 9.68 and 11.59 at 6 months and 12 months, with the 95% confidence intervals (6.54, 14.32) and (7.53, 17.84), respectively. Disease subtype violates the proportional odds assumption. Compared to patients with unknown reasons, the small vessel patients had lower Rankin scales, and the conditional cumulative odds ratio is $exp(3.49)$ for $Y \leq 1$, and is $exp(3.77)$ and $exp(6.14)$ for $Y \leq 2$ and $Y \leq 3$. Note that the estimate 6.14 may not be reliable due to the fact that there are only 4 patients with $Y = 4$ in the stratum small vessel. Patients with large vessel or cardioembolic stroke tended to have higher Rankin scales than patients with unknown reasons. The treatment is not as effective for large vessel or cardioembolic stroke patients as for patients with unknown reasons, and there is no significant difference in the treatment effects between patients with small vessel and those with unknown reasons. For patients with unknown reasons, the conditional cumulative odds ratio is $exp(1.48) = 4.39$ for $Y \leq 1$, 2, and 3 comparing rt-PA to placebo (the 95% confidence interval (2.30, 8.39)). In contrast, among large vessel or cardioembolic stroke patients, the conditional cumulative odds ratio is $exp(1.48-2.27) = 0.45$ (the 95% confidence interval (0.09, 2.31)).

No significant treatment effects are observed at the survival endpoint for dropout or death/treatment failure. There appears to be a higher risk of death or treatment failure among patients with high baseline Rankin scales. On the

Table 5.4 *Joint analysis for the rt-PA stroke study*

	Estimate (SE)
Longitudinal outcome	
proportional odds (PO)	
(cumulative prob of $Y \leq k$, $k = 1, 2, 3$)	
group	$1.48^\dagger$ (0.33)
modified Rankin scale prior onset	$-1.67^\dagger$ (0.27)
time3	$2.12^\dagger$ (0.20)
time6	$2.27^\dagger$ (0.20)
time12	$2.45^\dagger$ (0.22)
small vessel $\times$ group	-0.74 (1.26)
large vessel or cardioembolic stroke $\times$ group	$-2.27^\dagger$ (0.76)
partial PO (cumulative prob of $Y \leq 1$)	
small vessel	$3.49^\dagger$ (0.68)
large vessel or cardioembolic stroke	$-1.04^\dagger$ (0.44)
partial PO (cumulative prob of $Y \leq 2$)	
small vessel	$3.77^\dagger$ (0.68)
large vessel or cardioembolic stroke	$-1.36^\dagger$ (0.39)
partial PO (cumulative prob of $Y \leq 3$)	
small vessel	$6.14^\dagger$ (1.15)
large vessel or cardioembolic stroke	-0.64 (0.49)
Cause-specific hazards	
Risk 1: dropout	
group	0.23 (0.47)
modified Rankin scale prior onset	0.06 (0.42)
small vessel	0.55 (0.57)
large vessel	-0.29 (0.51)
small vessel $\times$ group	0.04 (1.14)
large vessel or cardioembolic stroke	0.30 (1.02)
Risk 2: death or remaining in severe disability	
group	-0.46 (0.27)
modified Rankin scale prior onset	$0.53^\dagger$ (0.17)
small vessel	$-2.07^\dagger$ (0.79)
large vessel	0.37 (0.27)
small vessel $\times$ group	0.35 (1.49)
large vessel or cardioembolic stroke	0.81 (0.54)
Random effects	
σ_b^2	34.66 (3.94)
σ_u^2	0.51 (0.07)
ρ_{bu}	$-0.997^\dagger$ (0.19)
ν_2	$3.12^\dagger$ (0.51)

† p-value < 0.05

other hand, patients with small vessels tended to have a lower risk for death or treatment failure than those with unknown reasons. The estimate of ν_2 is positive, suggesting that the two risks are positively correlated, i.e., patients with a higher risk of dropout were more likely to experience death or treatment failure. There is a negative correlation ($\rho_{bu} < 0$) between the random intercept b_i in (5.3) and frailty u_i in (5.2), which indicates that patients with higher Rankin scales tended to have a higher risk of dropout, death, or treatment failure. □

5.4 Bayesian Joint Models with Heterogeneous Random Effects

The joint models we have discussed thus far assume identical random effects covariance (matrix) for all subjects, so the model estimation and statistical inference may not be robust when there is heterogeneity in the covariance structure across study subjects. The impact of heterogeneous covariance on parameter estimation and statistical inference has been observed in analysis of longitudinal measurements. In this section we discuss extensions of the joint model in Section 5.1 to allow the joint multivariate random effects covariance matrix to be dependent on covariates. Specifically, a modified Cholesky decomposition is used to decompose the covariance matrix into a lower-triangular matrix and a diagonal matrix, and these matrix entries are linked to covariates using regression models. The methods can be found in Huang, Li, and Elashoff (2010)[103] and Huang, Li, Elashoff, and Pan (2011)[104].

Accommodating heterogeneous random effects in joint models has several advantages. First of all, the covariance model enables dimension reduction. With different choices of regression covariates, it provides a flexible means to model the heterogeneity and reduce the number of variance-covariance parameters. Second, the resulting estimated covariance matrices of the multivariate random effects are guaranteed to be positive definite, which is not always the case for other joint models. Finally, as the model includes homogeneous random effects as a special case, it provides a useful framework to assess the homogeneous covariance assumption.

Likelihood-based inference for joint models with heterogeneous random effects is rather challenging with high-dimensional random effects because the computational burden increases exponentially in terms of the number of random effects, as long as the estimation procedure involves numerical integration. Therefore, a Bayesian MCMC algorithm is developed to fit the joint model. A Gibbs sampling technique, together with Metropolis–Hastings sampling and adaptive rejection sampling methods, is used to draw random samples from the full conditional distribution of parameters. With the Bayesian approach, prior information can be incorporated in a natural way. If no prior information is available, noninformative priors for parameters are recommended since they allow data to dominate the determination of posterior distributions.

5.4.1 Model Specification

The joint model developed in Huang, Li, Elashoff, and Pan (2011)[104] assumes the same functional form as specified in (5.1) and (5.2) to specify the distribution of longitudinal and competing risks failure time data. Specifically, suppose there are n subjects in the study. For the ith subject at time t, the longitudinal outcome $Y_i(t)$ follows the linear mixed effects model

$$Y_i(t) = X_i^{(1)}(t)^T \beta + \tilde{X}_i^{(1)}(t)^T b_i + \epsilon_i(t), \tag{5.5}$$

where $X_i^{(1)}(t)$ and $\tilde{X}_i^{(1)}(t)$ are vectors of covariates associated with the fixed effects β and random effects b_i, respectively. The measurement error $\epsilon_i(t)$ is assumed to be distributed as $N(0, \sigma^2)$ and independent of b_i. Further assume $\epsilon_i(t_1) \perp \epsilon_i(t_2)$ for any $t_1 \neq t_2$.

The competing risks survival data $C_i = (T_i, D_i)$ are specified by

$$\lambda_k(t; X_i^{(2)}(t), u_i, \gamma_k, \nu_k)$$
$$= lim_{h \to 0} \frac{P[t \leq T_i < t + h, D_i = k | T_i \geq t, X_i^{(2)}(t), u_i, \gamma_k, \nu_k]}{h}$$
$$= \lambda_{0k}(t) \exp\{X_i^{(2)}(t)^T \gamma_k + \nu_k u_i\}. \tag{5.6}$$

The function $\lambda_k(t; X_i^{(2)}, u_i, \nu_k, \gamma_k)$ is the instantaneous failure rate from cause k at time t, given covariates $X_i^{(2)}(t)$ and the latent unknown factor u_i, in the presence of all other failure types. The regression coefficient ν_k represents the effect of the latent variable u_i, with ν_1 set to 1 to ensure identifiability. The parameter γ_k represents the effects of covariates $X_i^{(2)}(t)$ on cause k. Different from likelihood approaches, the kth baseline hazard is assumed to be a step function $\lambda_{0k}(t) = \lambda_{0k}^{(s)}$ for $t_k^{(s-1)} < t \leq t_k^{(s)}$ at prespecified points $t_k^{(s)}$, where $0 < t_k^{(1)} < ... < t_k^{(S^k)} < \infty$ is a partition of $(0, \infty)$ and S^k indicates the number of steps for the kth baseline hazard. Therefore, the baseline hazards are piecewise exponential with pre-selected change points. This strategy is commonly used in Bayesian inference for joint models.

To model the association between (5.5) and (5.6), assume that b_i and u_i jointly have a multivariate normal distribution:

$$a_i = \begin{pmatrix} b_i \\ u_i \end{pmatrix} \sim N_{q+1}(0, \Sigma_i) = N_{q+1}\left(0, \begin{pmatrix} \Sigma_{b_i} & \Sigma_{bu_i} \\ \Sigma_{bu_i}^T & \sigma_{u_i}^2 \end{pmatrix}\right),$$

where q is the dimension of b_i. Note that the covariance matrices Σ_i are allowed to be subject-specific. In this heterogenous random-effects joint model, Σ_i is modeled through a modified Cholesky decomposition $M_i \Sigma_i M_i^T = H_i$, where H_i is a diagonal matrix with positive entries and M_i is a lower triangular matrix with $-\phi_{i,jl}$ as its $(j, l)^{th}$ entry. This decomposition has a clear statistical interpretation: the below-diagonal entries of M_i are the negatives of generalized autoregressive parameters (GARP) , $\phi_{i,jl}$, in the autoregressive model

$$a_{ij} = \sum_{l=1}^{j-1} \phi_{i,jl} a_{jl} + e_{ij}, j = 1, \ldots, q + 1. \tag{5.7}$$

The diagonal entries of H_i are the innovation variances (IV) $h_{ij}^2 = var(e_{ij})$ and $cov(e_{ij}, e_{jk}) = 0$ if $j \neq k$ $(1 \leq j, k \leq q + 1$ and $i = 1, \ldots, n)$. The GARPs and the logarithms of the IVs are modeled with linear and log link functions:

$$\begin{cases} \phi_{i,jl} = x_{i,jl}^T \eta_1 & \text{for } i = 1, \ldots, n \\ \log h_{ij}^2 = z_{ij}^T \eta_2 & j = 1, \ldots, q + 1, l = 1, \ldots, j - 1 \end{cases} \tag{5.8}$$

where $x_{i,jl}$ and z_{ij} are covariates, and η_1 and η_2 are low-dimensional parameter vectors. For example, $x_{i,jl}$ and z_{ij} may contain group indicators, implying that the random effects covariances are heterogeneous between groups. Homogeneity of random effects in previous joint models becomes a testable assumption within this modeling framework. Furthermore, the resulting estimated covariance matrix is guaranteed to be positive definite.

Remark: Choice of design vectors for GARP/IV parameters. As we mentioned earlier, the choice of covariate vectors $x_{i,jl}$ and $z_{i,j}$ is flexible. For example, a 3-dimensional random effects variance-covariance matrix has 6 parameters. We can model the homogeneous unstructured covariance matrix by setting $x_{i,jl} = z_{ij} = 1$ for all $j = 1, \ldots, 3$, $l = 1, \ldots, j-1$. If we assume the design vectors contain a subject-dependent covariate, say, a group indicator (G), the unstructured heterogeneous covariance matrix can be modeled with $x_{i,jl} = z_{ij} = (1, G_i)$ for all $j = 1, \ldots, 3$, $l = 1, \ldots, j-1$; that is,

$$\begin{cases} x_i = (x_{i,jl}) = (1, G_i, 1, G_i, 1, G_i)^T; \eta_1 = (\eta_{11}^{Int}, \eta_{11}^G, \eta_{12}^{Int}, \eta_{12}^G, \eta_{13}^{Int}, \eta_{13}^G)^T \\ z_i = (z_{ij}) = (1, G_i, 1, G_i, 1, G_i)^T; \eta_2 = (\eta_{21}^{Int}, \eta_{21}^G, \eta_{22}^{Int}, \eta_{22}^G, \eta_{23}^{Int}, \eta_{23}^G)^T. \end{cases}$$

When there are high-dimensional random effects with limited data, one can impose a restricted covariance structure and assume some of the GARPs are identical to reduce the number of parameters.

5.4.2 Estimation and Inference

This joint model uses a Bayesian estimation procedure and a Markov chain Monte Carlo (MCMC) method for estimation and inference, to avoid the computational burden in maximum likelihood methods via EM algorithms that involve integrals with respect to random effects.

Suppose the longitudinal outcome $Y_i(t)$ is observed at time points t_{ij} for $j = 1, \ldots, n_i$, and denote $Y_i = (Y_{i1}, \ldots, Y_{in_i})$. Let $\Psi = \{\beta, \sigma^2, \gamma, \nu, \lambda_0, \eta_1, \eta_2\}$, where $\gamma = (\gamma_1, \gamma_2, ..., \gamma_g)$, $\nu = (\nu_2, ..., \nu_g)$, and $\lambda_0 = (\lambda_{01}^{(1)}, \lambda_{01}^{(2)}, ..., \lambda_{0g}^{(S^g)})$. To facilitate the MCMC implementation, it is convenient to work directly with the joint distribution of the observed data (Y, C) and unobservable random effects a, conditional on Ψ. The conditional joint density of (Y, C) and a is:

$$p(Y, C, a|\Psi) = \prod_{i=1}^{n} p(Y_i|a_i, \Psi)p(C_i|a_i, \Psi)p(a_i|\Psi)$$

$$\propto \prod_{i=1}^{m} (2\pi\sigma^2)^{-\frac{n_i}{2}} \exp\{-\frac{(Y_i - X_i^{(1)}\beta - \tilde{X}_i^{(1)}b_i)^T(Y_i - X_i^{(1)}\beta - \tilde{X}_i^{(1)}b_i)}{2\sigma^2}\}$$

$$\times \prod_{k=1}^{g} ((\lambda_k(T_i))^{I(D_i=k)} \exp\{-\Lambda_k(T_i)\})$$

$$\times \exp\{-\frac{1}{2}\sum_{j=1}^{q+1}[z_{ij}^T\eta_2 + (a_{ij} - \sum_{l=1}^{j-1} x_{ijl}^T\eta_1 a_{il})^2 \exp(-z_{ij}^T\eta_2)]\},$$

where

$$\lambda_k(T_i) = \lambda_{0k}(T_i)\exp\{X_i^{(2)}(T_i)\gamma_k + \nu_k u_i\}$$

and

$$\Lambda_k(T_i) = \int_0^{T_i} \lambda_{0k}(t)\exp(X_i^{(2)}(t)\gamma_k + \nu_k u_i)dt.$$

Under the piecewise constant hazard assumption,

$$\Lambda_k(T_i) = \exp(\nu_k u_i)\sum_{s=1}^{S^k} I(T_i > t_k^{(s-1)})\lambda_{0k}^{(s)} \int_{t_k^{(s-1)}}^{min(T_i,t_k^{(s)})} \exp(X_i^{(2)}(t)\gamma_k)dt.$$

Independent priors for Ψ can be used. Normal priors are used for the parameters β, γ, ν, η_1, and η_2, leading to conjugate posteriors for β and some components of η_1. An inverse Gamma prior is used for the measurement error variance σ^2 and a gamma prior for each step of the kth baseline hazard function λ_{0k} by which conjugate posterior distributions are easy to obtain.

Markov Chain Monte Carlo (MCMC) methods are used for posterior sampling. It involves sampling directly from the full conditional distribution, Metropolis–Hastings (MH) sampling, and adaptive rejection sampling (ARS). Since the full conditional distributions of β, σ^2, and $\lambda_{0k}^{(s)}$, $(s = 1, ..., S^g, k = 1, ..., g)$ are standard distributions, drawing random variates from their full conditional distributions is straightforward. For the rest of the parameters and random effects (b_i, u_i), either a Metropolis–Hastings step is used with normal approximation to the full conditional distributions as a candidate distribution or the adaptive rejection sampling technique is applied.

The initial values for parameter sampling are obtained by analyzing the longitudinal data and survival data separately using a linear mixed model (5.5) and a Cox proportional hazards model (5.6). The initial value for $\lambda_{0k}^{(s)}$ $(s = 1, ..., S^k, k = 1, ..., g)$ can be obtained by drawing a random variate from the Gamma full conditional distribution. The parameters are estimated using posterior medians and their approximate 95% probability intervals are based on the 2.5th and 97.5th percentiles. Standard errors are estimated using standard deviations of posterior samples. Convergence of the Gibbs sampler is monitored by examining time series plots of the parameters over iterations and using multiple chains.

Example 5.4. *The Scleroderma Lung Study (continued)*

As has been shown in Chapter 2, the beneficial effects of CYC on %FVC continued to increase after stopping treatment at 12 months and eventually began to wane at 18 months. Therefore, the following linear spline mixed effects model with a change point at month 18 was fit for longitudinal measurements %FVC:

$$
\begin{aligned}
\%FVC_{ij} = {} & \beta_0 + \beta_1 FVC_{0i} + \beta_2 FIB_{0i} + \beta_3 CYC_i + \beta_4 Time_{ij} + \beta_5 (Time_{ij} - 18)_+ \\
& + \beta_6 FVC_{0i} \times CYC_i + \beta_7 FIB_{0i} \times CYC_i + \beta_8 Time_{ij} \times CYC_i \\
& + \beta_9 (Time_{ij} - 18)_+ \times CYC_i + \tilde{X}_i^{(1)T} b_i + \epsilon_{ij},
\end{aligned}
\tag{5.9}
$$

where $\tilde{X}_i^{(1)}$ is a set of baseline covariates and ϵ_{ij} are mutually independent measurement errors.

Multiple choices for random effect covariates $\tilde{X}_i^{(1)}$ were considered and model selection was based on the Deviance information criterion (DIC) which is straightforward to compute using output from a Gibbs sampler. It has a similar form to the Akaika information criterion (AIC): a goodness-of-fit term measured by the deviance evaluated at the posterior mean of model parameters, and a penalty term defined by twice the effective number of parameters. The effective number of parameters is computed as the mean deviance minus the deviance evaluated at the posterior mean; that is,

$$
DIC = dev(\overline{\Psi}) + 2p_D,
$$

where $\overline{\Psi}$ is the posterior mean of Ψ, $p_D = \overline{dev} - dev(\overline{\Psi})$, where $\overline{dev}$ is the posterior mean of the deviance (i.e., the average of deviances calculated using estimated parameters at each step of the Markov chain Monte Carlo sampler). It is clear that models with a smaller DIC fit the data better.

The cause-specific competing risks model (5.6) was used to characterize disease-related dropout (risk 1) and treatment failure or death (risk 2):

$$
\begin{aligned}
\lambda_1(t) = {} & \lambda_{01}(t) \exp(\gamma_{11} FVC_{0i} + \gamma_{12} FIB_{0i} + \gamma_{13} CYC_i + \gamma_{14} FVC_{0i} \times CYC_i \\
& + \gamma_{15} FIB_{0i} \times CYC_i + u_i)
\end{aligned}
\tag{5.10}
$$

and

$$
\begin{aligned}
\lambda_2(t) = {} & \lambda_{02}(t) \exp(\gamma_{21} FVC_{0i} + \gamma_{22} FIB_{0i} + \gamma_{23} CYC_i + \gamma_{24} FVC_{0i} \times CYC_i \\
& + \gamma_{25} FIB_{0i} \times CYC_i + \nu_2 u_i).
\end{aligned}
\tag{5.11}
$$

The random effects at the longitudinal and survival endpoints were assumed to have a multivariate normal distribution with mean zero and variance-covariance matrix Σ_i, and the assumption of homogeneous covariance was tested by considering subject-dependent covariates for x_{ijl} and z_{ij}. Specifically, these vectors were chosen to be $(1, CYC_i)$, which allows heterogeneous covariance matrices for different treatments and enables testing of the homogeneous covariance assumption (i.e., all the GARP and IV parameters are zero).

Three-step baseline hazard functions, with change points at equally split percentiles of the observed event times, were utilized for disease-related dropout and treatment failure or death. Sensitivity analysis with 4- and 5-step baseline hazard functions showed no significant differences in results. Independent noninformative prior distributions were applied to all the parameters assumed to have relatively large variances. Specifically, the priors are: $\beta_0 \sim N(70, 10^3)$ and $\beta_l \sim N(0, 10^3)$ for $l = 1, \ldots, 9$; $\sigma^2 \sim IG(10^{-3}, 10^{-3})$; $\gamma_{kr} \sim N(0, 10^3)$ for $k = 1, 2$ and $r = 1, \ldots, 5$; $\lambda_{0k}^{(s)} \sim \Gamma(10^{-3}, 10^{-3})$ for $s = 1, \ldots, S^k$ and $S^1 = S^2 = 3$; $\nu_2 \sim N(0, 10^5)$; and each element of η_1 and $\eta_2 \sim N(0, 10^5)$.

Table 5.5 summarizes the covariance parameters of different models, each of which was based on 30,000 iterations of MCMC sampling chains following a 15,000-iteration "burn-in" period. Three models were considered: a one-random-slope (before 18 months) model, a structured two-random-slope model assuming the last row entries in matrix M_i (from the decomposition) are the same, and an unstructured two-random-slope model. The structured covariance model might be useful when dealing with a high-dimensional random effects model for limited data. It is clear that none of the 95% credible intervals for CYC exclude zero. Therefore, there is no sufficient evidence to reject the homogeneous covariance assumption. The two-random-slope model with unstructured covariance matrix has the smallest DIC, indicating that it might provide the best fit for the SLS data. Combining the earlier results, the homogenous two-random-slope model with unstructured covariance is chosen as the final model and its covariance parameters and DIC are given in the last column of Table 5.5.

Parameter estimates of the final model are given in Table 5.6. For comparison purposes, separate analysis of the two endpoints was performed by fitting a linear mixed model (5.9) with two random slopes for %FVC and a cause-specific hazards frailty model (5.10)–(5.11) for the competing risks failure time data, respectively. The two methods produce similar point estimates and credible intervals for baseline %FVC, lung fibrosis, and their interactions with CYC. In the joint model, the significant interaction between CYC and time trend indicates that trajectories of %FVC were different between the two treatments: during the first 18 months, %FVC declined in the placebo group ($\beta_4 = -0.12$) but increased in the CYC group ($\beta_4 + \beta_8 = 0.14$); after 18 months, the CYC group had a steep decrease ($\beta_4 + \beta_5 + \beta_8 + \beta_9 = -0.45$), whereas the placebo group rebounded ($\beta_4 + \beta_5 = 0.15$). However, the interaction between CYC and time trend is not significant in the separate analysis. This difference might be explained by the significant covariances $\Sigma_{b_1 u}$ and $\Sigma_{b_2 u}$ which indicate that the longitudinal measurements of %FVC and survival process were inter-correlated. The negative sign of $\Sigma_{b_1 u}$ and positive sign of $\Sigma_{b_2 u}$ together with positive ν_2 indicate that in the first 18 months, there tended to be a lower risk for both treatment failure or death and disease-related dropout among patients with higher than average increasing rate in %FVC; after 18 months, the trend was reversed due to the negative association between the two *slopes. The overall effect of treatment CYC on %FVC scores is tested using the null hypothesis $H_0 : \beta_3 = \beta_6 = \beta_7 = \beta_8 = \beta_9 = 0$, which yields a p-value of 0.01 for the joint model and 0.03 for the separate model.*

At the competing risks survival endpoint, the two methods produce similar point estimates and CIs for most parameters and identify the same set of significant effects. The joint model performs better than the separate analysis in estimation of ν_2, since extra information from the longitudinal endpoint helps with estimation of u_i, and thus increases the identifiability of ν_2. No significant overall CYC effect is found for treatment failure or death by testing the null hypothesis $H_{02} : \gamma_{23} = \gamma_{24} = \gamma_{25} = 0$. □

5.4.3 A Robust Joint Model with Heterogeneous Random Effects and t-Distributed Random Errors

A robust joint model with heterogeneous random effects was developed by incorporating t-distributed random errors to reduce the impact of outliers and influential data points in longitudinal measurements (Huang, Li, and Elashoff, 2010[103]). In this robust joint model, the same formulation as specified in (5.5) and (5.6) is used, except that the measurement error $\epsilon_i(t)$ is distributed as $t(0, \sigma^2, \kappa)$. More technical details about t-distributions are given in Section 5.2.

Parameter estimation and statistical inference can proceed via a Bayesian approach similar to what is outlined in the last section. Note that the t-distribution can be derived by mixing the sample ϵ_{ij} with a scaling variate τ_{ij}, such that $\epsilon_{ij} = \tau_{ij}^{-1/2} \varepsilon_{ij}$, where ε_{ij} are i.i.d. normal variables. The full conditional distribution of τ_{ij} under this complex joint model has a known form if we assume κ is prespecified. Further details of model estimation and inference can be found in Huang, Li, and Elashoff (2010)[103].

Example 5.5. *The Scleroderma Lung Study (continued)*

The longitudinal profiles of %FVC over time (Figure 5.1) indicate potential outliers. This analysis examines how these data points would affect the inference of joint models.

Firstly, in the robust joint model with heterogeneous random effects, the homogeneous covariance assumption was tested via incorporation of subject-dependent covariates x_{ijl} and z_{ij} in (5.7) and (5.8). To be specific, set $x_{ijl} = z_{ij} = (1, CYC_i)$, which corresponds to heterogeneous covariance matrices between treatment groups. The results (not shown) suggest that there is no sufficient evidence to reject the homogeneous covariance assumption. Therefore, joint models assuming a homogeneous covariance were used in the following analyses.

Seven possible outlying data points were identified by examining residuals from

Table 5.5 *Random effects covariance matrix parameters for four different models*

	$[Time_{ij}]$ Est.(95%CI)	$[Time_{ij}, time18_{ij}]^a$ Est.(95%CI)	$[Time_{ij}, Time18_i]^b$ Est.(95%CI)	$[Time_{ij}, Time18_i]^c$ Est.(95%CI)
Generalized Autoregressive Parameters				
η_{11} Intercept	−0.27(−1.02, 0.18)	−1.24(−2.08, −0.38)	−1.01(−1.81, −0.20)	−1.17(−1.74, −0.58)
η_{11} CYC	−0.71(−1.65, 0.08)	−0.67(−1.82, 0.93)	−0.26(−1.45, 0.92)	
η_{12} Intercept		0.23(0.03, 0.71)	−0.27(−1.23, 0.29)	−0.51(−1.23, −0.01)
η_{12} CYC		0.44(−1.47, 2.00)	−1.48(−2.64, 0.15)	0.34(0.08, 0.85)
η_{13} Intercept			0.36(0.10, 0.96)	
η_{13} CYC			−0.65(−1.49, 0.13)	
Innovation Variances				
η_{21} Intercept	−1.49(−1.87, −1.09)	−1.29(−1.67, −0.90)	−1.32(−1.69, −0.91)	−1.31(−1.59, −1.03)
η_{21} CYC	−0.06(−0.63, 0.49)	0.01(−0.58, 0.59)	−0.01(−0.59, 0.57)	−0.10(−0.68, 0.38)
η_{22} Intercept	−4.72(−7.21, −2.19)	0.23(−0.53, 0.84)	0.24(−0.48, 0.84)	−4.62(−7.26, −1.60)
η_{22} CYC		−0.66(−3.73, 0.45)	−0.68(−1.95, 0.37)	
η_{23} Intercept		−5.11(−7.55, −2.08)	−4.58(−7.38, −1.79)	
Model Fit				
DIC	5661.09	5565.38	5549.32	5540.80

Note: a, Structured heterogeneous two-random-slope model; b, Unstructured heterogeneous two-random-slope model; c, Unstructured homogeneous two-random-slope model.

Table 5.6 *Analysis of SLS data using the unstructured homogeneous two-random-slope model.*

	Joint Analysis Estimate (95%CI)	Separate Analysis Estimate (95%CI)
Longitudinal outcome %FVC		
Int (β_0)	65.33(64.72, 67.87)	65.94(64.41, 67.47)
FVC_0 (β_1)	0.89(0.80, 0.99)†	0.89(0.79, 0.99)†
FIB_0 (β_2)	$-1.85(-2.94, -0.79)^\dagger$	$-1.86(-2.94, -0.78)^\dagger$
CYC (β_3)	$-0.98(-3.18, 1.26)$	$-0.76(-2.94, 1.42)$
$Time$ (β_4)	$-0.12(-0.29, 0.06)$	$-0.05(-0.23, 0.13)$
$Time18$ (β_5)	0.27(-0.17, 0.72)	0.11(-0.34, 0.56)
$FVC_0 \times CYC$ (β_6)	0.14(0.00, 0.28)†	0.14(0.00, 0.28)†
$FIB_0 \times CYC$ (β_7)	1.74(0.13, 3.27)†	1.78(0.23, 3.33)†
$Time \times CYC$ (β_8)	0.26(0.01, 0.50)†	0.21(-0.04, 0.46)
$Time18 \times CYC$ (β_9)	$-0.72(-1.33, -0.08)^\dagger$	$-0.64(-1.29, 0.00)$
σ^2	21.55(19.23, 24.25)	21.28(18.80, 23.76)
$\Sigma_{b_{11}}$	0.27(0.20, 0.36)	0.25(0.18, 0.32)
$\Sigma_{b_{12}}$	$-0.31(-0.53, -0.14)$	$-0.31(-0.49, -0.12)$
$\Sigma_{b_{22}}$	1.29(0.70, 2.14)	1.34(0.67, 2.00)
p-value for $H_0 : \beta_3 = \beta_6 = \beta_7 = \beta_8 = \beta_9 = 0$	0.01	0.03
Cause-specific hazards		
(time to informative dropout)		
FVC_0 (γ_{11})	$-0.06(-0.12, -0.01)^\dagger$	$-0.06(-0.12, -0.00)^\dagger$
FIB_0 (γ_{12})	0.22(-0.27, 0.78)	0.20(-0.35, 0.75)
CYC (γ_{13})	0.23(-0.60, 1.12)	0.40(-0.46, 1.26)
$FVC_0 \times CYC$ (γ_{14})	0.10(0.03, 0.18)†	0.09(0.03, 0.15)†
$FIB_0 \times CYC$ (γ_{15})	0.13(-0.60, 0.83)	0.07(-0.64, 0.76)
p-value for $H_{01} : \gamma_{13} = \gamma_{14} = \gamma_{15} = 0$	0.08	0.07
Cause-specific hazards		
(time to treatment failure or death)		
FVC_0 (γ_{21})	0.02(-0.07, 0.09)	0.03(-0.07, 0.13)
FIB_0 (γ_{22})	0.29(-0.62, 1.19)	0.28(-0.80, 1.36)
CYC (γ_{23})	$-1.33(-3.44, 0.21)$	$-1.14(-3.26, 0.98)$
$FVC_0 \times CYC$ (γ_{24})	$-0.07(-0.21, 0.06)$	$-0.08(-0.24, 0.08)$
$FIB_0 \times CYC$ (γ_{25})	$-0.58(-2.31, 0.91)$	$-0.88(-2.78, 1.02)$
p-value for $H_{02} : \gamma_{23} = \gamma_{24} = \gamma_{25} = 0$	0.39	0.48
Random effects for survival endpoint		
ν_2	3.04(1.27, 7.65)	$-0.31(-79.80, 81.16)$
σ_u^2	0.38(0.07, 1.42)	0.04(0.00, 0.40)
Covariance of b_i and u_i		
$\Sigma_{b_1 u}$	$-0.25(-0.51, -0.09)$	-
$\Sigma_{b_2 u}$	0.60(0.21, 1.33)	-

Note: $\dagger$ p-value <0.05

the robust joint model. Table 5.7 compares the results from joint models assuming normal measurement errors based on data with and without the seven outliers. When the outliers are excluded, a fair amount of changes are observed in parameter estimates at the longitudinal endpoint. There was a significant time trend in the placebo group before 18 months ($\beta_1 = -0.18$), which is a steeper decrease in %FVC scores than that estimated from the joint model with all data points. A significant interaction between the slope (before 18 months) and treatment is also identified when the outliers are excluded. Possibly due to the fact that those outliers introduce extra noises to the data, the estimated standard error for β is larger in the model with all data points. Comparable estimates at the survival endpoint are obtained. Both models identify a negative association between the random slope before 18 months and the frailty u_i ($\Sigma_{b_1 u}$), and a positive association between the random slope after 18 months and u_i ($\Sigma_{b_2 u}$). These comparisons suggest that inference from the joint model with a normal distribution for measurement errors is not robust against potential outliers in the longitudinal data, although the outliers may not have substantial impact on parameter estimation at the survival endpoint.

The last column of Table 5.7 shows the estimated robust joint model with t-distributed ($\kappa = 3$) measurement errors. All data points were used when fitting this model. The model indicates that there was a significant decrease in %FVC measurements in the placebo group before 18 months (β_1) and this time trend was different from the CYC group (β_8). The estimates are similar to their counterparts in the normal joint model without outliers. Testing the overall CYC effect on %FVC gives a p-value of 0.003. All the three methods generate similar results for the competing risks parameters and random effects covariances. The overall fit is assessed using DIC, which suggests that the robust joint model provides the best fit. $\square$

5.5 Accelerated Failure Time Models for Competing Risks

The previously discussed joint models in this chapter use Cox regression to characterize the cause-specific hazards of competing risks. When the proportional hazards assumption is violated, accelerated failure time models could be an appealing alternative. For example, the joint model discussed in Section 4.4.2 can be extended to the setting of competing risks. Given that we know the entirely covariate history $\bar{Y}(t)$, the cause-specific hazard of risk k, $k = 1, \ldots, g$, can be specified as

$$\lambda_k\{t|\bar{Y}(t), \gamma\} = \lambda_{0k}[\int_0^t exp\{\gamma_k Y(s)\}ds]exp\{\gamma_k Y(t)\},$$

where $\lambda_{0k}(\cdot)$ and γ_k, $k = 1, \ldots, g$, are cause-specific baseline hazard functions and regression coefficients, respectively. Denote $\gamma = (\gamma_1, \ldots, \gamma_k)^T$. The above model may also include other baseline covariates with possibly cause-specific

Table 5.7 Analysis of 6–24 months scleroderma lung study data

	Normal Distribution		t-distribution ($\kappa = 3$)
	Include the outliers	Exclude the outliers	Include the outliers
	Estimate (95%CI)	Estimate (95%CI)	Estimate (95%CI)
Longitudinal outcome %FVC			
$Time$ (β_1)	-0.13(-0.30, 0.05)	**-0.18(-0.33, -0.02)**	**-0.20(-0.36, -0.03)**
$Time18$ (β_2)	0.23(-0.25, 0.74)	0.15(-0.25, 0.53)	0.22(-0.13, 0.56)
FVC_0 (β_3)	0.92(0.83, 1.03)	0.88(0.79, 0.98)	0.93(0.85, 1.01)
FIB_0 (β_4)	-2.05(-3.22, -0.94)	-1.83(-2.84, -0.81)	-1.88(-2.75, -0.99)
CYC (β_5)	-1.38(-3.66, 1.00)	-1.00(-2.89, 0.88)	-1.12(-2.83, 0.59)
$FVC_0 \times CYC$ (β_6)	0.11(-0.04, 0.25)	0.15(-0.02, 0.27)	0.09(-0.01, 0.20)
$FIB_0 \times CYC$ (β_7)	2.03(0.43, 3.69)	1.74(0.32, 3.19)	2.25(0.92, 3.52)
$Time \times CYC$ (β_8)	0.26(-0.01, 0.51)	**0.23(0.01, 0.45)**	**0.24(0.01, 0.47)**
$Time18 \times CYC$ (β_9)	-0.64(-1.33, 0.07)	-0.43(-0.96, 0.13)	-0.41(-0.92, 0.09)
p-value for H_0:Overall CYC Effect=0	**0.040**	**0.022**	**0.003**
Cause-specific hazards			
(informatively censored events)			
FVC_0 (γ_{11})	-0.06(-0.13, -0.01)	-0.06(-0.12, -0.01)	-0.06(-0.12, -0.01)
FIB_0 (γ_{12})	0.21(-0.28, 0.77)	0.21(-0.29, 0.76)	0.21(-0.27, 0.79)
CYC (γ_{13})	0.24(-0.61, 1.20)	0.29(-0.55, 1.21)	0.25(-0.57, 1.18)
$FVC_0 \times CYC$ (γ_{14})	0.11(0.03, 0.18)	0.10(0.03, 0.18)	0.11(0.04, 0.19)
$FIB_0 \times CYC$ (γ_{15})	0.13(-0.58, 0.83)	0.12(-0.61, 0.81)	0.08(-0.63, 0.78)

Table 5.7 (continued.)

| | Normal Distribution | | t-distribution ($\kappa = 3$) |
| | Include the outliers | Exclude the outliers | Include the outliers |
	Estimate (95%CI)	Estimate (95%CI)	Estimate (95%CI)
Cause-specific hazards (treatment failure of death)			
FVC_0 (γ_{21})	0.01(−0.07, 0.11)	0.02(−0.06, 0.10)	0.01(−0.07, 0.09)
$F1B_0$ (γ_{22})	0.25(−0.68, 1.22)	0.22(−0.62, 1.13)	0.25(−0.67, 1.20)
CYC (γ_{23})	−1.24(−3.20, 0.35)	−1.19(−3.29, 0.22)	−1.20(−3.50, 0.34)
$FVC_0 \times CYC$ (γ_{24})	−0.06(−0.20, 0.08)	−0.07(−0.20, 0.07)	−0.05(−0.19, 0.09)
$F1B_0 \times CYC$ (γ_{25})	−0.55(−2.26, 1.07)	−0.52(−2.12, 0.94)	−0.51(−2.22, 1.02)
Random effects			
ν_2	3.34(1.34, 8.35)	3.28(1.42, 8.81)	3.25(1.18, 7.84)
$\Sigma_{b_{11}}$	0.27(0.20, 0.36)	0.28(0.21, 0.37)	0.25(0.19, 0.33)
$\Sigma_{b_{12}}$	−0.36(−0.61, −0.18)	−0.32(−0.53, −0.17)	−0.27(−0.45, −0.15)
$\Sigma_{b_{22}}$	1.60(0.89, 2.59)	0.93(0.51, 1.61)	0.73(0.39, 0.1.25)
σ_u^2	0.40(0.07, 1.59)	0.31(0.05, 1.16)	0.35(0.06, 1.31)
Covariance of b_i and u_i			
$\Sigma_{b_1 u}$	−0.25(−0.53, −0.09)	−0.25(−0.50, −0.09)	−0.23(−0.47, −0.08)
$\Sigma_{b_2 u}$	0.69(0.24, 1.50)	0.42(0.11, 1.02)	0.39(0.11, 0.93)
Model fit			
DIC	5693.08	5295.18	5089.35

effects. When $Y(s)$ is intermittently measured and thus the entire history $\bar{Y}(t)$ is not observable, a longitudinal sub-model similar to (4.50) could be used to characterize the underlying trajectory of $Y(s)$.

Similar to the approach adopted by Tseng, Hsieh, and Wang (2005)[212], the cause-specific baseline hazards $\lambda_{0k}(\cdot)$ can be step functions that are constant between two adjacent estimated baseline failure times, and the maximum likelihood estimation and inference would then be done via the EM algorithm.

Chapter 6

Joint Models for Multivariate Longitudinal and Survival Data

This chapter considers extensions of joint models to multidimensional longitudinal and/or survival data. The approaches covered here are useful for studies that collect information on more than one longitudinal outcome or event on each participant. For example, when studying the profiles of cognitive aging in the elderly, cognition is measured by several psychometric tests and its association with the risk of dementia is of interest. In a Phase III clinical trial of second-line therapy for malignant pleural mesothelioma, repeated measurements of multi-item patient-reported outcomes were used to predict patient survival. An example of multiple event times is given by a study to investigate the impact of air quality on respiratory symptoms, in which recurrence of respiratory symptoms including runny nose, cough, and sore throat was monitored daily. Addition to recurrent events of the same cause, multivariate survival data are also commonly observed in studies where the events emerge in clusters, for example, twins, families, and different anatomical sites on the same patient, and it is often of interest to assess the association between the response variables and multivariate survival times.

In Section 6.1 we review joint modeling approaches that handle multivariate longitudinal outcomes. Methods for recurrent and multivariate survival data are discussed in Sections 6.2 and 6.3, respectively.

6.1 Joint Models for Multivariate Longitudinal Outcomes and an Event Time

There have been several attempts to extend joint analysis for a single longitudinal outcome to the situation where multiple outcomes are simultaneously recorded together with the event times. A key issue in modeling multivariate longitudinal data and their association with event times is to formulate the joint evolution of these multiple endpoints. Of note, the model for longitudinal outcomes needs to take into account two sources of data correlations: (1) the correlation within repeated measurements of each single outcome over time, and (2) the correlation between different outcomes collected at the same and different occasions. These data correlations are usually characterized by latent variables, either continuous (random effects) or discrete (latent classes), which are also used to link together the longitudinal outcomes and survival data.

Parameter estimation and statistical inference have been developed under both likelihood and Bayesian paradigms, and the estimation methods discussed previously can be generally applied here. The main approaches and examples discussed in this section can be found in Rizopoulos and Ghosh (2011)[186] and Proust–Lima et al. (2009)[178]. Li et al. (2012)[139] developed a shared-parameter model for bivariate ordinal longitudinal outcomes, assuming that the random effects at the longitudinal endpoint are shared with the event process. See Hatfield, Boye, and Carlin (2011)[92] and Luo (2014)[157] for other joint models via random effects. Extensions to multivariate event times include Huang et al. (2001)[102] and Chi and Ibrahim (2006)[40]. Deslandes and Chevret (2010)[53] considered multivariate longitudinal outcomes and competing risks survival data. Albert and Shih (2010)[9] proposed a two-stage regression calibration approach to jointly modeling of discrete time-to-event data and multiple longitudinal measurements. In what follows, we attempt to go through existing methods with an emphasis on model structure and formulation.

6.1.1   Random-Effects Models

We first look at a class of models that use continuous latent variables (random effects) to model the association between longitudinal and survival endpoints. Suppose there are K response variables. For $k = 1, \ldots, K$, let Y_{ik} be a $n_{ik} \times 1$ vector of repeated measures for the kth outcome collected on subject i at time points t_{ijk}, $i = 1, \ldots, n$, $j = 1, \ldots, n_{ik}$. Note that it is possible the measurement occasions t_{ijk} are different from subject to subject. A multivariate generalized linear mixed effects model would be an appropriate choice to describe the distribution of different types of longitudinal responses. The model assumes that given random effects b_{ik}, the distribution of Y_{ik} is a member of exponential families whose linear predictor is given by

$$g_k\{E(Y_{ik}(t)|b_{ik})\} = f_{ik}(t), \tag{6.1}$$

where $g_k(\cdot)$ is a known monotonic link function, $Y_{ik}(t)$ the kth longitudinal response measured at time t on subject i, and $f_{ik}(t)$ a time-dependent function to describe the true, underlying longitudinal profile for response k. Within the mixed effects model framework, a natural choice for $Y_{ik}(t)$ is

$$f_{ik}(t) = X_{ik}^T(t)\beta_k + Z_{ik}(t)^T b_{ik}, \tag{6.2}$$

where β_k is a vector of fixed effects, and $X_{ik}(t)$ and $Z_{ik}(t)$ are covariates measured at time t. To allow flexible trajectories in the longitudinal responses, the components in $X_{ik}(t)$ and $Z_{ik}(t)$ can be further classified into time-fixed or time-dependent covariates, and the latter may contain spline functions to characterize the time trend.

If a Cox proportional hazards model is assumed for the survival data, a general formulation to characterize its association with the longitudinal outcomes can be expressed as

$$h(t|H_i(t), W_i, u_i) = h_0(t)exp[W_i^T\gamma + \sum_{k=1}^{K} m_{ik}\{f_{ik}(t), u_i; \alpha_k\}], \qquad (6.3)$$

where $H_i(t) = \{f_{ik}(s), 0 \le s < t, 1 \le k \le K\}$ denotes the history of underlying longitudinal processes up to time t, W_i is a vector of time-fixed covariates with regression coefficients γ, $m_{ik}(\cdot)$ specifies which components of $f_{ik}(t)$ are associated with the hazard at time t, u_i is a frailty on subject i, and α_k is a vector of outcome specific regression coefficients in function m_{ik}. Some examples of $m_{ik}(\cdot)$ are given in Rizopoulos and Ghosh (2011)[186]:

$$m_{ik}\{f_{ik}(t), u_i; \alpha_k\} = \sum_{\nu=0}^{q} \alpha_{\nu k} \frac{d^\nu f_{ik}(t)}{dt^\nu}, with \frac{d^0 f_{ik}(t)}{dt^0} = f_{ik}(t), \quad (6.4)$$

$$m_{ik}\{f_{ik}(t), u_i; \alpha_k\} = \alpha_k^T b_{ik}, \qquad (6.5)$$

$$m_{ik}\{f_{ik}(t), u_i; \alpha_k\} = u_i. \qquad (6.6)$$

Equation (6.4) in its simplest form ($q = 0$) models the effect of the underlying trajectory of the kth longitudinal outcome on event times. This parameterization is frequently used in joint models with interest to evaluate impact of longitudinal biomarkers on the risk of clinically meaningful milestones. When $q > 0$, the formulation assumes that not only the longitudinal outcome at time t, but also its slope and curvature at time t, affects the event risk. To facilitate model parsimony and interpretability, values of q no greater than 2 are recommended. Such parametrization is often used in connection with spline functions when modeling $f_{ik}(t)$, which guarantee tractable quantification of the derivatives. Equation (6.5) represents a commonly used strategy for longitudinal measurements with nonignorable missing data caused by some terminating events such as death or dropout. This parameterization assumes that the risk of death or dropout at time t depends on deviation of the ith subject from the overall mean (e.g., deviation of subject-specific slope from the population slope). In contrast to the previous two parameterizations, formulation (6.6) does not directly include any components in $f_{ik}(t)$ to characterize its association with the event risk, but rather assumes that the dependence between the longitudinal and survival endpoints is modeled by the joint distribution (e.g., multivariate normal distribution) between a frailty u_i and the random effects b_{ik}. This is a more flexible framework that allows extra variation at the survival endpoint that cannot be explained by longitudinal data. The model reduces to (6.5) if u_i can be expressed as a linear function of b_{ik}.

Note that the latent variables in (6.1)–(6.3) include random effects b_{ik} and frailty u_i at the longitudinal and survival endpoints, respectively. The model assumes that the latent variables account for all dependencies in observed data. This implies conditional independence of longitudinal and survival processes, and conditional independence of the multivariate, repeatedly measured longitudinal outcomes. In a likelihood approach, it is natural to posit a multivariate normal distribution for b_{ik} and u_i. In a Bayesian framework, a Dirichlet process (DP) prior has been used:

$$\mathbb{B}_i \sim DP(\rho, \mathfrak{G}_0), \qquad \mathfrak{G}_0 \sim N(\mathbf{0}, \Sigma),$$

where $\mathbb{B}_i$ is a vector that contains $(b_{i1}, \ldots, b_{iK})$ and u_i, $\rho \geq 0$ a scalar precision parameter, and $\mathfrak{G}_0$ a parametric baseline distribution, which is assumed to be a multivariate normal with mean zero and covariance matrix Σ. An illustration of this Bayesian approach is given in Example 6.1.

The modeling strategy we consider next is appropriate for studies in which the multiple longitudinal outcomes jointly measure a latent process $U_i(t)$ of interest from different perspectives, and $U_i(t)$ is regarded as the main factor related to event development. If the longitudinal outcomes are continuous, the model can be specified as

$$Y_{ik}(t) = \beta_{0k} + \beta_{1k}U_i(t) + b_{ik} + \epsilon_{ik}(t), \qquad (6.7)$$

where $\beta_k = (\beta_{0k}, \beta_{1k})$ is a vector of regression coefficients for the kth outcome, $\epsilon_{ik}(t)$ is distributed as $N(0, \tau_k^2)$ with $\epsilon_{ik}(t) \perp \epsilon_{ik}(t')$ for $t \neq t'$, and the random intercept b_{ik} follows $N(0, \xi_k^2)$ and is independent of $\epsilon_{ik}(t)$. It is appropriate to assume $b_{ik}, k = 1, \ldots, K$, are mutually independent, which implies conditional independence of the multiple outcomes given $U_i(t)$, so that the cross-sectional correlation among $Y_{ik}, k = 1, \ldots, K$, at time t is induced by the shared latent process $U_i(t)$. Conditional on $U_i(t)$, the correlation of repeated measures on $Y_{ik}(t)$ within subject i is thus modeled by the random intercept b_{ik}. Note that β_{1k} can be interpreted as the factor loading of the kth outcome on $U_i(t)$. The higher the factor loading, the more contribution of that particular outcome to $U_i(t)$. For a mixture of continuous and discrete outcomes, generalized linear mixed effects models can be used to replace (6.7).

The latent process $U_i(t)$, which is continuous in nature, may be characterized by the following linear mixed effects model:

$$U_i(t) = X_i(t)^T \alpha + Z_i(t)^T a_i + e_i(t),$$

where $X_i(t)$ and $Z_i(t)$ are vectors of covariates that could be time-varying, α is a vector of regression coefficients, $a_i \sim N(0, D(\theta))$ is a vector of random effects, and $e_i(t)$ is normally distributed measurement error independent of

a_i. If $e_i(t) \perp e_i(t')$ for $t \neq t'$, it implies that the correlation of $U_i(t)$ over time is captured by a_i. To make the model identifiable, $X_i(t)$ should not include an intercept and the variance of $e_i(t)$ is set to 1.

Under the formulation of (6.7), it is natural to assume that $U_i(t)$ is the main factor that drives the event process of interest. Their interdependence is captured by the parameter ϕ in the following Cox proportional hazards model:

$$h(t|W_i, U_i(t)) = h_0(t)exp(W_i^T\gamma + \phi U_i(t)). \tag{6.8}$$

This framework can be extended to other regression models for survival data such as AFT models.

Example 6.1. *The Renal Graft Failure Study*

The model (6.1)–(6.3) is illustrated using a renal graft failure study that consists of 407 patients with chronic kidney disease who received renal transplantations in the hospital of the Catholic University of Leuven (Belgium) between 1983 and 2000 (Rizopoulos and Ghosh, 2011[186]). Patients were followed until graft failure, and three markers were measured periodically to test kidney conditions during follow-up: a continuous variable GFR that measures the kidney filtration rate, the blood hematocrit level (continuous) that indicates whether there is adequate amount of erythropoietin produced by the kidney that regulates red blood cell production, and a binary variable proteinuria that indicates whether the kidney is preventing important proteins from leaking from the blood stream into the urine. These markers are endogenous, stochastic, and measured with error. They reflect different aspects of kidney functions and are also biologically interrelated. Therefore, improved prediction of the risk of graft failure may be achieved by modeling the joint evolution of the three longitudinal markers. Figure 6.1 shows marker profiles measured on randomly selected five patients, suggesting nonlinear time trends and substantial heterogeneity among subjects. To characterize the nonlinear trajectories flexibly, a natural cubic spline-based approach was used to model the marker processes.

Of the 407 patients, 126 experienced graft failure. The Kaplan–Meier estimate of survival function for graft failure was obtained and compared to the fitted survival function of a Weibull model. Although the Weibull distribution provides a satisfactory fit, a piecewise-constant baseline hazard was used in the joint model to allow for more flexibility.

Three baseline covariates, age, gender, and weight, were considered in the multivariate longitudinal model specified in (6.1)–(6.2):

$$g_k\{E(y_{ik}(t)|b_{ik})\} = (\beta_{0k} + b_{i0,k}) + \beta_{1k}AGE_i + \beta_{2k}MALE_i$$

$$+\beta_{3k}WEIGHT_i + \sum_{l=1}^{3}(\tilde{\beta}_{lk} + b_{il,k})\mathcal{N}(t; \lambda_{lk}),$$

where $k = 1$ for GFR, $k = 2$ for hematocrit, and $k = 3$ for proteinuria, with

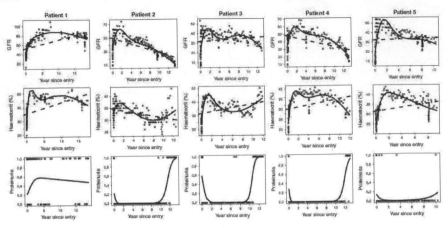

Figure 6.1 *Longitudinal response measurements for GFR, hematocrit, and protein-uria, for five randomly selected patients from the renal graft failure study. The solid lines depict the fitted subject-specific longitudinal profiles based on the multivariate joint model. The dashed lines depict the ordinary least squares fit.*

$g_k(\cdot)$ *being the identify function for $k = 1, 2$, and the logit function for $k = 3$, and $\mathcal{N}(\cdot)$ denotes the natural cubic splines basis. In the survival model (6.3), the same set of baseline covariates were considered and a piecewise constant function was assumed for $h_0(t)$ with knots at 2.87, 5.99, and 10.82 years which correspond to the 25th, 50th, and 75th percentiles of uncensored event times, respectively. The priors of model parameters were specified as follows: β and γ had $N(0, 100)$, and ρ had Gamma(2,1). The baseline risks ξ_t, $t = 1, 2, 3, 4$, were independent Gamma(0.1, 0.1). Parameterizations (6.4) and (6.6) were considered since parameterization (6.5) does not have intuitive interpretation for the random effects in the spline model. For (6.4), q was set to zero and a $N(0, 10)$ normal prior was used for α. For (6.6), the association between longitudinal and event processes was modeled by the joint distribution of b_i and u_i via a DP prior.*

Table 6.1 shows parameter estimates, standard errors, and 95% credibility intervals that were obtained after running the MCMC for 100,000 iterations with the first 50,000 as burn-in. The two models generated similar results for the longitudinal markers. At the survival endpoint, the estimates of α_1, α_2, and α_3 under parameterization (6.4) indicate that lower GFR, hematocrit, and higher proteinuria were associated with an increased risk of graft failure. Among the baseline covariates, only gender showed statistically significant effect, with a higher risk in males. The DIC criterion was used to compare model fit between (6.4) and (6.6). With a value of 1,382,119 and 1,395,714 for (6.4) and (6.6), respectively, it seemed the joint model using (6.4) provided a better fit to the data. Figure 6.1 suggests that the spline functions captured the main feature of observed trajectories on five randomly selected patients.

As a comparison, joint models were also fit for each marker individually using a simpler structure with random intercept and slope. A stronger association between each marker and the risk of graft failure was obtained, compared to its counterpart in the joint model with three markers simultaneously. This difference is expected because the markers were inter-correlated and the individual effect would be attenuated when other markers were included in the model as well. $\square$

Table 6.1 *Parameter estimates, standard errors, and 95% credibility intervals for the multivariate joint models fitted to the renal graft failure data.*

	Param(6.4)			Param(6.6)		
	Mean	SE	95% CI	Mean	SE	95% CI
Longitudinal process						
$Intercept_1$	22.79	2.02	(20.48; 26.95)	25.78	3.22	(17.86; 33.78)
Age_1	−0.31	0.01	(−0.32; −0.30)	−0.34	0.05	(−0.44; −0.23)
$Male_1$	0.10	0.15	(−0.21; 0.39)	0.05	1.39	(−2.83; 2.56)
$Weight_1$	0.38	0.01	(0.37; 0.39)	0.47	0.06	(0.35; 0.59)
$\ddot{\beta}_{11}$	−1.80	0.97	(−3.62; −0.13)	−2.07	0.25	(−2.55; −1.64)
$\ddot{\beta}_{12}$	4.17	1.63	(1.38; 7.79)	4.72	2.54	(−0.54; 9.81)
$\ddot{\beta}_{13}$	−6.60	0.75	(−8.00; −4.65)	−5.62	1.01	(−7.88; −3.61)
σ_1	13.03	0.04	(12.95; 13.10)	14.56	0.92	(12.74; 16.36)
$Intercept_2$	25.10	0.18	(24.74; 25.40)	23.89	1.06	(21.88; 25.95)
Age_2	0.04	0.001	(0.04; 0.04)	0.08	0.01	(0.05; 0.10)
$Male_2$	0.95	0.26	(0.46; 1.57)	1.18	0.35	(0.44; 1.84)
$Weight_2$	0.01	0.01	(0.01; 0.02)	0.02	0.02	(−0.01; 0.05)
$\ddot{\beta}_{21}$	−1.77	0.57	(−2.58; −0.35)	−2.27	0.96	(−4.03; −0.34)
$\ddot{\beta}_{22}$	27.53	0.62	(26.64; 28.81)	27.40	1.09	(25.41; 29.55)
$\ddot{\beta}_{23}$	6.53	0.72	(5.09; 7.51)	7.70	1.71	(4.30; 11.00)
σ_2	5.33	0.02	(5.30; 5.36)	5.44	0.08	(5.30; 5.64)
$Intercept_3$	−2.99	0.15	(−3.24; −2.66)	−3.02	0.14	(−3.29; −2.75)
Age_3	−0.01	0.01	(−0.02; −0.01)	−0.03	0.01	(−0.03; −0.01)
$Male_3$	0.03	0.04	(−0.05; 0.11)	0.03	0.03	(−0.01; 0.09)
$Weight_3$	0.03	0.01	(0.02; 0.03)	0.02	0.02	(0.00; 0.04)
$\ddot{\beta}_{31}$	0.01	0.57	(−0.81; 1.25)	0.08	0.61	(−1.12; 1.30)
$\ddot{\beta}_{32}$	−0.34	0.37	(−1.07; 0.28)	−0.56	0.44	(−1.46; 0.32)
$\ddot{\beta}_{33}$	2.66	0.57	(1.56; 3.71)	3.72	0.77	(2.12; 5.24)
Survival process						
α_1	−0.04	0.01	(−0.05; −0.02)	–	–	–
α_2	−0.03	0.01	(−0.04; −0.01)	–	–	–
α_3	0.66	0.08	(0.50; 0.81)	–	–	–
Age	−0.01	0.01	(−0.03; 0.01)	−0.02	0.01	(−0.03; 0.00)
Male	0.64	0.20	(0.26; 1.03)	0.52	0.20	(0.16; 0.94)
Weight	0.01	0.01	(−0.01; 0.03)	0.01	0.01	(0.00; 0.03)
ξ_1	0.80	0.44	(0.22; 1.85)	1.10	0.63	(0.44; 2.12)
ξ_2	0.85	0.51	(0.21; 2.05)	0.97	0.58	(0.19; 2.56)
ξ_3	0.32	0.20	(0.08; 0.76)	0.35	0.29	(0.13; 0.81)
ξ_4	0.57	0.35	(0.12; 1.56)	0.42	0.31	(0.08; 1.12)

The subscripts k=1,2, and 3 correspond to GFR, hematocrit, and proteinuria, respectively. The $\ddot{\beta}$'s denote the coefficients of the natural cubic spine for the three outcomes.

6.1.2 Latent Pattern Mixture Models

Estimation of the models discussed in Section 6.1.1 can be computationally intensive because the latent variables that are used to characterize the association between longitudinal and survival data are continuous in nature. As an alternative, latent pattern mixture models characterize class-specific evolution profiles of longitudinal and survival data based on the assumption that the population consists of heterogeneous sub-populations. Thus, discrete latent variables are used to specify the association between longitudinal and survival data. Such a model has been studied by Lin, McCulloch, and Rosenheck (2004)[148] (Section 4.5.1) to handle informative observation times in longitudinal studies. Another advantage of latent pattern mixture models is that it is straightforward to accommodate heterogeneous random effects across class patterns at the longitudinal endpoint. In the context of multiple longitudinal outcomes, the approach is illustrated using the following example in which quantitative random effects are used to characterize correlation among repeated measures of multiple responses, whereas the association between longitudinal and survival endpoints are captured by latent classes.

Model Formulation

We describe a latent pattern mixture model applied to a study of cognitive aging and dementia (Proust–Lima et al., 2009[178]). The profile of cognition is not directly observed, but is measured by several psychometric tests for which the scores are non-normally distributed. Suppose there are G unobserved sub-populations in the study. A latent variable $c_i = g$ if subject i belongs to class g, $i = 1, \ldots, n$ and $g = 1, \ldots, G$. A multinomial logistic regression is used to model the dependence of c_i on a vector of time-invariant covariates X_{1i}:

$$P(c_i = g | X_{1i}) = \pi_{ig} = \frac{exp(\gamma_{0g} + X_{1i}^T \gamma_{1g})}{\sum_{l=1}^{G} exp(\gamma_{0l} + X_{1i}^T \gamma_{1l})}, \tag{6.9}$$

where γ_{0g} is the intercept for class g and γ_{1g} is a vector of class-specific parameters associated with X_{1i}. For the sake of identifiability, $\gamma_{01} = \gamma_{11} = 0$.

Within each latent class, the multiple psychometric markers are assumed to be influenced by a shared latent process in continuous time $\{U_i(t)\}_{t \geq 0}$ which is interpreted as a measure of cognitive level on subject i. The latent cognitive level $U_i(t)$ is described by a linear mixed effects model specific to each class g:

$$U_i(t)|_{c_i=g} = X_{2i}(t)^T \beta + Z(t)^T b_{ig},$$

where $X_{2i}(t)$ is a vector of covariates with fixed effects β that are common to all classes, and $Z(t)$ is a vector of time-dependent covariates which can be polynomial functions to model the time trend. The random effects b_{ig} are assumed to have a class-specific normal distribution $N(\mu_g, \omega_g^2 \Sigma)$, where $\omega_1 = 1$ for identifiability and Σ is an unstructured variance-covariance matrix. Note the model can be generalized to allow class-specific β and Σ without difficulty.

The latent process $U_i(t)$ is then linked to the kth longitudinal outcome Y_{ik} via a flexible nonlinear measurement model

$$h_k(Y_{ik}(t); \eta_k) = U_i(t) + \alpha_{ik} + \epsilon_{ik}(t), \qquad (6.10)$$

where $h_k(y; \eta_k)$ is a Beta cumulative density function with parameters $\eta_k = (\eta_{1k}, \eta_{2k})$:

$$\tilde{Y}_{ik}(t) = h_k(Y_{ik}(t); \eta_k) = \frac{\int_0^y x^{\eta_{1k}-1}(1-x)^{\eta_{2k}-1}dx}{\int_0^1 x^{\eta_{1k}-1}(1-x)^{\eta_{2k}-1}dx}.$$

The Beta transformations are flexible and parsimonious, but require rescaling of Y_{ik} in $[0, 1]$ beforehand. The random intercept α_{ik} is subject- and marker-specific, characterizing additional within-individual correlation in each marker conditional on the latent cognitive level $U_i(t)$. Assume $\alpha_{ik} \sim N(0, \sigma_{\alpha_k}^2)$ and are independent of measurement errors $\epsilon_{ik}(t)$ which are distributed as $N(0, \sigma_{\epsilon_k}^2)$.

The third component is a class-specific proportional hazard model. Let T_i denote the event time and C_i the censoring time. We observe $(\tilde{T}_i, \Delta_i)$, where $\tilde{T}_i = min(T_i, C_i)$ and Δ_i is set to 1 if $T_i \leq C_i$ and 0 otherwise. The hazard function is specified as

$$\lambda(t|c_i = g, X_{3i}; \theta_g, \phi_g) = \lambda_{0g}(t; \theta_g)exp(X_{3i}^T\phi_g), \qquad (6.11)$$

where ϕ_g are class-specific parameters associated with covariates X_{3i} and $\lambda_{0g}(t; \theta_g)$ is the baseline hazard function for class g parameterized by θ_g. The baseline hazard can be modeled using a parametric distribution such as Weibull, a piecewise constant function, a semiparametric model through a spline basis, or completely unspecified. The simplest case is $\lambda_{0g}(t) = \lambda_0(t)exp(\phi_{0g})$ which assumes proportionality of hazard functions across classes.

Parameter Estimation

Parameter estimation can be done via a maximum likelihood method when the number of latent class G is given. The likelihood function is written out based on the assumption that longitudinal and survival endpoints are independent given the latent class membership. Let Ψ denote a vector of all parameters that appear in the model. The likelihood for subject i is

$$L_i(\Psi) = \sum_{g=1}^{G} P(c_i = g; \Psi)f(Y_i|c_i = g; \Psi)\lambda(\tilde{T}_i|c_i = g; \Psi)^{\Delta_i} S(\tilde{T}_i|c_i = g; \Psi),$$

$$(6.12)$$

where each component's density function can be written out based on (6.9)–(6.11). Note that the density $f(Y_i|c_i = g; \Psi)$ is a product of the multivariate normal density of transformed $\tilde{Y}_i$ and Jacobian of Beta transformation. A penalized likelihood approach can be used when the baseline hazard is estimated by splines. Maximum likelihood estimates are obtained via an EM algorithm or some Newton–Raphson type of algorithm to maximize the likelihood using the gradient and Hessian matrix. The EM algorithm relies on computation of the posterior probability of class membership in each E-step conditional on the observed data and current parameter estimates $\Psi^{(t)}$:

$$P^{(t+1)}(c_i = g | Y_i, \tilde{T}_i, \Delta_i; \Psi^{(t)})$$
$$= \frac{P(c_i = g; \Psi^{(t)}) f(Y_i, \tilde{T}_i, \Delta_i | c_i = g; \Psi^{(t)})}{\sum_{l=1}^{G} P(c_i = l; \Psi^{(t)}) f(Y_i, \tilde{T}_i, \Delta_i | c_i = l; \Psi^{(t)})}.$$

The posterior class membership of subject i can be determined using the class with the highest posterior probability.

The assumption of conditional independence between longitudinal and survival endpoints can be tested using a residual analysis. We refer the reader to Proust–Lima et al. (2009)[178] for further details. At last, the number of latent classes may be selected using the Bayes Information Criterion (BIC), which has been shown to work reasonably well compared to other criteria when determining the number of components in mixture models.

Example 6.2. *The PAQUID study*

The French prospective cohort study PAQUID was initiated in 1988 to evaluate normal and pathological aging among subjects 65 and older. Longitudinal measurements of cognitive impairment were taken at the initial visit and then at 1, 3, 5, 8, 10, 13 years. Occurrence of dementia was monitored during follow-up. The objective is to investigate the association between dementia and cognitive decline, with the latter being measured by three psychometric tests: the Isaacs Set Test (IST) to evaluate verbal fluency, the Benton Visual Retention Test (BVRT) to evaluate visual memory, and the Digit Symbol Substitution Test (DSSTW) of Wechsler to evaluate attention and logical reasoning; for all tests lower values indicate a more severe impairment. The analytic sample included 2383 subjects free of dementia at the study entry, 355 of which developed dementia during follow-up. Measurements after dementia were not considered in the analysis. The median and interquartile range of the number of measurements per participant was 4 (2–6) for IST, 3 (2–6) for BVRT, and 2 (1–4) for DSSTW. Three covariates were considered: age, gender, and educational level (those who graduated from primary school, e.g., obtained the CEP, the first French diploma, versus who did not). Out of the 2383 subjects, 1382 were women (58%) and 692 (29%) did not graduate from primary school.

The latent cognitive level $U_i(t)$ was characterized as a quadratic function of age to account for a nonlinear cognitive decline:

$$U_i(t)|_{c_i = g} = b_{0ig} + b_{1ig} \times AGE_i + b_{2ig} \times AGE_i^2 + \beta I_{t=T_{0i}},$$

where $b_{ig} = (b_{0ig}, b_{1ig}, b_{2ig})^T \sim N((\mu_{0g}, \mu_{1g}, \mu_{2g})^T, \omega_g^2 \Sigma)$, and $I_{t=T_{0i}}$ is a binary variable indicating whether the measurements were made at the initial visit to take into account the first passing effect. As specified previously, the longitudinal measurements of psychometric tests were linked to the latent process $U_i(t)$ via $h_k(Y_{ik}(t); (\eta_{1k}, \eta_{2k})) = U_i(t) + \alpha_{ik} + \epsilon_{ik}(t)$. Gender and education (binary, CEP versus not) were included in the class membership model as follows:

$$P(c_i = g | GENDER_i, CEP_i)$$
$$= \frac{exp(\gamma_{0g} + GENDER_i\gamma_{1g} + CEP_i\gamma_{2g})}{\sum_{l=1}^{G} exp(\gamma_{0l} + GENDER_i\gamma_{1l} + CEP_i\gamma_{2l})}.$$

In preliminary analyses, a common random effect variance across classes was assumed at the longitudinal endpoint. Three survival models were compared: a Weibull model and a semiparametric model, both of which assumed proportional hazards between classes, and a Weibull model stratified on the latent classes. The Weibull model assuming proportional hazards provided adequate fit compared to the other two based on the AIC selection criterion. This model was then expanded by including covariates gender and CEP:

$$\lambda(t)|_{c_i=g} = \lambda_0(t)exp(\phi_{0g} + GENDER_i\phi_1 + CEP_i\phi_2),$$

$g = 1, \ldots, G$, for G varying from 2 to 6. The baseline hazard $\lambda_0(t)$ had a Weibull distribution parameterized by θ_1 and θ_2. The smallest BIC was obtained when $G = 5$ $(BIC = 134733.60)$.

Results from the above model with five latent classes are given in Table 6.2. Education has a significant impact on class membership (likelihood ratio test (LRT) p<0.0001, df = 4), but gender does not (p = 0.084). Subjects with CEP are less likely in class 2 compared to those without CEP (the ratio of probability = $exp(-5.535)$ = 0.0039). Similarly, the ratio of probability is $exp(-7.163)$ = 0.0008 for being in class 4 and is $exp(-7.163)$ = 0.0119 for being in class 5 comparing the two education groups. This indicates that classes 2, 4, and 5 primarily consist of subjects without CEP and subjects with CEP are mostly in classes 1 and 3. Differential age effects on cognitive profiles across classes (the multivariate longitudinal model in Table 6.2) are presented more intuitively in Figure 6.2 (A). The cognitive level starts high in classes 1 and 3, but declines more rapidly in classes 3 and 4, which, as a consequence, leads to a higher probability of dementia (Figure 6.2 (B)). Class 5 has the most dramatic cognitive decline and the highest risk of developing dementia among all latent classes. At last, conditional on cognitive profiles, the risk of dementia is higher in subjects with CEP (Wald test p = 0.0055). □

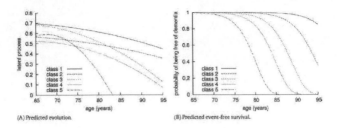

Figure 6.2 *(A) Predicted cognitive evolution according to age and (B) predicted survival curves without dementia according to age in the five-class model for a woman without CEP.*

Table 6.2 *Estimates (standard-errors) of the joint latent pattern mixture model with 5 classes.*

Parameter	Common estimates	Estimates specific to the latent classes				
		1	2	3	4	5
Class membership probability:						
Intercept		0	4.338	−10.944	3.714	2.104
			(0.942)	(88.28)	(0.947)	(0.975)
Gender[a]		0	−0.991	−0.155	−0.503	−0.245
(p=0.084)			(0.307)	(0.230)	(0.392)	(0.315)
CEP[b]		0	−5.535	9.932	−7.163	−4.435
(p < 0.0001)			(0.983)	(88.29)	(1.272)	(0.960)
Risk of dementia:						
θ_1	0.099					
	(0.001)					
θ_2	5.302					
	(0.284)					
ϕ_{0g}		1	1.879	3.686	4.927	6.572
			(0.337)	(0.337)	(0.418)	(0.401)
Gender[a]	−0.129					
	(0.145)					
CEP[b]	0.787					
	(0.269)					
Longitudinal multivariate model:						
Intercept		0.696	0.565	0.684	0.521	0.574
		(0.0096)	(0.012)	(0.016)	(0.018)	(0.031)
Age[c]		−0.0289	−0.0300	−0.0374	−0.0034	0.129
		(0.0075)	(0.012)	(0.0223)	(0.0197)	(0.057)
Age^{2}[c]		−0.018	−0.0135	−0.0497	−0.0489	−0.245
		(0.0026)	(0.0039)	(0.111)	(0.0083)	(0.032)
First visit TO	−0.017					
	(0.001)					

[a] Reference: Women.
[b] Reference: Subjects without CEP.
[c] Age in decades from 65 years old ($\frac{age-65}{10}$).

6.2   Joint Models for Recurrent Events and Longitudinal Data

Extension of joint models to recurrent events and multivariate survival times requires careful considerations about model formulation for the survival endpoint. Most of the work extends existing methods for recurrent events or multivariate survival data by incorporating longitudinal information. In this section we will look at methods for recurrent events. Multivariate survival data will be discussed in the next section.

The methods that have appeared in the literature for joint models with recurrent events are based on similar ideas discussed in Section 6.1, in which the association between longitudinal and survival data is specified by either continuous random effects or latent classes. Conditional on the latent variables, the recurrent event times can be characterized by transition models in which the transition intensity takes the function form of a Cox regression (Zhang *et al.*, 2008[251]). Han, Slate, and Peña (2007)[87] adopted a flexible recurrent event model in which the risk of recurrence is a function of accumulated events in the past. These approaches are described below in more detail.

6.2.1   Random-Effects Models

As mentioned previously, random effects or processes are naturally used to model the association between several outcomes of interest. Here we focus on the method developed by Zhang et al. (2008)[251] to illustrate the random-effects approach. The work was motivated by data from the Yale Mother and Infant Health study to assess effects of air quality on respiratory symptoms. Specially, the recurrent symptoms include runny nose, cough, and sore throat for mothers and runny nose, cough, and general sickness for infants. In this approach, each recurrent symptom is coded by a binary variable Z to indicate a normal state ($Z = 0$) and an abnormal state ($Z = 1$). The recurrent event process is then specified by a transition model, namely, transition from a normal state to an abnormal state ($0 \to 1$ with event intensity λ_1) and from an abnormal state to a normal state ($1 \to 0$ with event intensity λ_2). Air quality measures include the highest daily temperature (MTMP), humidity (MHUM), COARSE (the difference between PM_{10} and $PM_{2.5}$), and SO_4^{-2} (SO4). These longitudinal outcomes are denoted as Y_1, Y_2, Y_3, and Y_4, respectively. Thus, multiple outcomes at the longitudinal endpoint are another feature of this joint model.

The model is formulated to evaluate the association between the four longitudinal air quality measures and one respiratory symptom. The longitudinal measurements on subject i, $i = 1, \ldots, n$, are specified by

$$Y_{ik}(t) = \mu_{ik}(t) + W_{ik}(t), \tag{6.13}$$

where $\mu_{ik}(t)$ is the marginal mean of the kth air quality measure, $k = 1, 2, 3, 4$, which could be a function of time-varying covariates and some parametric or non-parametric functions of time. The random process $W_{ik}(t)$ has a zero mean and is decomposed into

$$W_{ik}(t) = q_k U_i(t) + \sigma_k \mathcal{E}_{ik}(t),$$

where $U_i(t)$ and $\mathcal{E}_i(t) = (\mathcal{E}_{i1}(t), \mathcal{E}_{i2}(t), \mathcal{E}_{i3}(t), \mathcal{E}_{i4}(t))$ are independent zero mean Gaussian processes with unit variance, and the coefficients q_k and σ_k are non-negative. The independence assumption is imposed here for the sake of uniqueness of the decomposition. The process $U_i(t)$ represents the underlying air pollution index that is shared by all four air quality measures, whereas each of $\mathcal{E}_{ik}(t)$, $k = 1, \ldots, 4$, is additional data variation that is unique to their associated air quality measure. The power exponential correlation function $\rho(\alpha, t) = exp(-\alpha|t|^\delta)$, $t \geq 0$, $0 < \delta \leq 2$, is used to describe the within-process correlations for $U_i(t)$ and $\mathcal{E}_{ik}(t)$. In particular, their t-lag correlation functions are written as $\rho_1(\alpha_1, t)$ and $\rho_{2k}(\alpha_{2k}, t)$, respectively.

In this study, it is hypothesized that air quality affects the transitions from a normal state to an abnormal state (with intensity λ_1) and from an abnormal state to a normal state (with intensity λ_2) through the latent process $U_i(t)$. For subject i and transition s, $s = 1, 2$,

$$\lambda_{is}(t) = exp\{X_i(t)^T \beta_s + \mathcal{B}_{is}(t)\}\lambda_s, \tag{6.14}$$

where $X_i(t)$ are possibly time-varying covariates, $\mathcal{B}_{is}(t) = \gamma_{0s}a_i + \gamma_s U_i(t)$ with $a_i \sim i.i.d.$ $N(0, 1)$ being a frailty independent of $U_i(t)$ and $\mathcal{E}_{ik}(t)$, and λ_s is a transition-specific parameter. This model indicates that the transition intensity for recurrent respiratory symptoms is affected by covariates $X_i(t)$, the latent air quality index $U_i(t)$, and the subject-specific frailty a_i that cannot be explained by $U_i(t)$.

Let Ψ denote all the parameters, and $N = \{(N_i^{(1)}(t), N_i^{(2)}(t)) : 0 < t \leq T, i = 1, \ldots, n\}$ in which the two counting processes are defined as

$$N_i^{(1)}(t) = \#\{0 < u \leq t : Z_i(u) = 1, Z_i(u-) = 0\},$$
$$N_i^{(2)}(t) = \#\{0 < u \leq t : Z_i(u) = 0, Z_i(u-) = 1\}.$$

Note that $N_i^{(1)}(0) = N_i^{(2)}(0) = 0$. Further, denote $L_1(\Psi, Y)$ the density of the marginal multivariate normal distribution of Y and $L_2(\Psi, N|U, a)$ the conditional density of the county process N given U and a. For the sake of simplicity, we drop the index i. The likelihood for Ψ is then

$$L(\Psi) = L_1(\Psi, Y)E_{(U,a)|Y}[L_2(\Psi, N|U, a)], \tag{6.15}$$

where $E_{(U,a)|Y}$ denotes the expectation with respect to U and a conditional on Y.

A two-stage strategy is proposed to estimate Ψ. In stage I, the marginal mean function $\mu_k(t)$ is pre-estimated by a weighted moving average,

$$\hat{\mu}_k(t) = \sum_{s=-m_0}^{m_0} w(s)Y_k(t+s),$$

using pre-specified weights $\{w(s) : s = -m_0, -m_0 + 1, \ldots, 0, \ldots, m_0 - 1, m_0\}$.

The first component in (6.15), $L_1(\Psi, Y)$, is then maximized to estimate α_1, α_{2k}, q_k, and σ_k. In stage II, the maximum likelihood estimates from stage I are treated as known and an EM algorithm is used to maximize $E_{(U,a)|Y}[L_2(\Psi, N|U, a)]$ for estimation of parameters in the recurrent process model. Note that the E-step could be computationally intensive due to integration with respect to U and a. One solution is to use the MCEM algorithm via a Gibbs sampler to approximate the integrals.

Example 6.3. *The Yale Mother and Infant Health Study*

As introduced previously, the Yale Mother and Infant Health (YMIH) study had four air quality measures, MTMP, MHUM, COARSE, and SO4. Their effects on each of the six respiratory symptoms (mother: running nose, cough, and sore throat; infant: running nose, cough, and general sickness) were evaluated using the joint model specified in (6.13) and (6.14).

The normality assumption was examined for the four air quality measures and transformation was applied to MTMP and MHUM using the function $(e^{\kappa y} - 1)/\kappa$, where $\kappa = 0.35$ and 0.45 for MTMP and MHUM, respectively. In stage I, estimates of model parameters in the marginal distribution of air quality measures were obtained. Figure 6.3 shows the mean processes estimated by the moving average method. Specifically, the parameter m_0 was set to 10 and constant weights were given to all points falling in the moving window. To check the fit of estimated latent process U, the study duration (0–83 days) was split into eight intervals. Although U is one component of $W_k(t)$, the density of U at the center of each time interval was found to be consistent with the histogram of pooled residuals (calculated as $\hat{W}_k(t) = Y_k(t) - \hat{\mu}_k(t)$) except in the interval between days 11 and 20 (results not shown).

In stage II, the parameters estimated in stage I were treated as known and an EM algorithm augmented by the Gibbs sampler was employed to obtain maximum likelihood estimates of the transition model parameters for recurrent respiratory symptoms. In particular, 500, 2,000, 10,000, and 40,000 repetitions were used in the Gibbs sampler in iterations 1–20, 21–40, 41–50, and over 50, respectively. In addition to U, the mean responses $\mu_k(t)$, $k = 1, \ldots, 4$, were considered in the model as fixed effects, and in each model only one of them was included to avoid inter-correlation of the four $\mu_k(t)$'s. It turned out the choice of air quality measures (i.e., which $\mu_k(t)$ to use, $k = 1, \ldots, 4$) had little impact on the effects of other covariates in $X_i(t)$.

Table 6.3 shows the estimated parameters for mothers' symptoms. The effects of $U_i(t)$, a_i, and baseline covariates were estimated from the model when the mean response of COARSE was included. The latent air quality index $U_i(t)$ does not seem to have a significant impact on symptoms, but each symptom shows substantial between-subject variability in their event risk (a_i). The mean response of COARSE is associated with an elevated risk of running nose and cough, whereas MHUM is related to a lower risk of cough. Among the baseline covariates, allergy and having pets (PET) predict an increased risk of running

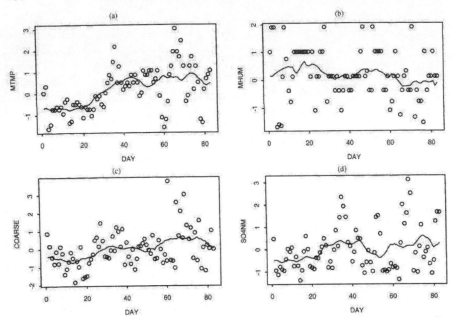

Figure 6.3 *Time series plots for the four air quality measures in the YMIH study. The dots represent the air quality data and the lines are moving average estimates of the mean process*

nose, married women (MS) have more frequent sore throat, and women with children in daycare or school (CHDC) are less likely to have sore throat. The second part of Table 6.3 reports the estimated transition model $\lambda_2(t)$, i.e., recovery from the symptoms. None of the effects are statistically significant. This might be due to the fact that respiratory symptoms usually are alleviated by medications and go away in about one week or so, which potentially reduces between-subject variability.

Different from the estimated model for mothers' symptoms, the latent air quality index $U_i(t)$ has a significant impact on infants' running nose symptom (Table 6.4). The highest daily temperature (MTMP) and Sulfate level (SO4) predict a deceased risk of running nose and cough, whereas COARSE and MHUM are not associated with the symptoms. There is also considerable between-subject variability in recovery from running nose. These differences from the findings for mothers' symptoms may deserve further investigation. □

Table 6.3 *Effects of air quality and covariates on mothers' symptoms*

Variable	Runny Nose Coefficient estimate	Runny Nose Standard error	Cough Coefficient estimate	Cough Standard error	Throat Coefficient estimate	Throat Standard error
$\lambda_1(t)$						
$U(t)$	.025	.082	−.043	.119	−.019	.095
a	1.092*	.135	1.571*	.199	1.010*	.147
COARSE	.404*	.202	.595*	.285	.232	.218
MTMP	.146	.140	.195	.195	.046	.151
SO4	.226	.238	.642	.334	.111	.261
MHUM	−.644	.356	−1.029*	.504	−.368	.392
ALLERGY	.598*	.241	.444	.354	.368	.247
PETS	.526*	.244	.245	.377	.139	.249
MS	.584	.379	.080	.515	1.073*	.434
CHDC	−.252	.154	−.366	.241	−.315*	.159
$\lambda_2(t)$						
$U(t)$	.065	.082	.074	.111	−.166	.096
a	.004	.139	.115	.163	−.052	.119
COARSE	−.267	.202	.228	.301	−.150	.237
MTMP	−.185	.147	.109	.226	−.095	.168
SO4	−.231	.252	.194	.382	−.267	.274
MHUM	.544	.358	−.480	.527	.288	.418
ALLERGY	−.255	.182	.032	.262	.063	.203
PETS	.209	.172	.163	.307	.150	.200
MS	−.576	.312	−.290	.423	−.469	.402
CHDC	.046	.133	−.009	.214	−.090	.153

NOTE: COARSE, MTMP, SO4, and MHUM represent the effects of their mean trends, and they were included in the model one at a time. Inclusion of which means air quality in the model had very little effect on the estimates of the other parameters, and this table is based on the model with COARSE included.
* Significant effects at the .05 level.

6.2.2   Latent Pattern Mixture Models

As stated previously, latent pattern mixture models are an appealing alternative of random-effects models if it is hypothesized that the whole population consists of heterogeneous sub-populations. In latent pattern mixture models, the association of longitudinal and event time data is usually simplified by the conditional independence assumption given class membership. In what follows, we look at the latent pattern mixture joint model proposed by Han, Slate, and Peña (2007)[87] to handle recurrent event times. The model has three components: a multinomial regression to characterize the marginal distribution of latent classs, a class-specific linear mixed effects model for the longitudinal outcome of interest, and a class-specific recurrent event time model. This approach extends the method by Lin, McCulloch, and Rosenheck (2004)[148] (Section 4.5.1) to the situation of recurrent event times.

Specifically, the class membership is modeled by a multinomial logistic regression with covariates X_i for subject i:

$$\pi_{ik} = P(c_{ik} = 1) = \frac{exp(X_i^T \eta_k)}{\sum_{l=1}^{G} exp(X_i^T \eta_l)},$$

where $i = 1, \ldots, n$, $k = 1, \ldots, G$ is the class membership with G being

Table 6.4 *Effects of air quality and covariates on infants' symptoms*

	Runny Nose		Cough		Throat	
Variable	Coefficient estimate	Standard error	Coefficient estimate	Standard error	Coefficient estimate	Standard error
$\lambda_1(t)$						
$U(t)$	−.188*	.081	.038	.109	.027	.077
a	.811*	.107	1.000*	.153	.596*	.118
COARSE	−.159	.157	−.425	.222	.031	.172
MTMP	−.220*	.107	−.321*	.151	.002	.120
SO4	−.419*	.188	−.653*	.266	−.024	.206
MHUM	−.025	.284	.676	.401	−.032	.307
PETS	−.018	.176	.092	.248	.192	.165
MS	.372	.254	−.341	.311	.362	.246
CHDC	−.110	.109	−.245	.159	−.050	.098
$\lambda_2(t)$						
$U(t)$	.033	.070	−.131	.109	−.041	.075
a	.152*	.076	.031	.131	−.110	.113
COARSE	.170	.156	.167	.225	.045	.181
MTMP	.105	.110	.112	.156	.068	.127
SO4	.101	.189	.079	.269	.077	.212
MHUM	−.023	.285	.143	.430	.173	.326
PETS	−.169	.138	.150	.199	.028	.155
MS	−.361	.199	−.246	.235	−.226	.229
CHDC	.038	.098	.059	.144	.065	.101

NOTE: COARSE, MTMP, SO4, and MHUM represent the effects of their mean trends, and they were included in the model one at a time. Inclusion of which means air quality in the model had very little effect on the estimates of the other parameters, and this table is based on the model with COARSE included.
* Significant effects at the .05 level.

the total number of latent classes, and X_i and η_k are vectors of covariates and class-specific regression coefficients, respectively. Set $\eta_1 = 0$ for the sake of identifiability. Note that $\sum_{k=1}^{G} \pi_{ik} = 1$ and $c_i = (c_{i1}, \ldots, c_{iG})^T \sim$ multinomial$(\pi_{i1}, \ldots, \pi_{iG})$.

The distribution of the longitudinal outcome $Y_i = (Y_{i1}, \ldots, Y_{in_i})$ is given by

$$Y_i = Z_i \beta + \tilde{Z}_i b_i + W_i(Mc_i) + \epsilon_i, \tag{6.16}$$

where Z_i and $\tilde{Z}_i$ are matrices of covariates, β is a vector of fixed effects, b_i are random effects distributed as $N(0, \Sigma)$, W_i is a matrix of covariates with class-specific effects, and $M = (\mu_1, \ldots, \mu_G)$ are class-specific effects so we have $Mc_i = \mu_k$ if $c_{ik} = 1$. At last, the measurement error ϵ_i is assumed to follow $N(0, \sigma^2 I_{n_i})$. The first component in (6.16), $Z_i \beta$, characterizes the common fixed effects shared by all study subjects, whereas $W_i(Mc_i)$ quantifies the class-specific deviation of effects from $Z_i \beta$. For the ease of estimation, no constraints are posited for M, but the model requires no overlap in the covariates of W and Z to ensure identifiability.

The recurrent event process can be expressed using the counting process framework:

$$\{(N_i^\dagger(s), R_i^\dagger(s), x_i(s), \mathscr{F}_{is}, s \geq 0\},$$

where $N_i^\dagger(s)$ is the number of events observed over $[0, s]$, $R_i^\dagger(s)$ is the at-risk indicator at time s, and $x_i(s)$ is a vector of possibly time-dependent covariates hypothesized to be associated with recurrence. Define $\mathscr{E}_i(s)$ as the effective age of subject i at calendar time s. The natural filtration generated by the data is $\mathscr{F}_{is} = \sigma\{(N_i^\dagger(v), R_i^\dagger(v+), x_i(v+), \mathscr{E}_i(v+)) : v \leq s\}$, with respect to which $R_i^\dagger(\cdot)$, $x_i(\cdot)$, and $\mathscr{E}_i(\cdot)$ are predictable processes.

The class-specific recurrent event model is given by

$$P(dN_i^\dagger(s) = 1|\mathscr{F}_{is-}, c_{ik} = 1, \omega_i)$$
$$= \omega_i R_i^\dagger(s)\lambda_k^0(\mathscr{E}_i(s))\rho(E_i(N_i^\dagger(s-)), \alpha_k)\psi(\gamma^T x_i(s))ds,$$

where ω_i is a latent frailty variable assumed to follow a gamma distribution with mean 1, $\lambda_k^0(\mathscr{E}_i(s))$ is the class-specific baseline hazard function, $E_i(N_i^\dagger(s-))$ is the number of accumulated events just before time s, $\rho(j, \alpha)$ is the event accumulation effect function of known form with $\rho(0, \alpha) = 1$, and $\psi(\cdot)$ is a nonnegative link function of known form. Different from (6.14), this model assumes that the past history of recurrence may have an impact on the recurrence yet to occur.

The effective age $\mathscr{E}_i(s)$ is an observable, nonnegative, and nondecreasing process. It could be a piecewise linear or nonlinear function of calendar time. The function $\rho(\cdot, \alpha)$, which characterizes the effect of accumulating events, can be either increasing or decreasing, depending on whether the event occurrence worsens or improves the subject's condition. A simple example is given by the exponential function $\rho(j, \alpha) = \alpha^j$, $j = 1, 2, \ldots$.

It is reasonable to assume that the longitudinal and recurrent event processes are independent of each other if the class membership is known. Not specific to the topic discussed in this section, the conditional independence assumption is commonly used in latent pattern mixture joint models. Based on this assumption, the likelihood on subject i is then written as

$$f(Y_i, N_i^\dagger, R_i^\dagger|O_i, c_{ik} = 1) = f(Y_i|O_i, c_{ik} = 1)f(N_i^\dagger, R_i^\dagger|O_i, c_{ik} = 1),$$

where O_i denotes all covariates on subject i. Model estimation can be carried out using an EM algorithm. See Section 6.1.2 for more details.

6.3 Joint Models for Multivariate Survival and Longitudinal Data

Multivariate survival data arise in studies with a clustered design (e.g., twins, families), and are also seen in cancer research, such as time to relapse in different organs, disease-free survival, and overall survival. It is often of interest to investigate the inter-correlation between these multiple failure times and their association with longitudinal outcomes. Similar to joint models for recurrent event times, the association between longitudinal and survival data can be specified by either random effects or latent classes. The methods in Section 6.2 can be easily extended to studies with multivariate survival data.

In this section we describe in detail the model proposed by Chi and Ibrahim (2006)[40] for bivariate survival data and multiple longitudinal outcomes. One distinguishing feature of this joint model is that the survival endpoint accommodates a non-zero cure fraction. The work was motivated by a clinical trial designed to study the duration of adjuvant chemotherapy and reintroduction of delayed chemotherapy in premenopausal women with node-positive breast cancer (the IBCSG study). Repeated measurements were available on four quality of life (QOL) indicators, which were self-assessed and subject to missing data and measurement error. Two failure times, disease-free survival (DFS) and overall survival (OS), were monitored for cancer progression. The Kaplan–Meier curve of DFS shows a plateau after 12 years, suggesting a possible cure fraction in the patients which might be a result of advances in breast cancer medications. In this joint analysis, the survival model uses a shared frailty to induce the correlation between DFS and OS, and each marginal survival function incorporates zero and non-zero cure fractions for the event time.

Since this study has multiple QOL outcomes, a multivariate normal mixed effects model is used to characterize the data distribution. Let $Y_{ik}(t_{ij})$ be the kth outcome measured at time t_{ij}, $k = 1, \ldots, K$ with K being the total number of longitudinal outcomes. The model for $Y_{ik}(t_{ij})$ is

$$Y_{ik}(t_{ij}) = Y_{ik}^*(t_{ij}) + \epsilon_{ijk},$$

where $Y_{ik}^*(t_{ij})$ is the trajectory function for the kth outcome and ϵ_{ijk} are measurement errors. The trajectory $Y_{ik}^*(t_{ij})$ is expressed as a function of $X_{ik}(t_{ij})$ which is a vector of covariates for the kth outcome measured at time t_{ij} and its subset $\tilde{X}_{ik}(t_{ij})$:

$$Y_{ik}^*(t_{ij}) = X_{ik}(t_{ij})\beta_k + \tilde{X}_{ik}(t_{ij})b_{ik},$$

where β_k and b_{ik} are fixed and random effects, respectively.

Let $\epsilon_{ij.} = (\epsilon_{ij1}, \ldots, \epsilon_{ijK})^T$, a vector of measurement errors for all K outcomes for subject i at time t_{ij}. Assume that $\epsilon_{ij.} \sim N(0, \Sigma_\epsilon)$ and are independent of each other for different i and t_{ij}. The structure of Σ_ϵ captures the association between multivariate longitudinal outcomes measured at the same occasion. The random effects b_{ik} are assumed to be i.i.d. $N(0, \Sigma_k)$. Note that since b_{ik} are independent for different i and k, they are used solely to characterize the association among the repeated measurements within each outcome over time. At last, assume $\epsilon_{ijk} \perp b_{ik}$ to ensure identifiability. One implicit assumption of this model is that the longitudinal outcomes are uncorrelated at different occasions.

To characterize the association between the multivariate QOL outcomes and bivariate survival times (DFS and OS), as well as the inter-correlation between DFS and OS, a bivariate survival model is developed on the basis of nonhomogeneous Poisson processes that are extended to incorporate covariates and latent QOL trajectories $Y_{ik}^*(t_{ij})$. As is seen in the following, the model is developed to reflect the carcinogenic mechanism in cancer progression. This approach is flexible in that it provides the possibility of accommodating both nonzero and zero cure fractions in survival functions.

Let $T = (T_1, T_2)$ be the bivariate survival variable. In the IBCSG example, T_1 is time to progression and T_2 is time to death. Assume for each T_m, $m = 1, 2$, there are latent precursors which accumulate over time and T_m manifests itself when any precursor develops into an event. In the context of the IBCSG data, the precursors can be conceived as metastasis-competent tumor cells. Let $N(t) = (N_1(t), N_2(t))$ be the number of latent precursors generated at time t. Define

$$N_m^* = \int_0^{t_m} N_m(\mu)d\mu$$

as the number of precursors accumulated up to time t_m for T_m, $m = 1, 2$. Assume that conditional on a latent variable w (frailty), the precursor generating process follows a Poisson distribution:

$$N_m(t)|w \sim Pois(w\lambda_m(t)),$$

where $w\lambda_m(t)$ is the mean of the Poisson process at time t, and $N_1(t)$ and $N_2(t)$ are independent given w. That is, w induces the correlation between the two event processes. As a result, N_1^* and N_2^* are also Poisson variables with means $w\Lambda_1(t_1)$ and $w\Lambda_2(t_2)$, respectively, where $\Lambda_m(t_m) = \int_0^{t_m} \lambda_m(\mu)d\mu$, $m = 1, 2$.

Assume each precursor has a latent event time denoted by U_{ml}, $l = 1, \ldots, N_m^*$, and occurrence of any event leads to an observed T_m. Conditional on N_m^*, the latent event times U_{ml} are assumed to be i.i.d. random variables with distribution function $F_m(t) = 1 - S_m(t)$, and this distribution function is independent of N_m^*. The independence assumption is reasonable in the context of cancer development because N_m^* may not have any impact on the progression of each precursor. The joint survival function of T_1 and T_2 conditional on w is

$$S^*(t_1, t_2|w) = \prod_{m=1}^{2} [P(N_m^* = 0) + \sum_{n_m^*=1}^{\infty} P(T_m > t_m|N_m^*)P(N_m^* = n_m^*)]$$

$$= exp\{-w[\int_0^{t_1} \lambda_1(t)F_1(t_1 - t)dt + \int_0^{t_2} \lambda_2(t)F_2(t_2 - t)dt]\}.$$

The frailty w is taken to follow a positive stable law distribution with density

$$f_s(w|\rho) = \rho^* w^{-(\rho^*+1)} \int_0^1 s(u)exp[-\frac{s(u)}{w^{\rho^*}}]du$$

for $w > 0$ and $0 < u < 1$, where $\rho^* = \frac{\rho}{1-\rho}$ and $s(u) = [\frac{sin(\rho\pi u)}{sin(\pi u)}]^{\rho^*}[\frac{sin[(1-\rho)\pi u]}{sin(\pi u)}]$.

The parameter ρ determines the strength of association between T_1 and T_2 with a small ρ indicating a high association.

The positive stable law distribution is chosen because of its desirable properties. The resultant unconditional bivariate survival function has a simple form:

$$S^*(t_1, t_2) = exp\{-[\int_0^{t_1} \lambda_1(\mu)F_1(t_1 - \mu)d\mu$$

$$+ \int_0^{t_2} \lambda_2(\mu)F_2(t_2 - \mu)d\mu]^\rho\}.$$

Based on the above equation, the marginal survival functions are given by

$$S^*(t_m) = exp\{-[\int_0^{t_m} \lambda_m(\mu)F_m(t_m - \mu)d\mu]^\rho\},$$

for $m = 1, 2$. The marginal cure fraction is then

$$S_m^*(\infty) = exp\{-[\lim_{t\to\infty} \int_0^\infty \lambda_m(\mu)F_m(t - \mu)d\mu]^\rho\}.$$

It is clear that the cure fraction is nonzero if $\lim_{t\to\infty} \int_0^\infty \lambda_m(\mu)F_m(t - \mu)d\mu$ is bounded and thus the marginal survival function is improper. Proper marginal survival functions are obtained when $S_m^*(\infty) = 0$. The bivariate survival function can accommodate a mixture of proper and improper marginal survival functions since each event type has its own parameters to determine the cure fraction.

The impact of longitudinal trajectories $Y_k^*(t)$ and baseline covariates Z on the event risks is modeled through $\lambda_m(t)$, the mean number (which is time-varying) of latent precursors. To be specific, $\lambda_m(t)$ is assumed to take the following form:

$$\lambda_m(t) = exp\{\sum_{k=1}^K \gamma_{mk}Y_k^*(t) + Z\delta_m\}, \tag{6.17}$$

for $m = 1, 2$. Equation (6.17) implies that the latent trajectories $Y_k^*(t)$, which are shared by $\lambda_1(t)$ and $\lambda_2(t)$, induce additional correlation between T_1 and T_2. Thus, the association between the two failure types is captured by the frailty w and latent longitudinal trajectories.

Let T denote the bivariate survival data, Y the longitudinal QOL outcomes, and Z and X the covariates associated with T and Y, respectively. Based on the assumption that the bivariate event times are independent of repeated measurements of multivariate QOL outcomes given the latent QOL trajectories (denoted by Y^*), the likelihood of the observed data is

$$P(T, Y|Z, X) = \int p(T|Z, Y^*)P(Y|Y^*)P(Y^*|X)dY^*.$$

We refer the reader to Chi and Ibrahim (2006)[40] for more details about the functional form of each component in the above likelihood. In the context of the IBCSG study, a Bayesian approach is adopted for estimation and inference, assuming non-informative priors for all model parameters. The Gibbs sampler is used for parameters with closed form full conditional distributions, including parameters in the multivariate longitudinal model and N_m^*, $m = 1$, 2. The adaptive rejection algorithm is used for parameters without closed form full conditional distributions, and an extra Metropolis step is incorporated for those without log concave full conditionals.

Example 6.4. *The IBCSG Study*

In the IBCSG trial, premenopausal women with node-positive breast cancer were randomized according to a 2 × 2 factorial design to receive either six initial courses of CMF (oral cyclophosphamide, methotrexate, and fluorouracil) from months 1 to 6 with or without three single courses of reintroduction CMF given on months 9, 12, and 15; or three initial courses of CMF from months 1 to 3 with or without three single courses of reintroduction CMF given on months 6, 9, and 12. This example focuses on 832 patients from Switzerland, Sweden, and New Zealand/Australia. The study participants received QOL questionnaires at baseline, 3 months, and 18 months to self-assess their physical well-being (lousy-good), mood (miserable-happy), appetite (none-good), and perceived coping ("How much effort does it cost you to cope with your illness?" [a great deal-none]). The scores were between 0 and 100 with a higher value indicating a better perceived QOL. Median QOL scores over time (Figure 6.4) suggest an improvement in mood and perceived coping at 18 months compared to baseline. However, these two items were consistently scored lower on average than appetite and physical well-being throughout the study. During follow-up, patients were monitored for their DFS and OS, with DFS defined as the time from randomization to any relapse, occurrence of a second primary cancer, or death. The median DFS is 7.61 years with a censoring rate of 46.39%, and the median OS is 9.26 years with a censoring rate of 63.10%. The Kaplan–Meier curve for DFS indicates a nonzero cure fraction (∼ 40%) after about 12 years of follow-up.

The previously described joint model was applied to study the association between QOL, DFS, and OS. Transformation $(100 - QOL)^{1/2}$ was applied to normalize QOL measurements, so the range became 0 to 10 after transformation, with a lower value indicating a better condition. A random intercept and random slope model hypothesizing a linear time trend was used to specify the latent QOL trajectories. Baseline covariates considered in the QOL measurement model included adjuvant therapy (# initial cycle and reintroduction), age, and residency. Adjuvant therapy, age, number of positive nodes, and ER status were considered for DFS and OS in the bivariate survival model.

Posterior means and their 95% highest probability density (HPD) intervals for parameters in the QOL measurement model are presented in Table 6.5. Patients who had six initial CMF courses reported a worse QOL in the domains of

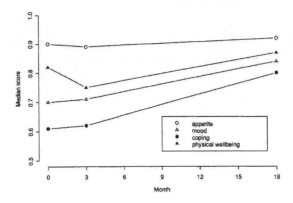

Figure 6.4 *Median QOL scores over time.*

coping with the disease, mood, and physical well-being, compared to those with three initial courses. Reintroduction of CMF as well as its interaction with the number of initial cycles does not seem to have a significant impact on QOL. Older patients and those who lived in Switzerland or Sweden tended to report a lower QOL. There is a negative correlation between the random intercept and random slope (the off-diagonal element of Σ_k; results not shown), implying that patients with better QOL scores at baseline would achieve less improvement over time. The four QOL domains measured at the same occasion are positively correlated as indicated by the estimated off-diagonal elements of Σ_ϵ. The empirical correlations of estimated b_{ik} between the QOL domains have a range of (0.004, 0.093), suggesting that the independence assumption for b_{ik} across k may be plausible.

Table 6.5 *Posterior means (with 95% HPD intervals in parentheses) for regression coefficients in the longitudinal model of the IBCSG data*

	Appetite	Coping	Mood	Physical well-being
Intercept	3.494	5.276	4.278	3.945
	(3.227, 3.764)	(4.880, 5.624)	(4.008, 4.544)	(3.739, 4.176)
Time(in years)	−0.578	−0.974	−0.725	−0.515
	(−0.687, −0.465)	(−1.112, −0.852)	(−0.845, −0.586)	(−0.637, −0.368)
#Initial cycle	0.0173	0.367	0.460	0.268
	(−0.265, 0.251)	(0.045, 0.691)	(0.185, 0.747)	(0.027, 0.570)
Reintroduction	−0.064	0.124	0.182	−0.059
	(−0.378, 0.263)	(−0.189, 0.439)	(−0.097, 0.441)	(−0.314, 0.212)
#Initial cycle × reintroduction	−0.025	−0.278	−0.403	−0.054
	(−0.411, 0.388)	(−0.718, 0.192)	(−0.772, 0.007)	(−0.474, 0.322)
Age > 40	0.483	0.295	0.561	0.701
	(0.266, 0.744)	(0.016, 0.601)	(0.360, 0.777)	(0.497, 0.900)
Residency: Swiss	0.084	0.374	0.304	0.070
	(−0.144, 0.327)	(0.105, 0.641)	(0.083, 0.527)	(−0.147, 0.308)
Residency: Sweden	0.199	0.502	0.993	0.681
	(−0.080, 0.462)	(0.211, 0.781)	(0.733, 1.243)	(0.446, 0.926)

Table 6.6 *Posterior means and 95% HPD intervals for parameters in the survival model.*

	DFS	OS
α	0.030(0.007, 0.061)	0.007(0.001, 0.014)
Appetite	0.196(−0.009, 0.423)	0.157(−0.087, 0.413)
Coping score	0.115(−0.095, 0.318)	0.087(−0.134, 0.290)
Mood	0.095(−0.209, 0.380)	0.161(−0.178, 0.489)
Physical well-being	0.145(−0.283, 0.539)	0.176(−0.235, 0.581)
# Initial cycle	0.232(−0.438, 0.874)	0.405(−0.306, 1.155)
Reintroduction	−0.270(−0.948, 0.412)	−0.272 (−1.011, 0.474)
# Initial cycle × reintroduction	−0.314(−1.294, 0.600)	−0.157(−1.207, 0.918)
Age>40	−1.185(−1.779, −0.600)	−0.957(−1.575, −0.307)
# Positive nodes > 4	2.309(1.750, 2.856)	2.492(1.913, 3.076)
ER(1= positive)	−0.060(−0.569, 0.490)	−0.436(−1.018, 0.132)
ρ	0.396(0.352, 0.439)	

Table 6.6 summarizes estimated parameters for the survival model. For both DFS and OS, the posterior means of the four time-varying QOL measures are all positive, suggesting that patients with a better QOL were less likely to relapse or die, but the 95% HPD intervals of these effects do not exclude zero. The number of initial cycles, reintroduction of CMF, and ER status do not seem to affect DFS or OS. Older patients showed a lower risk of relapse and death; this suggests that patients older than 40 might have different cancer progression mechanisms compared to those under 40. Increased positive nodes (> 4) at baseline are associated with an increased risk of DFS and OS. The parameter ρ has a posterior mean of 0.396 with a 95% HPD interval (0.352, 0.439), suggesting a moderate, positive association between DFS and OS.

Incorporating covariates into the survival model yields subject-specific cure fractions for DFS and OS. The marginal cure fraction has a posterior mean of 0.303 (SD = 0.133) and 0.363 (SD = 0.168) for DFS and OS, respectively, indicating that on average 30.3% patients are not susceptible to cancer relapse and 36.6% would not die of the cancer after surgery. □

Chapter 7

Further Topics

This chapter reviews topics in specific areas of joint modeling of longitudinal and time-to-event data, including model assumption assessment (i.e., sensitivity analysis and model diagnostics), variable selection, multistate models, cure rate survival data, and sample size estimation for joint models. Some of these areas, such as variable selection and sample size estimation, have not been fully explored and additional research is necessary to investigate their applications in different studies.

7.1 Joint Models and Missing Data: Assumptions, Sensitivity Analysis, and Diagnostics

As discussed in Chapter 2, missing data generated under the *missing completely at random* (MCAR) and *missing at random* (MAR) mechanisms are *ignorable*, meaning that if the response variable model and missingness mechanism have distinct parameters, valid statistical inference about the response variable can be obtained based on the likelihood of observed data if missingness is MCAR or MAR. On the other hand, under the *missing not at random* (MNAR) assumption, the probability of missingness is dependent on missing, unobserved measurements. As a result, ignoring the missing data could lead to biased estimates.

As has been discussed in previous chapters, a great body of research on non-ignorable missing data in longitudinal studies employs selection models to characterize the association between one or more response variables and missing data mechanism. One potential problem with selection models is that the observed data provide little evidence about the appropriate functional form of the linkage between missingness and unobserved measurements under the MNAR assumption. In such models, estimation and inference are typically model-driven instead of data-driven. Therefore, tests of ignorability have to be conducted given specific model assumptions, which are unverifiable using the observed data only. This problem is not unique to selection models. Pattern mixture models for longitudinal measurements with nonignorable missing data also posit important assumptions about data structure that can be difficult to verify.

The problem of untestable MNAR assumptions has led to development of sensitivity analysis to investigate the stability of parameter estimation in the neighborhood of an MAR model towards non-ignorability. A local influence approach to sensitivity analysis was proposed by Verbeke et al. (2001)[223] to evaluate the impact of individual subjects on parameter estimation by perturbing an MAR model in the direction of nonrandom dropout. The method was developed for normally distributed repeated measures, and extended to ordinal longitudinal data by Van Steen et al. (2001)[222]. A general index of sensitivity to nonignorability (ISNI) was proposed by Troxel et al. (2004)[210] for cross-sectional data and discussed in Ma et al. (2005)[158] and Viviani et al. (2014)[227] for repeated measures with discrete- and continuous-time dropout processes, respectively. Note that sensitivity analysis surveyed in this section focuses on selection models. We refer the reader to Daniels and Hogan (2008)[49] for sensitivity analysis in pattern-mixture models.

This section also discusses diagnosis of joint models to evaluate how well the proposed model fits observed data, thus focusing on assumptions that can be assessed. We review the residual and graphical methods for model adequacy evaluation developed by Dobson and Henderson (2003)[57] and Rizopoulos et al. (2010)[187].

7.1.1   Sensitivity Analysis

A Local Influence Approach

The local influence approach to sensitivity analysis developed by Verbeke et al. (2001)[223] is applicable to studies with discrete dropout times in which the probability for subject i ($i = 1, \ldots, n$) to drop out at occasion j, denoted as $p(\bar{H}_{ij}, Y_{ij})$, is modeled by

$$
\begin{aligned}
logit[p(\bar{H}_{ij}, Y_{ij})] &= logit[P(D_i = j | D_i \geq j, \bar{H}_{ij}, Y_{ij})] \\
&= \psi \bar{H}_{ij} + \omega Y_{ij},
\end{aligned} \tag{7.1}
$$

where $\bar{H}_{ij}$ contains covariates and all Y's observed prior to occasion j, D_i is the occasion at which dropout occurs, and ψ and ω are the dropout model parameters. Note that a probit link function can also be used here. Given the assumption that the model is correctly specified, when $\omega = 0$, the missing data due to dropout are ignorable, whereas when $\omega \neq 0$, the missing data are MNAR and dropouts are nonrandom.

A perturbed version of (7.1) is considered to investigate how sensitive parameter estimation could be to the dropout assumption:

$$
\begin{aligned}
logit[p(\bar{H}_{ij}, Y_{ij})] &= logit[P(D_i = j | D_i \geq j, \bar{H}_{ij}, Y_{ij})] \\
&= \psi \bar{H}_{ij} + \omega_i Y_{ij}.
\end{aligned} \tag{7.2}
$$

It is different from model (7.1) because ω_i is no longer a population parameter; instead, it can be interpreted as local, individual-specific perturbations around the null model that corresponds to the MAR assumption, i.e., $\omega = 0$. If an individual drives the model toward nonrandom dropouts, then the posterior distribution of missing values conditional on observed data may be quite different from that under the MAR assumption. This will, in turn, affect not only the dropout model parameters, but also those in the longitudinal model for Y. Therefore, the local influence approach aims to identify individuals for whom small perturbations in ω_i lead to nonnegligible changes in the dropout and longitudinal model parameters.

The local influence measures are defined based on ω_i. Denote the log-likelihood function that corresponds to (7.2) by $l(\gamma|\omega) = \sum_{i=1}^{n} l_i(\gamma|\omega_i)$, where γ is a $s \times 1$ vector containing the longitudinal and dropout model parameters not including $\omega = (\omega_1, \ldots, \omega_n)^T$. It is assumed that ω belongs to an open subset Ω of $\mathbb{R}^n$. When $\omega = \omega_0 = (0, \ldots, 0)^T$, $l(\gamma|\omega_0)$ is the log-likelihood function for an MAR dropout model. The local influence compares $\hat{\gamma}_\omega$ with $\hat{\gamma}$, where $\hat{\gamma}_\omega$ is the maximum likelihood estimator for γ obtained by maximizing $l(\gamma|\omega)$, and $\hat{\gamma}$ is the maximum likelihood estimator for γ when ω is set to ω_0. The difference between $\hat{\gamma}_\omega$ and $\hat{\gamma}$ can be measured by the likelihood displacement defined by $LD(\omega) = 2[l(\hat{\gamma}|\omega_0) - l(\hat{\gamma}_\omega|\omega)]$. Note that $LD(\omega)$ is large if $l(\gamma|\omega_0)$ is strongly curved at $\hat{\gamma}$. The geometric surface formed by $\xi(\omega) = (\omega^T, LD(\omega))^T$ as ω changes in Ω conveys the information on how influential the perturbations are. Its local influences, i.e., the normal curvatures C_h of $\xi(\omega)$ in ω_0 in the direction of an n-dimensional vector h of unit length can be calculated by

$$C_h = 2|h^T \Delta^T \ddot{L}^{-1} \Delta h|,$$

where $\ddot{L}$ is the $(s \times s)$ matrix of second-order derivatives of $l(\gamma|\omega_0)$ with respect to γ, evaluated at $\gamma = \hat{\gamma}$, and Δ is a $(s \times n)$ matrix with its ith column defined as

$$\Delta_i = \frac{\partial^2 l_i(\gamma|\omega_i)}{\partial \omega_i \partial \gamma}\Big|_{\gamma=\hat{\gamma}, \omega_i=0}.$$

Note that the local influence measure C_h is a function of the direction h. One natural choice is the vector h_i that contains one in the ith position and zero elsewhere, and as a consequence, C_h becomes $C_i = 2|\Delta_i^T \ddot{L}^{-1} \Delta_i|$, which measures the influence by perturbing the ith individual toward the MNAR direction while assuming the other subjects drop out at random. The direction h_{max} that yields the largest local changes in the likelihood displacement is the eigenvector corresponding to the largest eigenvalue C_{max} of $-2\Delta^T \ddot{L}^{-1} \Delta$, and the maximal normal curvature is given by C_{max}. This local influence approach can also be applied to a subset of γ which is denoted as γ_1, and the log-likelihood would then be replaced by the profile log-likelihood of γ_1.

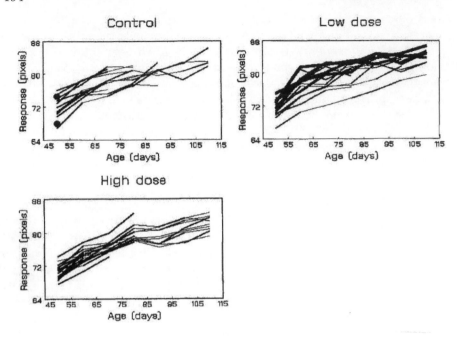

Figure 7.1 *Individual growth curves for the three treatment groups separately. Influential subjects are highlighted.*

Example 7.1. *The Rat Data*

The above local influence approach is illustrated by a rat study. A total of 50 male Wistar rats were randomized into three groups, control, low dose of cecapeptyl, and high dose of cecapeptyl, to evaluate the effect of inhibiting testosterone production in rats. The rats started receiving treatment at the age of 45 days, and a characterization of the skull height was repeatedly measured every 10 days since day 50. Because the response was measured under anesthesia and many rats did not survive it, only 22 (44%) completed all seven measurements.

Figure 7.1 shows individual profiles. When fitting the longitudinal model, a transformation of $ln(1 + (age - 45)/10)$ was applied to age in order to linearize the relationship. A common average intercept β_0 was assumed, and the treatments had group-specific slopes β_1, β_2, and β_3, respectively. Data correlation was characterized by a compound symmetry variance-covariance structure, with variance $\sigma^2 + \tau^2$ and covariance τ^2. Denote $\alpha = (\sigma^2, \tau^2)$. The first part of Table 7.1 summarizes parameter estimates and their standard errors for three dropout (death due to anesthesia) mechanisms: completely random (MCAR), random (MAR), and nonrandom (MNAR). The dropout mechanism might be MAR as suggested by the estimated ω.

Table 7.1 *Maximum likelihood estimates (standard errors) of completely random, random, and nonrandom dropout models fitted to the rat data set with and without modification.*

Effect	Parameter	MCAR	MAR	MNAR
		Original Data		
Measurement model				
Intercept	β_0	68.61(0.33)	68.61(0.33)	68.60(0.33)
Slope control	β_1	7.51(0.22)	7.51(0.22)	7.53(0.24)
Slope low dose	β_2	6.87(0.23)	6.87(0.23)	6.89(0.23)
Slope high dose	β_3	7.31(0.28)	7.31(0.28)	7.35(0.30)
Random intercept	γ^2	3.44(0.77)	3.44(0.77)	3.43(0.77)
Measurement error	σ^2	1.43(0.14)	1.43(0.14)	1.43(0.14)
Dropout model				
Intercept	ψ_0	−1.98(0.20)	−8.48(4.00)	−10.30(6.88)
Previous measurement	ψ_1		0.08(0.05)	0.03(0.16)
Current measurement	$\omega{=}\psi_2$			0.07(0.22)
-2 log likelihood		1100.4	1097.6	1097.5
		Modified Data		
Measurement model				
Intercept	β_0	70.20(0.92)	70.20(0.92)	70.25(0.92)
Slope control	β_1	7.52(0.25)	7.52(0.25)	7.42(0.26)
Slope low dose	β_2	6.97(0.25)	6.97(0.25)	6.90(0.25)
Slope high dose	β_3	7.21(0.31)	7.21(0.31)	7.04(0.33)
Random intercept	γ^2	40.38(0.18)	40.38(0.18)	40.71(8.25)
Measurement error	σ^2	1.42(0.14)	1.42(0.14)	1.44(0.15)
Dropout model				
Intercept	ψ_0	−1.98(0.20)	−0.79(1.99)	2.08(3.08)
Previous measurement	ψ_1		−0.015(0.03)	0.23(0.15)
Current measurement	$\omega{=}\psi_2$			−0.28(0.17)
-2 log likelihood		1218.0	1217.7	1214.8

The local influence C_i of each rat, as well as $C_i(\theta)$, $C_i(\beta)$, $C_i(\alpha)$, and $C_i(\psi)$ for subsets of the model parameters, is shown in Figure 7.2, where θ contains all parameters in the longitudinal model. The last panel also displays h_{max} that corresponds to the maximal local influence. Note that these influence measures are not unitless, so it is more meaningful to make comparisons based on relative magnitudes. Four rats in the low-dose group, labeled by IDs 10, 16, 35, and 41, have the largest C_i and $C_i(\psi)$. They are completers with relatively high responses and large variances of dropout probability $(v_{ij} = g(h_{ij})(1-g(h_{ij})))$, as computed using parameter estimates for the MAR dropout model in Table 7.1. All these factors contribute to their influence measures.

Since all deviations are rather moderate, in a second analysis, all responses of these four rats were artificially disturbed by an increment of 20 units, and the results are shown in the second part of Table 7.1. This analysis is done with the hope to show that these deviations would impact the model parameter estimates, and the local influence approach is adequately sensitive to detect such deviations. Estimates for the fixed effects stay virtually the same, but there is a dramatic increase in the random intercept variance (τ^2). The dropout model parameters are also affected, and the likelihood ratio statistic for MAR versus

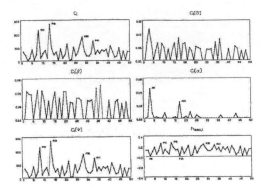

Figure 7.2 *Index plots of C_i, $C_i(\theta)$, $C_i(\beta)$, $C_i(\alpha)$, $C_i(\psi)$, and of the components of the direction h_{max} of maximal curvature.*

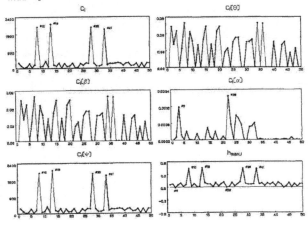

Figure 7.3 *Index plots of C_i, $C_i(\theta)$, $C_i(\beta)$, $C_i(\alpha)$, $C_i(\psi)$, and of the components of the direction h_{max} of maximal curvature, where four profiles have been shifted upward*

MCAR changes from 2.8 to 0.3 and for MNAR versus MAR changes from 0.1 to 2.9. Thus, the modified data tend to show stronger evidence towards MNAR than the original data, though these tests are not statistically significant. Figure 7.3 shows that the four extreme profiles have large influence measures as indicated by C_i, $C_i(\alpha)$, and $C_i(\psi)$. □

An Index of Sensitivity to Nonignorability

Different from the above discussed local influence approach that examines the impact of departures from ignorability in individual observations, a general index of sensitivity to nonignorability (ISNI) has been developed to measure overall sensitivity of longitudinal data inference in a neighborhood of the ignorable model (Ma et al., 2005[158]; Viviani et al., 2014[227]). Let θ denote parameters that describe the distribution of the longitudinal outcome Y. Similar to (7.1), given subject i is observed at occasion $j-1$, the probability that this subject drops out at occasion j is assumed to be

$$g\{P(D_i = j | D_i \geq j, \bar{H}_{ij}, Y_{ij})\} = \psi \bar{H}_{ij} + \omega Y_{ij},$$

where $\bar{H}_{ij}$ contains covariates and all Y's observed prior to occasion j, and $D_i = j$ if subject i drops out at occasion j. The link function $g(\cdot)$ may be logit or probit. ISNI measures the sensitivity of $\hat{\theta}(\omega)$, the maximum likelihood estimate of θ for a given value of ω, to small departures of ω from zero (the MAR model). To be specific, it is defined as

$$ISNI = \frac{\partial \hat{\theta}(\omega)}{\partial \omega}|_{\omega=0},$$

describing the approximate change in $\hat{\theta}$ for one unit change in the nonignorability parameter ω around $\omega = 0$. In particular, $\hat{\theta}(\omega)$ can be obtained from a Taylor-series expansion of the log-likelihood around the maximum likelihood estimate of θ and ψ when $\omega = 0$. Note that an ISNI can be defined for each individual parameter in the longitudinal model for Y. Since ISNI is dependent on the unit of Y, a scale-free sensitivity transformation c is defined as

$$c = |\frac{\sigma_Y SE_Y}{ISNI_Y}|,$$

where σ_Y is the standard deviation of Y conditional on the covariates in the longitudinal model, SE_Y is the standard error of a parameter of interest, and $ISNI_Y$ is the ISNI for that parameter. A small value of c indicates possibly strong sensitivity even for modest nonignorability, and a cutoff $c < 1$ has been recommended to identify important sensitivity (Ma et al., 2005[158]).

Example 7.2. *Milk Protein Trial*

This approach is illustrated by the milk protein trial discussed in Example 4.8. The missing data are concluded to be nonignorable based on the model specified in equation (4.27): cows with low protein content are more likely to drop out of the study. Table 7.2 summarizes results from the ISNI analysis to investigate the impact of nonignorability on the mean response parameters. The sensitivity transformation c is large for γ_1, γ_2, γ_3, and α, but relatively small for η and ξ, suggesting that estimation of the linear and quadratic trends in the mean response might be affected by nonignorable dropouts, but the treatment effects and time trend prior to week 3 are not. This is consistent with the fact that all dropouts occurred from week 15 onward. Nevertheless, the overall impact of the nonignorable missing data assumption seems to be small since all sensitivity transformations are above 1. $\square$

Table 7.2 *MLEs under ignorable and nonignorable models and ISNI analysis for the milk protein data.*

					Estimates of regression coefficients	
	γ_1	γ_2	γ_3	α	$\eta \times 100^*$	$\xi \times 100^*$
Ignorable model	4.16	4.05	3.94	-0.23	0.72	-0.06
SE of coefficients	0.052	0.051	0.051	0.015	0.009	0.0005
ISNI*1000	0.14	0.40	0.44	-0.11	0.58	-0.08
Sensitivity						
Transformation(c)	111.91	39.25	36.14	44.30	4.76	2.06
Nonignorable model	4.15	4.05	3.93	-0.23	0.51	-0.02
ISNI estimates	4.16	4.05	3.94	-0.23	0.40	-0.01
$(\text{Ign} + \text{ISNI} \times \hat{\beta}_1)^\dagger$						

The mean estimates of η and ξ are multiplied by 100.
† Ign stands for estimates under ignorable model; $\hat{\beta}_1 = -5.65$.

7.1.2 Joint Model Diagnostics

As mentioned previously, diagnostic procedures for joint models have been developed to evaluate how well the proposed model fits observed data, thus focusing on assumptions that can be assessed. In this section we review residual methods to evaluate the impact of individual cases on model estimation.

Use D and δ to denote the dropout data, where D is the dropout time and δ indicates the cause of dropout. For example, we may use $\delta = 1$ or 2 to indicate informative and noninformative dropouts, respectively. For complete cases without dropout, $\delta = 0$. In the conditional residual approach developed by Dobson and Henderson (2003)[57], the joint model is assumed to take the following form:

$$Y_i(t) = X_{1i}(t)^T \beta_1 + W_{1i}(t) + \epsilon_i(t), \tag{7.3}$$

and the risk of informative dropout is

$$\lambda_i(t|W_{2i}) = \lambda_0(t) exp(X_{2i}(t)^T \beta_2 + W_{2i}(t)), \tag{7.4}$$

where $W_{1i}(t)$ and $W_{2i}(t)$ are two potentially correlated zero-mean Gaussian processes characterized by a vector of random effects b_i that are assumed to be multivariate normal. When a continuous-time stochastic Gaussian process $V_i(t)$ is incorporated into $W_{1i}(t)$ and/or $W_{2i}(t)$, $V_i(t)$ needs to be defined only at distinct measurement and even times and thus can be stacked into b_i. This model has been discussed and illustrated in more detail in Section 4.1.1.

The residual of Y after removing fixed effects is defined as $R(t) = Y(t) - X_1(t)^T \hat{\beta}_1$, where individual subscripts are omitted for ease of discussion. Based on (7.3)–(7.4), the conditional mean of $R(t)$ given $D = d$ and $\delta = 1$ is given by

$$E\{R(t)|D = d, \delta = 1\} = \frac{\int W_1(t) f(d|b) f(b) db}{\int f(d|b) f(b) db},$$

where $0 \le t \le d$, $f(b)$ is the multivariate Gaussian density, and

$$
\begin{aligned}
f(d|b) \quad = \quad & \lambda_0(d)\exp\{X_2(d)^T\beta_2 + W_2(d)\} \\
& \times \exp[-\int_0^d \lambda_0(s)\exp\{X_2(s)^T\beta_2 + W_2(s)\}ds].
\end{aligned}
$$

For noninformative dropout ($\delta = 2$) and completion ($\delta = 0$), the conditional mean is

$$
E\{R(t)|D = d, \delta \neq 1\} = \frac{\int W_1(t)S(d|b)f(b)db}{\int S(d|b)f(b)db},
$$

where $0 \le t \le d$ and $S(d|b)$ is the survival function for informative dropout

$$
S(d|b) = \exp[-\int_0^d \lambda_0(s)\exp\{X_2(s)^T\beta_2 + W_2(s)\}ds].
$$

The conditional variance of $W_1(t)$ is calculated as $E\{W_1^2(t)\} - [E\{W_1(t)\}]^2$, where $E\{W_1^2(t)\}$ is obtained by substituting $W_1^2(t)$ for $W_1(t)$ in the above equations. Note that the conditional variance of $R(t)$ is $E\{W_1^2(t)\} - [E\{W_1(t)\}]^2 + \sigma^2$, where σ^2 is the variance of measurement errors.

Figure 7.4 shows expected residual profiles conditioning on informative dropout calculated from a hypothesized data set in which Y are measured at 0, 1, 2, 4, 6, and 8 units, and all measurements are truncated at 9. Four scenarios are considered, with $W_1(t)$ being b_1 (intercept), b_2t (slope), b_3t^2 (quadratic), and $V(t)$, where b_1, b_2, and b_3 are zero-mean normal random variables, and $V(t)$ is a zero-mean Gaussian process such that $Cov(V(t), V(t + s)) = \sigma_v^2\exp(-|s|/\phi)$. In the dropout model, $W_2(t)$ is posited to be $W_1(t)$. The parameter values are set in a way such that $Var(W_1(4)) = 2$ for all four models. In each panel the individual lines represent $E(R(t)|D = d, \delta = 1)$ conditional on different dropout times d. In the random intercept model, the expected residuals are constant for each d, with high values associated with early dropouts. The residual profiles are linear for the random slope model; late dropouts have a steeper decline in the profiles. A similar pattern is seen in the quadratic model, but the trend is nonlinear. The Gaussian process model has within-individual variability in the random effects, and the risk of dropout is more related to the expected value of $W_1(t)$ at the current moment rather than its history. Similar patterns are seen for residual profiles conditional on $d \neq 1$ (Figure 7.5), except that the expected residuals are all negative. This can be explained by the fact that individuals with positive values of random effects tend to leave the study early (informative dropout), so those remaining would have negative residuals.

Expected residual profiles can be derived in a similar way under other time trend assumptions for $W_1(t)$, and would be compared with observed residual profiles calculated from fitted joint models to assess goodness of fit.

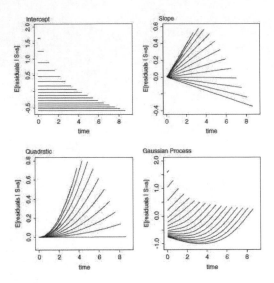

Figure 7.4 *Expected residual profiles conditional upon informative dropout at time d (endpoint of each line).*

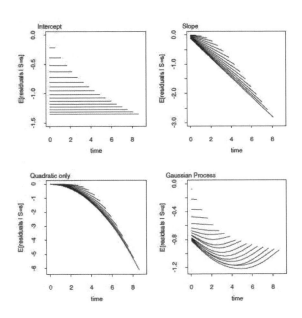

Figure 7.5 *Expected residual profiles conditional upon noninformative dropout at time d (endpoint of each line).*

Different from the above method that examines residuals for observed longitudinal data conditional on the dropout information, Rizopoulos et al. (2010)[187] proposed a multiple imputation approach to simulate residuals for missing longitudinal observations, so that the standard residual diagnostic tools for complete data can be applied. In this approach, multiple residuals are imputed for each missing observation. When weighted loess curves are used to check for systematic trend, weight one would be used for observed residuals and weight $1/L$ for imputed residuals, where L is the number of imputation. This method fits naturally well into the Bayesian framework for joint model inference since each missing longitudinal measurement is simulated from its posterior distribution conditional on the observed data and event time information.

Another area of model diagnosis is to identify influential data points that have undue effects on parameter estimation. Denote $\theta = (\beta_1, \beta_2, \gamma)$, where γ is the parameter to formulate $W_2(t)$ as a function of random effects b. The impact of individual i on parameter estimation can be measured by the difference between $\hat{\theta}$ and $\hat{\theta}_{(i)}$, which are the estimated θ based on the sample with and without individual i. Fitting joint models with each individual removed at a time is not computationally efficient. A one-step approximation is given by

$$\hat{\theta}_{(i)} - \hat{\theta} \simeq -I_{(i)}^{-1}(\hat{\theta})u_{(i)}(\hat{\theta})$$

via a Taylor series expansion of the log likelihood at $\hat{\theta}_{(i)}$, where $u_{(i)}(\hat{\theta})$ and $I_{(i)}(\hat{\theta})$ are the observed score and information with individual i omitted. A Cook-type distance can then be used to evaluate the influence of individual i:

$$CD_i = (\hat{\theta}_{(i)} - \hat{\theta})^T \hat{Var}(\hat{\theta})^{-1}(\hat{\theta}_{(i)} - \hat{\theta}).$$

In addition, a local influence measure, $u_{(i)}(\hat{\theta})^T \hat{Var}(\hat{\theta})^{-1} u_{(i)}(\hat{\theta})$, may also be useful.

Example 7.3. *The Schizophrenia Trial*

The conditional residual approach proposed by Dobson and Henderson (2003)[57] is applied to the schizophrenia trial analyzed in Example 4.1. The latent processes $W_1(t)$ and $W_2(t)$ that link together Y and (D, δ) are assumed to be $b_1 + b_2 t + b_3 t^2$ and $\gamma_1 b_1 + \gamma_2 b_2 t + \gamma_3 b_3 t^2 + \gamma_4 b_3$, respectively, where b_1, b_2, and b_3 are normally distributed subject-specific random effects. This model provides a slightly better fit to the data as measured by log-likelihood compared to Model X discussed in Example 4.1. Shown in Figure 7.6 are the residual profiles of this model, which suggest fairly different patterns between the informative and noninformative dropout groups. The observed residual profiles are in good agreement with the expected, especially for the experimental (risperidone) group which has the largest sample size. Some discrepancies are seen in the standard (haloperidol) and placebo groups for noninformative dropouts, which are probably due to small sample sizes.

Figure 7.7 shows case influence of the schizophrenia data. Cook-type distances were calculated using both the full case deletion and one-step approximation, and the latter took substantially shorter computation time. Three cases, 103, 241, and 447, stand out as influential, though in a different order (panels (a) and (b)). The correlation of CD_i between the two methods is 0.88, indicating that the approximation works reasonably well. Only case 447 has a high local influence (panel (c)). The correlation between full case deletion CD_i and local influence measures is 0.55. PANSS profiles for the three cases are shown in panel (d), together with their group means. Case 103 had a early steep decline in PANSS and was an informative dropout in the haloperidol group. This patient had the highest influence on β_2 and γ, and second highest influence on β_1. Case 241 had a fast increase in PANSS just before dropout and was most influential for β_1, but had almost no effect on β_2 and γ. The PANSS score for case 447, who was a completer, was steadily increasing over the study period. This case was influential for β_2 and γ, but not for β_1. However, there are no dramatic changes in the joint model results after deleting the three cases (results not shown), although a larger separation between treatment groups is observed in their dropout survival curves. □

7.2   Variable Selection in Joint Models

In biomedical studies it is often of interest to select important predictors for a scientifically meaningful response variable from a large pool of candidates for prognostic purposes. When the response variable is repeatedly measured and a mixed effects model is used, the variable selection often involves selecting both fixed and random effects. As we have discussed before, missing data due to dropout during follow-up in longitudinal studies may lead to invalid statistical inference if the data are missing not at random. It is clear that estimation bias due to missing data would compromise the validity of commonly used variable selection procedures. In other situations there is also interest to select predictors for event times that indicate clinical milestones, and quite often the event times are collected together with longitudinal data during follow-up.

These are the circumstances where a joint modeling approach of variable selection may play a role. However, research in this area has been limited. In this section we review two Bayesian approaches in which variable selection is implemented by positing mixture priors for regression coefficients of the predictors to be selected. Two types of mixture priors that have been used for variable selection in cross-sectional and longitudinal settings are employed in joint models. These priors are conjugate for models that are linear in parameters. The first is a spike-and-slab type of prior (Bao, 2011[19]) for regression coefficients β_k, $j = 1, \ldots, p$, assuming there are p candidate predictors. Conditional on a binary latent indicator τ_k, the prior of β_k is $(1 - \tau_k)N(0, c_k\sigma_k^2) + \tau_k N(0, \sigma_k^2)$. When $\tau_k = 1$ (i.e., the kth predictor is included in the model), β_k has a normal prior with mean zero and relatively large variance σ_k^2 (the slab), whereas when

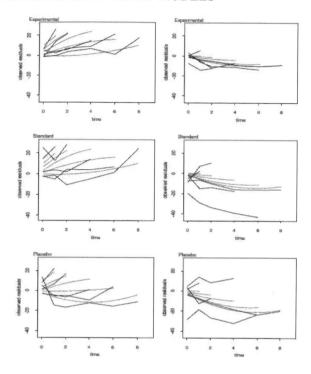

Figure 7.6 *Observed (solid line) and expected (broken line) residual profiles for the schizophrenia trial. The left column shows mean residuals for informative dropout groups, the right column for noninformative dropout groups.*

$\tau_k = 0$ (i.e., the kth predictor is not included), β_k has a normal prior with a suitably small variance $c_k \sigma_k^2$ (the spike), where $c_k \in (0, 1)$. Caution should be taken when choosing c_k and σ_k^2 to avoid selecting models with too few or too many predictors.

The second type is called the zero-inflated mixture prior, which is a mixture of a point mass at zero and a normal distribution. By setting a positive probability at zero, the prior allows effective exclusion of variables from the model. It is a proper prior, thereby avoiding possible impropriety of the posterior. Estimation bias and asymptotic behaviors of posterior selection probability with this prior have been studied for longitudinal measurements with missing data. It is shown that if data are missing not at random but the model ignores the missing data mechanism, the variable selection procedure asymptotically selects wrong effects. This problem has motivated a joint modeling framework

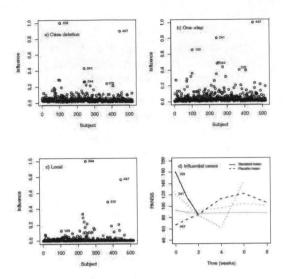

Figure 7.7 *Case influence for the schizophrenia trial. Cook distances under: (a) full case deletion, (b) a one-step approximation, (c) local influence measure. Panel (d) shows observed PANSS scores for the three most influential cases together with respective estimated group means (case 103, standard; cases 241 and 447, both placebo).*

for variable selection in the presence of nonignorable missing data (Li et al., 2013[136]).

7.2.1   Spike-and-Slab Priors

Bao (2011)[19] studied variable selection in joint models using the spike-and-slab priors. The approach assumes that the longitudinal outcome has a distribution in exponential families and there is a single failure type at the survival endpoint. Specifically, the joint model (4.1)–(4.3) discussed in Chapter 4 is used to specify the joint distribution of longitudinal and survival data. Variable selection can be done for the fixed effects β and random effects b_i at the longitudinal endpoint, and the regression coefficients γ at the survival endpoint. When the interest is to select predictors for the longitudinal outcome while adjusting for potentially nonignorable missing data caused by dropouts (or deaths), variable selection then takes place in the longitudinal model only.

Suppose there are p predictors in $X_{ij}^{(1)}$. Let $\tau_k = 1$ if the kth predictor is included in the model and $\tau_k = 0$ otherwise, $k = 1, \ldots, p$. The spike-and-slab prior for β_k is specified as

$$\beta_k | \tau_k \sim \tau_k N(0, \sigma_k^2) + (1 - \tau_k) N(0, c_1 \sigma_k^2), \qquad (7.5)$$

where c_1 is positive and suitably small. When the kth fixed effect is included,

β_k has a normal prior with mean zero and variance σ_k^2. When $\tau_k = 0$, i.e., the kth fixed effect is not included, β_k has a normal prior with a relatively small variance $c_1\sigma_k^2$, which usually leads to small posterior values of β_k, so the kth fixed effect tends to be removed from the model. At last, the prior of τ_k is a Bernoulli distribution with mean π_k.

In the approach by Bao (2011)[19], Dirichlet process (DP) priors, which are more flexible than parametric distributions, are used for the random effects b_i. Specifically, let $b_r = (b_{1r}, b_{2r}, \ldots, b_{nr})^T$ denote the rth random effect for a sample of n subjects, $r = 1, \ldots, q$. The DP prior is defined as

$$b_{ir} \sim DP(M_r, G_{0r}),$$
$$G_{0r}|\tau_{br} \sim \tau_{br}N(0, \sigma_{br}^2) + (1 - \tau_{br})N(0, c_2\sigma_{br}^2),$$
$$M_r \sim Gamma(a, b),$$

where $DP(M_r, G_{0r})$ is a Dirichlet process with concentration parameter M_r and base measure G_{0r}. A spike-and-slab prior is assumed for the base measure G_{0r}. It is a mixture of two normal distributions, $N(0, \sigma_{br}^2)$ and $N(0, c_2\sigma_{br}^2)$, with c_2 being a small positive scaler. Similar to (7.5), τ_{br} indicates whether the rth random effect is included in the model. The prior of τ_{br} is a Bernoulli distribution with mean π_{br}. For the hyperparameter σ_{br}, it has been shown that a uniform prior performs better than the inverse-gamma family of priors.

Posterior Distribution of Indicator Variables

On the basis of the likelihood function and the priors, a Gibbs sampler can be used to generate samples of model parameters from their posterior distributions. For the fixed effect β_k in the longitudinal model, the conditional distribution of τ_k (the selection indicator) has a Bernoulli distribution with mean $\hat{\pi}_k$:

$$\hat{\pi}_k = \frac{P(\beta_k|slab)P(slab)}{P(\beta_k|slab)P(slab) + P(\beta_k|spike)P(spike)}$$
$$= \frac{\pi_k exp(-\beta_k^2/2\sigma_k^2)}{\pi_k exp(-\beta_k^2/2\sigma_k^2) + (1 - \pi_k)c_1^{-\frac{1}{2}} exp(-\beta_k^2/2c_1\sigma_k^2)}.$$

It is the probability that β_k is from a normal distribution with mean zero and relatively large variance σ_k^2 (the slab), conditional on its sampled value. A high value of $\hat{\pi}_k$ suggests that the kth predictor be selected in the current iteration. If there is no prior information regarding the probability of selecting the kth predictor, π_k can be set to 0.5.

Similarly, the posterior distribution of τ_{br} for the rth random effect is a Bernoulli with the posterior selection probability

$$\hat{\pi}_{br} = \frac{\pi_{br} exp(-\sum b_{ir}^2/2\sigma_{br}^2)}{\pi_{br} exp(-\sum b_{ir}^2/2\sigma_{br}^2) + (1 - \pi_{br})c_2^{-\frac{n}{2}} exp(-\sum b_{ir}^2/2c_2\sigma_{br}^2)}.$$

Posterior Probability of Selecting an Effect

There are two ways to calculate the posterior probability of selecting a specific fixed or random effect using the Gibbs sampler. Over the N iterations, the marginal inclusion probability for the kth fixed effect, $k = 1, \ldots, p$, and the rth random effect, $r = 1, \ldots, q$, can be estimated by

$$P(\text{the } k\text{th fixed effect is included in the model}) \approx \frac{\sum_{t=1}^{N} \hat{\pi}_k^{(t)}}{N},$$

$$P(\text{the } r\text{th random effect is included in the model}) \approx \frac{\sum_{t=1}^{N} \hat{\pi}_{br}^{(t)}}{N},$$

where $\hat{\pi}_k^{(t)}$ and $\hat{\pi}_{br}^{(t)}$ are the posterior probability of selecting the kth fixed effect and the rth random effect in iteration t, respectively. These quantities can also be estimated using indicator variables τ_k and τ_{br} sampled over the N iterations:

$$P(\text{the } k\text{th fixed effect is included in the model}) \approx \frac{\sum_{t=1}^{N} I(\tau_k^{(t)} = 1)}{N},$$

$$P(\text{the } r\text{th random effect is included in the model}) \approx \frac{\sum_{t=1}^{N} I(\tau_{br}^{(t)} = 1)}{N},$$

where $\tau_k^{(t)}$ and $\tau_{br}^{(t)}$ are the sampled indicator variables from their posterior Bernoulli distributions in iteration t, so that the numerator is the frequency of selecting a specific fixed or random effect over the N iterations. Similarly, the posterior probability of selecting a model that contains a specific set of fixed and random effects can be calculated as

$$P(Model_j) \approx \frac{\text{the frequency of } Model_j \text{ over } N \text{ iterations}}{N}.$$

Example 7.4. *The AIDS Clinical Trial*

In this study a total of 467 HIV-infected patients were randomized into the di-danosine (ddI) and zalcitabine (ddC) treatment arms. Repeated measurements of CD4 counts were obtained at baseline, 2, 6, 12, and 18 months. Data on patient survival were recorded, with a censoring rate of around 60%. Due to dropouts and deaths, observations were available on 230, 182, 153, 102, and 22 patients at the five occasions in the ddI group and on 236, 186, 157, 123, and 14 patients in the ddC group.

The longitudinal model for the square-root transformed CD4 count Y_{ij} measured on subject i at occasion j is specified as

$$Y_{ij} = X_{ij}^{T(1)} \beta_1 + \tilde{X}_{ij}^{(1)T} b_i + \epsilon_{ij},$$

where the measurement errors ϵ_{ij} are i.i.d. $N(0, \sigma^2)$. The covariate vector $X_{ij}^{(1)}$

contains candidate predictors including Drug (ddI = 1, ddC = 0), Gender (male = 1, female = −1), PrevOI (previous opportunistic infection at the study entry; PrevOI = 1 for AIDS diagnosis and PrevOI = −1 otherwise), and Stratum (AZT failure = 1, AZT intolerance = −1). A linear time trend and its interaction with Drug are also considered. In this example, $\tilde{X}_{ij}^{(1)}$ is identical to $X_{ij}^{(1)}$, which is in line with the random effects selection purpose because there is no a priori knowledge which predictors have subject-specific effects on CD4 counts. The event intensity for survival at time t is given by

$$\lambda_i(t) = \lambda_0(t)exp(X_i^{(2)}\beta_2 + u_i),$$

where u_i is a linear combination of random effects $b_{i1}, \ldots, b_{ip}$ with coefficients $\phi_1, \ldots, \phi_p$. The same four baseline variables, Drug, Gender, PrevOI, and Stratum, are included in $X_i^{(2)}$.

Table 7.3 *Posterior means and 95% credible intervals of parameters in the joint and separate models for the AIDS Clinical Trial.*

Parameter	Joint model Posterior mean (95% CI) Longitudinal submodel	Separate model Posterior mean (95% CI) Longitudinal submodel
Intercept(β_{10})	7.592 (6.73, 8.39)	6.862 (4.99, 8.79)
Drug(β_{11})	0.845 (−0.04, 1.62)	0.332 (−1.25, 2.29)
Time(β_{12})	−0.169 (−0.25, −0.09)	−0.204 (−0.29, −0.12)
Time × Drug(β_{13})	−0.158(−0.35, 0.03)	0.07(−0.09, 0.25)
Gender(β_{14})	−0.231(−0.90, 0.51)	0.353 (−1.17, 1.94)
PrevOI(β_{15})	−2.483 (−3.10, −1.84)	−0.556 (−2.29, 0.16)
Stratum(β_{16})	−0.11 (−0.53, 0.59)	−0.037 (−1.91, 0.85)
σ^2	1.164 (0.93, 1.60)	2.11 (2.10, 2.12)
	Survival submodel	Survival submodel
Drug(β_{21})	0.113 (−1.09, 0.98)	0.229 (−0.37, 0.75)
Gender(β_{22})	−0.286(−1.35, 0.58)	−0.173 (−0.65, 0.34)
PrevOI(β_{23})	0.613 (−0.38, 1.39)	0.559 (−0.04, 0.85)
Stratum(β_{24})	0.035 (−0.87, 0.97)	0.017 (−0.42, 0.41)

The Gibbs sampler was run for 30,000 iterations following a 50,000-iteration "burn-in," and the Markov chain was then thinned by a factor of 5 to reduce sample autocorrelation. Therefore, statistical inference was based on a sample of 6000 draws from the posterior distribution. Geweke's statistic and Raftery and Lewis diagnostics were used to check convergence of the chain. Table 7.3 presents estimated posterior means and 95% credible intervals for the joint

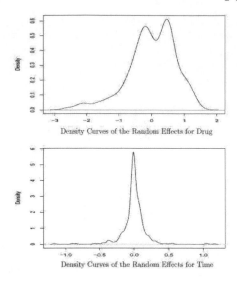

Figure 7.8 *Density curves for the random effects of Drug and Time*

and separate models. In the joint model, there is no difference in CD4 counts between the ddC and ddI groups at study entry. The estimated slope for ddC is −0.169 (95% credible interval [−0.25, −0.093]), indicating that CD4 counts decreased over time. A faster decline in CD4 counts is observed in the ddI group, with the slope being −0.169 − 0.158 = −0.327. The estimated PrevOI effect indicates that patients diagnosed with AIDS at baseline had lower CD4 counts compared to those without AIDS. Gender and Stratum do not seem to have an impact on CD4. However, in the separate analysis, the PrevOI effect and Time×Drug interaction are much smaller compared to their counterparts in the joint model. None of the four predictors seem to affect patient survival in the joint and separate models.

The fixed effects of Drug and PrevOI have a very high marginal inclusion probability in the joint model (>85%), but the selection probability for Time, Time×Drug, Gender, Stratum is only moderate (45.1% to 64.9%). The estimated density curve of the random effects for Drug (Figure 7.8) reveals a bimodal distribution, indicating possible heterogeneity in random effect distributions between the two treatment arms. The random effects for Time and Time×Drug have a sharp peak around zero with very short tails, suggesting small variability in time trends between individuals. □

7.2.2 Zero-Inflated Mixture Priors

As mentioned previously, selection of fixed and random effects can also be implemented via zero-inflated mixture priors with a point mass at zero. Zero-inflated mixture priors have been studied in longitudinal analysis by Chen and Dunson (2003)[37], Cai and Dunson (2006)[30], and Kinney and Dunson (2007)[116]. Li et al. (2013)[136] applied the priors in a joint model to address bias in variable selection when there are nonignorable missing values in longitudinal binary data.

In this approach, a logistic mixed effects model is used to characterize the longitudinal binary outcome:

$$logit(p_{ij}) = logit\{P(Y_{ij} = 1|X_{ij}^{(1)}, Z_{ij}, u_i, \beta, \Sigma)\} = X_{ij}^{(1)T}\beta + Z_{ij}^T u_i, \quad (7.6)$$

where Y_{ij} denotes the longitudinal binary outcome measured on subject i at time t_{ij}, $j = 1, \ldots, n_i$, $X_{ij}^{(1)}$ and Z_{ij} are $p \times 1$ and $q \times 1$ vectors of covariates, respectively, and β and u_i are associated fixed and random effects. In the context of variable selection, $X_{ij}^{(1)}$ and Z_{ij} consist of all candidate predictors of interest. The model is formulated for a study in which all subjects follow the same visit schedule. Because some subjects may drop out of the study early, $n_i \leq m$, where m is the maximum number of visits.

Assume the random effects u_i in (7.6) follow a multivariate normal distribution with mean zero and variance-covariance Σ. To facilitate random effects selection, Σ is reparameterized by a modified Cholesky decomposition:

$$\Sigma = \Lambda \Gamma \Gamma^T \Lambda,$$

where $\Lambda = diag(\lambda_1, \ldots, \lambda_q)$ with $\lambda_l \geq 0$ for $l = 1, \ldots, q$ and Γ is a lower triangular $q \times q$ matrix with the diagonal elements equal to 1 and $q(q-1)/2$ off diagonal elements $\gamma = (\gamma_{21}, \gamma_{31}, \gamma_{32}, \ldots, \gamma_{q1}, \ldots, \gamma_{qq-1})$. It can be shown that λ_l is proportional to the standard deviation of the lth random effect, so $\lambda_l = 0$ is equivalent to dropping the lth random effect from the model. Under this decomposition, model (7.6) can be rewritten in the following form:

$$logit\{P(Y_{ij} = 1|X_{ij}^{(1)}, Z_{ij}, b_i, \beta, \lambda, \gamma)\} = X_{ij}^{(1)T}\beta + Z_{ij}^T \Lambda \Gamma b_i, \quad (7.7)$$

where $b_i \sim N_q(0, I)$ with I being the $q \times q$ identity matrix.

This model is then augmented with a missing data (dropout) mechanism. Denote the response indicator $R_{ij} = I(Y_{ij}$ is observed) for subject i at time t_{ij}. That is, R_{ij} is equal to 1 if Y_{ij} is observed and 0 if Y_{ij} is missing. Set $R_{i0} = 1$ for all i. Given that the binary outcome is observed at time t_{ij-1}, the probability that it is observed at time t_{ij} is

$$logit\{P(R_{ij} = 1|R_{ij-1} = 1, Y_i, \eta)\} = h(\bar{Y}_{ij}; \eta),$$

where $h(\cdot)$ is a known function, $Y_i = \{Y_{ij} : j = 1, \ldots, n_i\}$, $\bar{Y}_{ij} = (Y_{i1}, \ldots, Y_{ij})$, and η is an unknown (possibly vector-valued) parameter associated with $\bar{Y}_{ij}$. The model assumes that the probability of observing Y_{ij} given the subject has not yet dropped out at time t_{ij-1} is related to the responses up to time t_{ij}, conditioning on all observations of Y_i. Various functional forms of $h(\bar{Y}_{ij}; \eta)$ have been proposed to characterize the relationship between the longitudinal outcome and dropout process.

An advantage of using a selection model formulation is that there is a direct correspondence between the functional form of $h(\bar{Y}_{ij}; \eta)$ and missing data mechanisms: (1) when $h(\bar{Y}_{ij}; \eta) \neq h(\bar{Y}_{ij-1}; \eta)$, which indicates that the dropout probability is related to the current (possibly missing) response Y_{ij}, the data are missing not at random (MNAR); (2) when $h(\bar{Y}_{ij}; \eta) = h(\bar{Y}_{ij-1}; \eta)$, the data are missing at random (MAR) because the dropout probability is a function of observed values, not the missing components. This model can be further generalized to incorporate a $1 \times \kappa$ vector of baseline covariates $X_i^{(2)}$ that may affect the dropout probability:

$$logit\{P(R_{ij} = 1 | R_{ij-1} = 1, Y_i, X_i^{(2)}, \eta, \alpha)\} = h(\bar{Y}_{ij}, X_i^{(2)}; \eta, \alpha), \qquad (7.8)$$

where $\alpha = (\alpha_1, \ldots, \alpha_\kappa)$ are unknown parameters associated with $X_i^{(2)}$.

Zero-inflated mixture priors are used for β and λ to allow a subset of fixed and random effects to be omitted from the model. Similar priors can also be used for the parameters η and α in the logistic model (7.8) for dropout hazard. To be specific, the prior for β is $\prod_{l=1}^{p} f(\beta_l)$, where $f(\beta_l)$ is a zero-inflated normal density $ZI\text{-}N(\beta_l | \pi_{0l}^\beta, \mu_{0l}^\beta, \sigma_{0l}^{\beta 2})$ defined as

$$f(\beta_l) = (1 - \pi_{0l}^\beta) I(\beta_l = 0) + \pi_{0l}^\beta I(\beta_l \neq 0) N(\beta_l; \mu_{0l}^\beta, \sigma_{0l}^{\beta 2}),$$

in which $\pi_{0l}^\beta \in [0, 1]$ and $N(\beta_l; \mu_{0l}^\beta, \sigma_{0l}^{\beta 2})$ is the normal density function with mean μ_{0l}^β and variance $\sigma_{0l}^{\beta 2}$. The prior probability that the lth predictor is selected into the model is thus π_{0l}^β. Because $\lambda_l \geq 0$, $l = 1, \ldots, q$, a zero-inflated positive normal density $f(\lambda_l) = ZI\text{-}N^+(\lambda_l | \pi_{0l}^\lambda, \mu_{0l}^\lambda, s_{0l}^\lambda)$ is chosen as the prior for λ_l. That is,

$$f(\lambda_l) = (1 - \pi_{0l}^\lambda) I(\lambda_l = 0) + \pi_{0l}^\lambda I(\lambda_l > 0) \frac{N(\lambda_l; \mu_{0l}^\lambda, s_{0l}^2)}{\Phi(0; -\mu_{0l}^\lambda, s_{0l}^2)},$$

where $\pi_{0l}^\lambda \in [0, 1]$ and Φ is the normal cumulative density function. The prior for λ is thus $p(\lambda) = \prod_{l=1}^{q} f(\lambda_l)$ assuming λ_l's are independent. Similar to π_{0l}^β, π_{0l}^λ is the prior probability that the lth random effect is selected. The variance-covariance parameters have the joint prior $p(\lambda, \gamma) = p(\gamma | \lambda) p(\lambda)$, in which the prior for γ is $p(\gamma | \lambda) = N(\gamma; \gamma_0, C_0) I(\gamma \in H_\lambda)$, where $N(\gamma; \gamma_0, C_0)$ is a multivariate normal prior with mean γ_0 and variance-covariance matrix C_0 and H_λ sets γ_{tk} to zero if $\lambda_t = 0$ or $\lambda_k = 0$. A similar zero-inflated normal density $ZI\text{-}N(\eta_l | \pi_{0l}^\eta, \mu_{0l}^\eta, \sigma_{0l}^{\eta 2})$ can be used to facilitate selection of parameters pertaining to missing data mechanisms. If one is also interested in selecting baseline covariates in model (7.8), a zero-inflated normal prior $ZI\text{-}N(\alpha_l | \pi_{0l}^\alpha, \mu_{0l}^\alpha, \sigma_{0l}^{\alpha 2})$, $l = 1, \ldots, \kappa$, can be specified for α.

The joint posterior distribution for $\Psi = (\beta, \lambda, \gamma, \eta, \alpha)$ has a complex form, particularly due to nonlinearity of parameters in the logistic function. To solve this problem, the logistic density is approximated by a t-density and a data augmentation approach is then used to obtain conditional linearity of Ψ. This strategy helps establish conditional conjugacy to simplify the Gibbs sampler.

The posterior probability of selecting each of the fixed (β) and random (λ) effects, as well as η and α, is estimated by the proportion of non-zero posterior samples. If the posterior selection probability is greater than a pre-specified threshold, the corresponding effect (fixed or random) is selected. A cutoff at 0.5 can be used as a general rule of thumb, but a more stringent selection criterion is obtained by increasing the threshold. The probability of visiting a particular model (with a specific set of fixed and random effects) over the space all possible candidate models is estimated by the proportion of the specific model that appears in the posterior samples. Those models with highest probabilities can be identified.

Example 7.5. *The rt-PA trial*

The method is illustrated using data from a double-blinded, randomized clinical trial of intravenous recombinant tissue plasminogen activator (rt-PA) in patients with acute ischemic stroke. A total of 624 patients were enrolled and randomized to receive either intravenous recombinant t-PA (N = 312) or placebo (N = 312). Repeated measurements of Barthel Index, a scale in the range of 0 to 100 to measure performance in daily living, were recorded at 7–10 days, 3 months, 6 months, and 12 months post stroke onset. An unfavorable outcome is defined as a score of less than 95 on Barthel Index to yield a dichotomized measure, which is the outcome of interest in this analysis. Out of the 624 patients, 25 dropped out before 12 months (14 and 11 in the rt-PA and placebo groups, respectively) and 168 died (78 and 90 in the rt-PA and placebo groups, respectively, including those who died after 12 months). The average number of measurements per patient was 3.2, and 30% data were missing at 12 months. Table 7.4 shows the number of patients with unfavorable Barthel Index at each follow-up time as well as the frequency of missing data. The placebo group has a higher rate of unfavorable Barthel Index and more missing data than the rt-PA group.

Variable selection for unfavorable Barthel Index (yes/no) was conducted using the joint model outlined previously and an ignorable analysis in which the missing data mechanism was ignored. In the zero-inflated mixture priors for the fixed and random effects, the variance was set to 10 and the prior selection probability $\pi_0 = 0.2$. Estimates were obtained using 60,000 iterations thinned by a factor of 10 after 40,000 burn-in iterations.

At the longitudinal endpoint, an unstructured time trend was posited: three binary variables time3, time6, and time12 were created to indicate if the outcome was measured at 3 months, 6 months, or 12 months post stroke onset,

Table 7.4 *The rt-PA stroke trial: frequency of patients with unfavorable Barthel Index at each follow-up time.*

	7-10 days		3 months		6 months		12 months	
rt-PA group (N, %)	179	60.6%	96	37.7%	86	35.5%	67	30.2%
Total observed	296		255		242		222	
Missing	16		57		70		90	
placebo group (N, %)	218	76.5%	129	52.0%	116	50.2%	96	44.4%
Total observed	285		248		231		216	
Missing	27		64		81		96	

respectively. Three models were fit, in each of which a random intercept was considered and a second random effect was assumed for one of the time indicator variables. All three models suggest that the time effect has minimal between-subject variability. Candidate baseline covariates considered in this analysis include treatment group (rt-PA versus placebo), age, gender (male versus female), smoking status, alcohol drinking, abnormal baseline CT, and history of diabetes, hypertension, and angina at baseline. The dropout hazard was initially specified as

$$logit\{P(R_{ij} = 1 | R_{ij-1} = 1, Y_i, X_i^{(2)}, \eta, \alpha)\} = \eta_0 + \eta_1 Y_{ij-1} + \eta_2 Y_{ij} + X_i^{(2)T}\alpha,$$

but the baseline covariates had negligible effects on dropout, so the term $X_i^{(2)T}\alpha$ was omitted.

For illustration purposes, the posterior mean, standard deviation, and selection probability (SP) from the model that assumes a random intercept and random time3 effect are shown in Table 7.5. The probability of seeing an unfavorable Barthel Index decreases over time in the placebo group. Conditional on the random effects, the odds ratio of unfavorable Barthel Index is 0.05 (95% credible interval (0.02, 0.09)), 0.05 (0.02, 0.09), and 0.02 (0.007, 0.05), comparing measurements at 3, 6, and 12 months post stroke onset with that at 7–10 days, respectively. The two groups have a similar trend over time (i.e., the interaction between group and time is close to zero). On average, the odds ratio of unfavorable Barthel index is 0.17 (95% credible interval (0.05, 0.53)) comparing the rt-PA group versus control. Among the baseline covariates, only history of hypertension shows a higher than 50% chance of being selected. There is a large variation in the intercept and its posterior selection probability is >0.99. However, the variation of time3 effect is relatively small, with a selection probability of 0.20. In the dropout model, the posterior selection probability for η_1 is >0.99, but is only 0.57 for η_2. The estimated η_1 is negative, indicating that patients with unfavorable Barthel Index had a higher probability of missing the next visit. Assuming the dropout process and full *data response have been modeled correctly, the results indicate that the missing data mechanism is likely MAR, which is consistent with the fact that the ignorable analysis yields similar results.* □

Table 7.5 *Analyses of unfavorable Barthel Index in the rt-PA stroke trial* ($\pi_0 = 0.2$).

	Joint Analysis			Ignorable Analysis		
	Mean	SD	Posterior SP	Mean	SD	Posterior SP
intercept	2.39	0.68	–	2.35	0.71	–
time3	−3.07	0.34	>0.99	−2.90	0.31	>0.99
time6	−3.07	0.33	>0.99	−2.96	0.31	>0.99
time12	−3.93	0.52	>0.99	−3.66	0.34	>0.99
t − PA	−1.78	0.58	0.97	−1.88	0.56	0.99
time3 × t − PA	0.004	0.07	0.03	0.003	0.08	0.03
time6 × t − PA	0.01	0.11	0.04	0.01	0.10	0.04
time12 × t − PA	0.02	0.15	0.05	0.02	0.13	0.05
age	<0.001	<0.001	<0.001	<0.001	<0.001	<0.001
gender	−0.46	0.66	0.39	−0.21	0.48	0.19
smoking	−0.05	0.22	0.08	−0.07	0.28	0.09
drinking	−0.13	0.37	0.15	−0.29	0.53	0.29
diabetes	0.56	0.82	0.38	0.63	0.86	0.41
hypertension	1.37	0.75	0.85	1.71	0.60	0.98
angina	−0.15	0.42	0.15	−0.24	0.56	0.21
abnormal CT	0.25	0.50	0.24	0.27	0.54	0.25
$\lambda_1(intercept)$	4.69	0.53	>0.99	5.00	0.44	>0.99
$\lambda_2\ (time3)$	0.20	0.53	0.20	0.12	0.31	0.18
η_0	3.37	0.22	–			
η_1	−2.19	0.55	>0.99			
η_2	0.94	0.93	0.57			

7.3 Joint Multistate Models

In some studies, a terminating event occurs after subjects go through several intermediate states, for example, from normal to severe disease, and from severe disease to death. In lung transplant studies, patients may develop chronic lung allograft dysfunction (CLAD), which is an important clinical event associated with an increased risk of death. In these scenarios, extending joint models to accommodate multistate event times is necessary if the interest is to predict a chain of events using a longitudinal marker. Dantan et al. (2011)[50] analyzed data from the PAQUID cohort to study the effect of cognitive decline on dementia and death. Specifically, a latent state was assumed in the longitudinal cognitive process to characterize the transition from a healthy state to a pre-diagnosis state. Proportional transition intensity models were used to specify transitions between states including heathy, pre-diagnosis (latent), illness, and death at the survival endpoint. The association between longitudinal cognitive scores and disease development was modeled by latent variables. Farewell and Tom (2014)[63] developed a joint multistate model for a clinical event $Y(t)$ and a time-dependent, ordinal response variable $W(t)$ of level K. Changes in the ordinal variable $W(t)$ are modeled by a multi-state process to characterize transitions between distinct categories (or states) over time. Suppose there are L states in the development of $Y(t)$. The association between $Y(t)$ and $W(t)$ is posited by an expanded multistate model with proportional transition intensities between $K \times L$ states. This approach is feasible when the total number of states $K \times L$ is small or moderate. It does not allow simultaneous transitions of $Y(t)$ and $W(t)$, which, however, is not necessarily a limitation if the processes are continuous in time.

7.4   Joint Models for Cure Rate Survival Data

Joint models that accommodate a cure fraction at the survival endpoint have been developed for clinical studies in which a subset of patients are believed to be free of disease recurrence or death after treatment. An example is given by the prostate carcinoma study conducted at the University of Michigan (Law et al., 2002[129]; Yu et al., 2004[244]) in which patients were treated with radiation therapy and followed for clinical recurrence including local recurrence and distant metastasis. A subgroup of patients may be cured by the treatment and thus would not experience the event of interest. During follow-up, one important biomarker, Prostate-Specific Antigen (PSA), was repeatedly measured to monitor disease progression. It is of interest to characterize PSA profiles and evaluate its association with recurrence.

Joint models for data with a cure fraction are extensions of cure survival models by characterizing the impact of longitudinal measurements on either the cure fraction or the event risk among uncured subjects, or both. One approach is based on a mixture model formulation in which a fraction p of the population are assumed to be susceptible to the event of interest and the remaining are cured (Law et al., 2002[129]; Yu et al., 2004[244]; Yu et al., 2008[245]). The patient susceptible status D is a latent binary indicator, with $P(D = 1) = p$ for the susceptibles and $P(D = 0) = 1 - p$ for the cured. The population survival function is thus $S(t) = pS_1(t) + (1 - p)$, where $S_1(t)$ is the survival function for the susceptibles and is assumed be dependent on the longitudinal outcome and covariates. Incorporating information from longitudinal biomarker data can relieve the identifiability problem in mixture cure models that is due to lack of information at the tail of $S_1(t)$ (Law et al., 2002[129]). The distribution of D is typically specified by a logistic regression conditional on baseline covariates. In this case, the marginal survival distribution $S(t)$ does not have the property of proportional hazards if $S_1(t)$ is specified by a proportional hazards model.

Joint analysis for cure data has also been studied using non-mixture models (Herring and Ibrahim, 2002[94]; Brown and Ibrahim, 2003[27]; Chen et al., 2004[34]). Specifically, this approach posits that there are N_i independent metastatis-competent tumor cells in subject i, each of which has a cumulative distribution function $F_i(t)$ for the time to develop detectable metastatic disease. Assuming a recurrence manifests itself when at least one metastatis-competent tumor cell develops detectable metastatic disease, the recurrence time on subject i is thus the minimum of the N_i latent event times. The number of latent metastatis-competent tumor cells N_i is assumed to follow a Poisson distribution with mean λ_i. It can been shown that the survival function for subject i is $S_i(t) = exp(-\lambda_i F_i(t))$. Since $F_i(t) \to 1$ as $t \to \infty$ for a proper distribution function, $S_i(t) \to exp(-\lambda_i)$ as $t \to \infty$, which is the cure fraction. Chen et al. (2004)[34] specified $F_i(t)$ by a piecewise exponential model and related λ_i to covariates and random effects of longitudinal measurements, whereas Brown and Ibrahim (2003)[27] assumed a proportional hazards model for $F_i(t)$ conditional on latent trajectories of longitudinal measurements and characterized the cure-rate parameter λ_i using baseline covariates. Chi and Ibrahim (2006)[40], Chi and Ibrahim (2007)[41], and Bakar et al. (2007, 2009)[15, 14] extended this class of joint models to allow the number of carcinogenic cells, denoted as $N_i(t)$, to change over time. It is assumed that $N_i(t)$ follows a non-homogeneous Poisson process with mean $\lambda_i(t)$ which is a function of the longitudinal trajectories.

7.5   Sample Size and Power Estimation for Joint Models

Research on the design aspects of joint modeling of longitudinal and time-to-event data is limited, although joint models have been an active area in the past two decades. Chen, Ibrahim, and Chu (2011)[33] extended Schoenfeld's ([198]) method to the setting of a joint model associating the longitudinal process and event times for estimation of the overall treatment effect in a randomized trial. They first derived a closed-form sample size formula assuming the variance-covariance matrix Σ of random effects for the longitudinal data is known, then extended this approach to the situation of unknown Σ based on the two-step inferential approach by Tsiatis et al.[218], and discussed the impact of within-subject variability and data collection strategies, such as spacing and frequency of repeated measurements, on the power of the joint model. Additional research is necessary to extend this method to different joint modeling settings and to investigate their applications.

Appendices

Appendix A

Software to Implement Joint Models

In Table A.1 we list the software packages and programs that have been developed to implement joint models. The codes are downloadable from our book website, http://publications.biostat.ucla.edu/gangli/jm-book.

Table A.1 *Software/Programs to fit joint models.*

Author	Reference	Programming Language	Book Example
Rizopoulos, D. [185]	Joint models for longitudinal and time-to-event data with applications in R. CRC Press, 2012	The R package JM	
Li, Z., Tosteson, T.D., and Bakitas, M. A. [140]	Joint modeling quality of life and survival using a terminal decline model in palliative care studies. Statistics in Medicine (2013) 32, 1394–1406.	SAS	The ENABLE II study (Example 4.7)
Diggle, P. and Kenward, M. G. [54]	Informative drop-out in longitudinal data analysis. Applied Statistics (1994) 43, 49–93.	SAS	The milk protein trial (Example 4.8)
Tseng, Y-K., Hsieh, F., and Wang, J-L. [212]	Joint modelling of accelerated failure time and longitudinal data. Biometrika (2005) 92, 587–603.	MATLAB	Medfly fecundity data (Example 4.14)
Sun, J., Sun, L., and Liu, D. [205]	Regression analysis of longitudinal data in the presence of informative observation and censoring times. Journal of the American Statistical Association (2007) 102, 1397–1406.	MATLAB and Fortran	The bladder cancer data (Example 4.16)
Elashoff, R., Li, G., and Li, N. [61]	A joint model for longitudinal measurements and survival data in the presence of multiple failure types. Biometrics (2008) 64, 762–771.	C	The scleroderma lung study (Example 5.1)
Rizopoulos, D. and Ghosh, P. [186]	A Bayesian semiparametric multivariate joint model for multiple longitudinal outcomes and a time-to-event. Statistics in Medicine (2011) 30, 1366–1380.	R and WinBUGS/JAGS	The renal graft failure study (Example 6.1)
Proust-Lima, C., et al. [178]	Joint modelling of multivariate longitudinal outcomes and a time-to-event: A nonlinear latent class approach. Computational Statistics and Data Analysis (2009) 53, 1142–1154.	Fortran90	The PAQUID study (Example 6.2)

Bibliography

[1] O Aalen. Nonparametric estimation of partial transition probabilities in multiple decrement models. *The Annals of Statistics*, 6(3):534–545, 1978.

[2] O Aalen. Nonparametric inference for a family of counting processes. *The Annals of Statistics*, 6(4):701–726, 1978.

[3] O Aalen. A model for nonparametric regression analysis of counting processes. *Lecture Notes in Statistics*, 2:1–25, 1980.

[4] OO Aalen. A linear regression model for the analysis of life times. *Statistics in Medicine*, 8(8):907–925, 1989.

[5] OO Aalen and S Johansen. An empirical transition matrix for non-homogeneous markov chains based on censored observations. *Scandinavian Journal of Statistics*, 5(3):141–150, 1978.

[6] JH Abbring and GJ Van den Berg. The identifiability of the mixed proportional hazards competing risks model. *Journal of the Royal Statistical Society: Series B (Statistical Methodology)*, 65(3):701–710, 2003.

[7] DI Abrams, AI Goldman, C Launer, JA Korvick, JD Neaton, LR Crane, M Grodesky, S Wakefield, K Muth, S Kornegay, et al. Comparative trial of didanosine and zalcitabine in patients with human immunodeficiency virus infection who are intolerant of or have failed zidovudine therapy. *New England Journal of Medicine*, 330(10):657–662, 1994.

[8] M Aerts, G Molenberghs, LM Ryan, and H Geys. *Topics in Modelling of Clustered Data*. CRC Press, 2002.

[9] PS Albert and JH Shih. An approach for jointly modeling multivariate longitudinal measurements and discrete time-to-event data. *The Annals of Applied Statistics*, 4(3):1517, 2010.

[10] PD Allison. *Survival Analysis Using SAS: A Practical Guide*. SAS Institute, 2010.

[11] PK Andersen, Ø. Borgan, RD Gill, and N Keiding. *Statistical Models Based on Counting Processes*. Springer Verlag, 1993.

[12] PK Andersen, O Borgan, RD Gill, and N Keiding. *Statistical Models Based on Counting Processes*. Springer Science & Business Media, 2012.

[13] PK Andersen and RD Gill. Cox's regression model for counting pro-

cesses: a large sample study. *The Annals of Statistics*, 10(4):1100–1120, 1982.

[14] MRA Bakar, KA Salah, NA Ibrahim, and K Haron. A semiparametric joint model for longitudinal and time-to-event univariate data in presence of cure fraction. *European Journal of Scientific Research*, 18(4):707–729, 2007.

[15] MRA Bakar, KA Salah, NA Ibrahim, and K Haron. Bayesian approach for joint longitudinal and time-to-event data with survival fraction. *Bulletin of the Malaysian Mathematical Sciences Society*, 32(1):75–100, 2009.

[16] M Bakitas, KD Lyons, MT Hegel, S Balan, KN Barnett, FC Brokaw, IR Byock, JG Hull, Z Li, E Mckinstry, et al. The project enable ii randomized controlled trial to improve palliative care for rural patients with advanced cancer: baseline findings, methodological challenges, and solutions. *Palliative and Supportive Care*, 7(01):75–86, 2009.

[17] MB Bakitas, KD Lyons, MT Hegel, S Balan, FC Brokaw, J Seville, JG Hull, Z Li, TD Tosteson, IR Byock, et al. Effects of a palliative care intervention on clinical outcomes in patients with advanced cancer: the project enable ii randomized controlled trial. *JAMA*, 302(7):741–749, 2009.

[18] S Bandyopadhyay, B Ganguli, and A Chatterjee. A review of multivariate longitudinal data analysis. *Statistical Methods in Medical Research*, 20(4):299–330, 2011.

[19] H Bao. Semiparametric Bayesian joint model with variable selection. 2011.

[20] R Beran. Nonparametric regression with randomly censored survival data. Technical report, Technical Report, Univ. California, Berkeley, 1981.

[21] N Breslow. Covariance analysis of censored survival data. *Biometrics*, 30(1):89–99, 1974.

[22] N Breslow and J Crowley. A large sample study of the life table and product limit estimates under random censorship. *The Annals of Statistics*, 2(3):437–453, 1974.

[23] NE Breslow. Contribution to the discussion of the paper by DR Cox. *Journal of the Royal Statistical Society: Series B*, 34(2):216–217, 1972.

[24] NE Breslow and DG Clayton. Approximate inference in generalized linear mixed models. *Journal of the American Statistical Association*, 88(421):9–25, 1993.

[25] NE Breslow and X Lin. Bias correction in generalised linear mixed models with a single component of dispersion. *Biometrika*, 82(1):81–91, 1995.

[26] G Broström. *Event History Analysis with R*. CRC Press, 2012.

[27] ER Brown and JG Ibrahim. Bayesian approaches to joint cure-rate and longitudinal models with applications to cancer vaccine trials. *Biometrics*, 59(3):686–693, 2003.

[28] ER Brown and JG Ibrahim. A Bayesian semiparametric joint hierarchical model for longitudinal and survival data. *Biometrics*, 59(2):221–228, 2003.

[29] J Buckley and I James. Linear regression with censored data. *Biometrika*, 66(3):429–436, 1979.

[30] B Cai and DB Dunson. Bayesian covariance selection in generalized linear mixed models. *Biometrics*, 62(2):446–457, 2006.

[31] JR Carey, P Liedo, HG Müller, J Wang, and J Chiou. Relationship of age patterns of fecundity to mortality, longevity, and lifetime reproduction in a large cohort of mediterranean fruit fly females. *The Journals of Gerontology Series A: Biological Sciences and Medical Sciences*, 53(4):B245–B251, 1998.

[32] K Chen, Z Jin, and Z Ying. Semiparametric analysis of transformation models with censored data. *Biometrika*, 89(3):659–668, 2002.

[33] LM Chen, JG Ibrahim, and H Chu. Sample size and power determination in joint modeling of longitudinal and survival data. *Statistics in Medicine*, 30(18):2295–2309, 2011.

[34] MH Chen, JG Ibrahim, and D Sinha. A new joint model for longitudinal and survival data with a cure fraction. *Journal of Multivariate Analysis*, 91(1):18–34, 2004.

[35] S Chen. Rank estimation of transformation models. *Econometrica*, 70(4):1683–1697, 2002.

[36] S Chen and S Khan. Semiparametric estimation of a partially linear censored regression model. *Econometric Theory*, 17(03):567–590, 2001.

[37] Z Chen and DB Dunson. Random effects selection in linear mixed models. *Biometrics*, 59(4):762–769, 2003.

[38] SC Cheng, LJ Wei, and Z Ying. Analysis of transformation models with censored data. *Biometrika*, 82(4):835–845, 1995.

[39] SC Cheng, LJ Wei, and Z Ying. Predicting survival probabilities with semiparametric transformation models. *Journal of the American Statistical Association*, 92(437):227–235, 1997.

[40] YY Chi and JG Ibrahim. Joint models for multivariate longitudinal and multivariate survival data. *Biometrics*, 62(2):432–445, 2006.

[41] YY Chi and JG Ibrahim. Bayesian approaches to joint longitudinal and survival models accommodating both zero and nonzero cure fractions. *Statistica Sinica*, 17(2):445, 2007.

[42] DR Cox. Regression models and life-tables. *Journal of the Royal Statistical Society: Series B (Methodological)*, 34(2):187–220, 1972.

[43] DR Cox. Regression models and life-tables. *Journal of the Royal Statistical Society: Series B (Methodological)*, 34:187–220, 1972.

[44] DR Cox. Partial likelihood. *Biometrika*, 62(2):269–276, 1975.

[45] DR Cox and D Oakes. *Analysis of Survival Data*, volume 21. CRC Press, 1984.

[46] DM Dabrowska. Non-parametric regression with censored survival time data. *Scandinavian Journal of Statistics*, 14(3):181–197, 1987.

[47] DM Dabrowska. Uniform consistency of the kernel conditional Kaplan-Meier estimate. *The Annals of Statistics*, 17(3):1157–1167, 1989.

[48] DM Dabrowska and KA Doksum. Partial likelihood in transformation models with censored data. *Scandinavian Journal of Statistics*, 15(1):1–23, 1988.

[49] MJ Daniels and JW Hogan. *Missing Data in Longitudinal Studies: Strategies for Bayesian Modeling and Sensitivity Analysis*. CRC Press, 2008.

[50] E Dantan, P Joly, JF Dartigues, and H Jacqmin-Gadda. Joint model with latent state for longitudinal and multistate data. *Biostatistics*, 12(4):723–736, 2011.

[51] V De Gruttola and XM Tu. Modelling progression of CD4-lymphocyte count and its relationship to survival time. *Biometrics*, 50(4):1003–1014, 1994.

[52] AP Dempster, NM Laird, and DB Rubin. Maximum likelihood from incomplete data via the EM algorithm. *Journal of the Royal Statistical Society: Series B (Methodological)*, 39(1):1–38, 1977.

[53] E Deslandes and S Chevret. Joint modeling of multivariate longitudinal data and the dropout process in a competing risk setting: application to icu data. *BMC Medical Research Methodology*, 10(1):69, 2010.

[54] P Diggle and MG Kenward. Informative drop-out in longitudinal data analysis. *Applied Statistics*, 43(1):49–93, 1994.

[55] PJ Diggle. An approach to the analysis of repeated measurements. *Biometrics*, 44:959–971, 1988.

[56] PJ Diggle, P Heagerty, K Liang, and SL Zeger. *Analysis of Longitudinal Data*. Oxford University Press, 2002.

[57] A Dobson and R Henderson. Diagnostics for joint longitudinal and dropout time modeling. *Biometrics*, 59(4):741–751, 2003.

[58] H Doss and RD Gill. An elementary approach to weak convergence for quantile processes, with applications to censored survival data. *Journal of the American Statistical Association*, 87(419):869–877, 1992.

[59] B Efron. Censored data and the bootstrap. *Journal of the American Statistical Association*, 76(374):312–319, 1981.

[60] B Efron and R Tibshirani. Bootstrap methods for standard errors, con-

fidence intervals, and other measures of statistical accuracy. *Statistical Science*, 1(1):54–75, 1986.

[61] RM Elashoff, G Li, and N Li. A joint model for longitudinal measurements and survival data in the presence of multiple failure types. *Biometrics*, 64(3):762–771, 2008.

[62] J Fan and I Gijbels. Censored regression: local linear approximations and their applications. *Journal of the American Statistical Association*, 89(426):560–570, 1994.

[63] VT Farewell and BDM Tom. The versatility of multi-state models for the analysis of longitudinal data with unobservable features. *Lifetime Data Analysis*, 20(1):51–75, 2014.

[64] CL Faucett, N Schenker, and RM Elashoff. Analysis of censored survival data with intermittently observed time-dependent binary covariates. *Journal of the American Statistical Association*, 93(442):427–437, 1998.

[65] CL Faucett and DC Thomas. Simultaneously modelling censored survival data and repeatedly measured covariates: a gibbs sampling approach. *Statistics in Medicine*, 15(15):1663–1685, 1996.

[66] JP Fine. Analysing competing risks data with transformation models. *Journal of the Royal Statistical Society: Series B (Statistical Methodology)*, 61(4):817–830, 1999.

[67] JP Fine. Regression modeling of competing crude failure probabilities. *Biostatistics*, 2(1):85–97, 2001.

[68] JP Fine and RJ Gray. A proportional hazards model for the subdistribution of a competing risk. *Journal of the American Statistical Association*, 94(446):496–509, 1999.

[69] JP Fine, Z Ying, and LG Wei. On the linear transformation model for censored data. *Biometrika*, 85(4):980–986, 1998.

[70] GM Fitzmaurice, NM Laird, and JH Ware. *Applied Longitudinal Analysis*. John Wiley & Sons, 2012.

[71] TR Fleming. Asymptotic distribution results in competing risks estimation. *The Annals of Statistics*, 6(5):1071–1079, 1978.

[72] TR Fleming. Nonparametric estimation for nonhomogeneous markov processes in the problem of competing risks. *The Annals of Statistics*, 6:1057–1070, 1978.

[73] TR Fleming and DP Harrington. *Counting Processes and Survival Analysis*, volume 169. John Wiley & Sons, 2011.

[74] S Gao. A shared random effect parameter approach for longitudinal dementia data with non-ignorable missing data. *Statistics in Medicine*, 23(2):211–219, 2004.

[75] FH Garre, AH Zwinderman, RB Geskus, and YWJ Sijpkens. A joint

latent class changepoint model to improve the prediction of time to graft failure. *Journal of the Royal Statistical Society: Series A (Statistics in Society)*, 171(1):299–308, 2008.

[76] EA Gehan. A generalized wilcoxon test for comparing arbitrarily singly-censored samples. *Biometrika*, 52(1-2):203–223, 1965.

[77] TA Gerds, TH Scheike, and PK Andersen. Absolute risk regression for competing risks: interpretation, link functions, and prediction. *Statistics in Medicine*, 31, 2012.

[78] A Gichangi and W Vach. The analysis of competing risks data: A guided tour. *Statistics in Medicine*, 31, 2005.

[79] RD Gill. Censoring and stochastic integrals. *Statistica Neerlandica*, 34(2):124–124, 1980.

[80] AI Goldman, BP Carlin, LR Crane, C Launer, JA Korvick, L Deyton, and DI Abrams. Response of CD4 lymphocytes and clinical consequences of treatment using ddI or ddC in patients with advanced HIV infection. *JAIDS Journal of Acquired Immune Deficiency Syndromes*, 11(2):161–169, 1996.

[81] G Gong and FJ Samaniego. Pseudo maximum likelihood estimation: theory and applications. *The Annals of Statistics*, 9(4):861–869, 1981.

[82] RJ Gray. A class of K-sample tests for comparing the cumulative incidence of a competing risk. *The Annals of Statistics*, 16(3):1141–1154, 1988.

[83] M Greenwood. The errors of sampling of the survivorship tables. *Reports on Public Health and Statistical Subjects*, 33(1):26, 1926.

[84] Stroke Study Group et al. Tissue plasminogen activator for acute ischemic stroke. *New England Journal of Medicine*, 333:1581–1587, 1995.

[85] X Guo and BP Carlin. Separate and joint modeling of longitudinal and event time data using standard computer packages. *The American Statistician*, 58(1):16–24, 2004.

[86] SM Hammer, DA Katzenstein, MD Hughes, H Gundacker, RT Schooley, RH Haubrich, WK Henry, MM Lederman, JP Phair, M Niu, et al. A trial comparing nucleoside monotherapy with combination therapy in HIV-infected adults with CD4 cell counts from 200 to 500 per cubic millimeter. *New England Journal of Medicine*, 335(15):1081–1090, 1996.

[87] J Han, EH Slate, and EA Peña. Parametric latent class joint model for a longitudinal biomarker and recurrent events. *Statistics in Medicine*, 26(29):5285–5302, 2007.

[88] M Han, X Song, L Sun, and L Liu. Joint modeling of longitudinal data with informative observation times and dropouts. *Statistica Sinica*, 24(4):1487–1504, 2014.

[89] DP Harrington and TR Fleming. A class of rank test procedures for

censored survival data. *Biometrika*, 69(3):553–566, 1982.

[90] D Harville. Extension of the gauss-markov theorem to include the estimation of random effects. *The Annals of Statistics*, 4(2):384–395, 1976.

[91] DA Harville. Maximum likelihood approaches to variance component estimation and to related problems. *Journal of the American Statistical Association*, 72(358):320–338, 1977.

[92] LA Hatfield, ME Boye, and BP Carlin. Joint modeling of multiple longitudinal patient-reported outcomes and survival. *Journal of Biopharmaceutical Statistics*, 21(5):971–991, 2011.

[93] R Henderson, P Diggle, and A Dobson. Joint modelling of longitudinal measurements and event time data. *Biostatistics*, 1(4):465–480, 2000.

[94] AH Herring and JG Ibrahim. Maximum likelihood estimation in random effects cure rate models with nonignorable missing covariates. *Biostatistics*, 3(3):387–405, 2002.

[95] JW Hogan and NM Laird. Model-based approaches to analysing incomplete longitudinal and failure time data. *Statistics in Medicine*, 16(3):259–272, 1997.

[96] JD Holt. Competing risk analyses with special reference to matched pair experiments. *Biometrika*, 65(1):159–165, 1978.

[97] P Hougaard. Life table methods for heterogeneous populations: distributions describing the heterogeneity. *Biometrika*, 71(1):75–83, 1984.

[98] P Hougaard. Survival models for heterogeneous populations derived from stable distributions. *Biometrika*, 73(2):387–396, 1986.

[99] F Hsieh, YK Tseng, and JL Wang. Joint modeling of survival and longitudinal data: likelihood approach revisited. *Biometrics*, 62(4):1037–1043, 2006.

[100] W Hu, G Li, and N Li. A Bayesian approach to joint analysis of longitudinal measurements and competing risks failure time data. *Statistics in Medicine*, 28(11):1601–1619, 2009.

[101] CY Huang, MC Wang, and Y Zhang. Analysing panel count data with informative observation times. *Biometrika*, 93(4):763–775, 2006.

[102] W Huang, SL Zeger, JC Anthony, and E Garrett. Latent variable model for joint analysis of multiple repeated measures and bivariate event times. *Journal of the American Statistical Association*, 96(455):906–914, 2001.

[103] X Huang, G Li, and RM Elashoff. A joint model of longitudinal and competing risks survival data with heterogeneous random effects and outlying longitudinal measurements. *Statistics and Its Interface*, 3(2):185, 2010.

[104] X Huang, G Li, RM Elashoff, and J Pan. A general joint model for longitudinal measurements and competing risks survival data with het-

erogeneous random effects. *Lifetime Data Analysis*, 17(1):80–100, 2011.

[105] FW Huffer and IW McKeague. Weighted least squares estimation for aalen's additive risk model. *Journal of the American Statistical Association*, 86(413):114–129, 1991.

[106] JG Ibrahim, MH Chen, and SR Lipsitz. Missing responses in generalised linear mixed models when the missing data mechanism is nonignorable. *Biometrika*, 88(2):551–564, 2001.

[107] JG Ibrahim and G Molenberghs. Missing data methods in longitudinal studies: a review. *Test*, 18(1):1–43, 2009.

[108] M Jacobsen. Existence and unicity of mles in discrete exponential family distributions. *Scandinavian Journal of Statistics*, 16(4):335–349, 1989.

[109] RI Jennrich and MD Schluchter. Unbalanced repeated-measures models with structured covariance matrices. *Biometrics*, 42(4):805–820, 1986.

[110] J Jiang. Asymptotic properties of the empirical blup and blue in mixed linear models. *Statistica Sinica*, 8(3):861–885, 1998.

[111] Z Jin, DY Lin, LJ Wei, and Z Ying. Rank-based inference for the accelerated failure time model. *Biometrika*, 90(2):341–353, 2003.

[112] S Johansen. An extension of Cox's regression model. *International Statistical Review/Revue Internationale de Statistique*, 51(2):165–174, 1983.

[113] JD Kalbfleisch and RL Prentice. *The Statistical Analysis of Failure Time Data*, volume 360. John Wiley & Sons, 2011.

[114] EL Kaplan and P Meier. Nonparametric estimation from incomplete observations. *Journal of the American statistical association*, 53(282):457–481, 1958.

[115] MG Kenward and G Molenberghs. Parametric models for incomplete continuous and categorical longitudinal data. *Statistical Methods in Medical Research*, 8(1):51–83, 1999.

[116] SK Kinney and DB Dunson. Fixed and random effects selection in linear and logistic models. *Biometrics*, 63(3):690–698, 2007.

[117] JP Klein. Modelling competing risks in cancer studies. *Statistics in Medicine*, 25(6):1015–1034, 2006.

[118] JP Klein and PK Andersen. Regression modeling of competing risks data based on pseudovalues of the cumulative incidence function. *Biometrics*, 61(1):223–229, 2005.

[119] JP Klein and ML Moeschberger. *Survival Analysis: Techniques for Censored and Truncated Data*. Springer Science & Business Media, 2003.

[120] MR Kosorok, BL Lee, and JP Fine. Robust inference for univariate proportional hazards frailty regression models. *Annals of Statistics*, 32(2):1448–1491, 2004.

[121] H Koul, V Susarla, and J Van Ryzin. Regression analysis with randomly

right-censored data. *The Annals of Statistics*, 9(6):1276–1288, 1981.

[122] SW Lagakos. A covariate model for partially censored data subject to competing causes of failure. *Applied Statistics*, 27(3):235–241, 1978.

[123] TL Lai and Z Ying. Large sample theory of a modified buckley-james estimator for regression analysis with censored data. *The Annals of Statistics*, 19(3):1370–1402, 1991.

[124] TL Lai, ZL Ying, and ZK Zheng. Asymptotic normality of a class of adaptive statistics with applications to synthetic data methods for censored regression. *Journal of Multivariate Analysis*, 52(2):259–279, 1995.

[125] NM Laird and JH Ware. Random-effects models for longitudinal data. *Biometrics*, 38(4):963–974, 1982.

[126] K Lange and JS Sinsheimer. Normal/independent distributions and their applications in robust regression. *Journal of Computational and Graphical Statistics*, 2(2):175–198, 1993.

[127] KL Lange, RJA Little, and JMG Taylor. Robust statistical modeling using the t distribution. *Journal of the American Statistical Association*, 84(408):881–896, 1989.

[128] MG Larson. Covariate analysis of competing-risks data with log-linear models. *Biometrics*, 40(2):459–469, 1984.

[129] NJ Law, JMG Taylor, and H Sandler. The joint modeling of a longitudinal disease progression marker and the failure time process in the presence of cure. *Biostatistics*, 3(4):547–563, 2002.

[130] L Letenneur, D Commenges, JF Dartigues, and P Barberger-Gateau. Incidence of dementia and alzheimer's disease in elderly community residents of south-western france. *International Journal of Epidemiology*, 23(6):1256–1261, 1994.

[131] MK Leung and RM Elashoff. Estimation of a generalized linear mixed-effects model with a finite-support random-effects distribution via Gibbs sampling. *Biometrical Journal*, 38(5):519–536, 1996.

[132] G Li. On nonparametric likelihood ratio estimation of survival probabilities for censored data. *Statistics & Probability Letters*, 25(2):95–104, 1995.

[133] G Li and H Doss. An approach to nonparametric regression for life history data using local linear fitting. *The Annals of Statistics*, 23(3):787–823, 1995.

[134] G Li and QH Wang. Empirical likelihood regression analysis for right censored data. *Statistica Sinica*, 13(1):51–68, 2003.

[135] G Li and Q Yang. Joint inference for competing risks survival data. *Journal of the American Statistical Association*, (just-accepted):00–00, 2015.

[136] N Li, MJ Daniels, G Li, and RM Elashoff. An exploration of fixed and random effects selection for longitudinal binary outcomes in the presence of nonignorable dropout. *Biometrical Journal*, 55(1):17–37, 2013.

[137] N Li, RM Elashoff, and G Li. Robust joint modeling of longitudinal measurements and competing risks failure time data. *Biometrical Journa*, 51(1):19, 2009.

[138] N Li, RM Elashoff, G Li, and J Saver. Joint modeling of longitudinal ordinal data and competing risks survival times and analysis of the ninds rt-pa stroke trial. *Statistics in Medicine*, 29(5):546–557, 2010.

[139] N Li, RM Elashoff, G Li, and CH Tseng. Joint analysis of bivariate longitudinal ordinal outcomes and competing risks survival times with nonparametric distributions for random effects. *Statistics in Medicine*, 31(16):1707–1721, 2012.

[140] Z Li, TD Tosteson, and MA Bakitas. Joint modeling quality of life and survival using a terminal decline model in palliative care studies. *Statistics in Medicine*, 32(8):1394–1406, 2013.

[141] KY Liang and SG Self. On the asymptotic behaviour of the pseudo-likelihood ratio test statistic. *Journal of the Royal Statistical Society: Series B (Methodological)*, 58(4):785–796, 1996.

[142] KY Liang and SL Zeger. Longitudinal data analysis using generalized linear models. *Biometrika*, 73(1):13–22, 1986.

[143] KY Liang and SL Zeger. Inference based on estimating functions in the presence of nuisance parameters. *Statistical Science*, 10(2):158–173, 1995.

[144] KY Liang, SL Zeger, and B Qaqish. Multivariate regression analyses for categorical data. *Journal of the Royal Statistical Society: Series B (Methodological)*, 54(1):3–40, 1992.

[145] Y Liang, W Lu, and Z Ying. Joint modeling and analysis of longitudinal data with informative observation times. *Biometrics*, 65(2):377–384, 2009.

[146] DY Lin and Z Ying. Semiparametric analysis of the additive risk model. *Biometrika*, 81(1):61–71, 1994.

[147] DY Lin and Z Ying. Semiparametric inference for the accelerated life model with time-dependent covariates. *Journal of Statistical Planning and Inference*, 44(1):47–63, 1995.

[148] H Lin, CE McCulloch, and RA Rosenheck. Latent pattern mixture models for informative intermittent missing data in longitudinal studies. *Biometrics*, 60(2):295–305, 2004.

[149] H Lin, DO Scharfstein, and RA Rosenheck. Analysis of longitudinal data with irregular, outcome-dependent follow-up. *Journal of the Royal Statistical Society: Series B (Statistical Methodology)*, 66(3):791–813, 2004.

[150] X Lin and NE Breslow. Bias correction in generalized linear mixed models with multiple components of dispersion. *Journal of the American Statistical Association*, 91(435):1007–1016, 1996.

[151] DV Lindley and ND Singpurwalla. Multivariate distributions for the life lengths of components of a system sharing a common environment. *Journal of Applied Probability*, 32(2):418–431, 1986.

[152] RJA Little. Modeling the drop-out mechanism in repeated-measures studies. *Journal of the American Statistical Association*, 90(431):1112–1121, 1995.

[153] RJA Little and DB Rubin. *Statistical Analysis with Missing Data*. John Wiley & Sons, 2014.

[154] L Liu and X Huang. Joint analysis of correlated repeated measures and recurrent events processes in the presence of death, with application to a study on acquired immune deficiency syndrome. *Journal of the Royal Statistical Society: Series C (Applied Statistics)*, 58(1):65–81, 2009.

[155] TA Louis. Finding the observed information matrix when using the EM algorithm. *Journal of the Royal Statistical Society: Series B (Methodological)*, 44(2):226–233, 1982.

[156] M Lunn and D McNeil. Applying Cox regression to competing risks. *Biometrics*, 51(2):524–532, 1995.

[157] S Luo. A Bayesian approach to joint analysis of multivariate longitudinal data and parametric accelerated failure time. *Statistics in Medicine*, 33(4):580–594, 2014.

[158] G Ma, AB Troxel, and DF Heitjan. An index of local sensitivity to nonignorable drop-out in longitudinal modelling. *Statistics in Medicine*, 24(14):2129–2150, 2005.

[159] S Ma and P Du. Variable selection in partly linear regression model with diverging dimensions for right censored data. *Statistica Sinica*, 22(3):1003, 2012.

[160] N Mantel. Evaluation of survival data and two new rank order statistics arising in its consideration. *Cancer Chemotherapy Reports. Part 1*, 50(3):163–170, 1966.

[161] CA McGilchrist and CW Aisbett. Regression with frailty in survival analysis. *Biometrics*, 47(2):461–466, 1991.

[162] IW McKeague and PD Sasieni. A partly parametric additive risk model. *Biometrika*, 81(3):501–514, 1994.

[163] IW McKeague and KJ Utikal. Inference for a nonlinear counting process regression model. *The Annals of Statistics*, 18(3):1172–1187, 1990.

[164] JJ Miller. Asymptotic properties of maximum likelihood estimates in the mixed model of the analysis of variance. *The Annals of Statistics*, 5(4):746–762, 1977.

[165] RG Miller. Least squares regression with censored data. *Biometrika*, 63(3):449–464, 1976.

[166] CJ Mode. A large sample investigation of a multiple decrement life table estimator. *Mathematical Biosciences*, 32(1):111–123, 1976.

[167] G Molenberghs, H Thijs, I Jansen, C Beunckens, MG Kenward, C Mallinckrodt, and RJ Carroll. Analyzing incomplete longitudinal clinical trial data. *Biostatistics*, 5(3):445–464, 2004.

[168] SA Murphy. Consistency in a proportional hazards model incorporating a random effect. *The Annals of Statistics*, 22(2):712–731, 1994.

[169] SA Murphy. Likelihood ratio-based confidence intervals in survival analysis. *Journal of the American Statistical Association*, 90(432):1399–1405, 1995.

[170] E Parner. Asymptotic theory for the correlated gamma-frailty model. *The Annals of Statistics*, 26(1):183–214, 1998.

[171] M Parzen, SR Lipsitz, GM Fitzmaurice, JG Ibrahim, and A Troxel. Pseudo-likelihood methods for longitudinal binary data with non-ignorable missing responses and covariates. *Statistics in Medicine*, 25(16):2784, 2006.

[172] L Peng and JP Fine. Competing risks quantile regression. *Journal of the American Statistical Association*, 104(488):1440–1453, 2009.

[173] MS Pepe. Inference for events with dependent risks in multiple endpoint studies. *Journal of the American Statistical Association*, 86(415):770–778, 1991.

[174] M Pintilie. *Competing Risks: A Practical Perspective*. John Wiley & Sons New York:, 2006.

[175] JL Powell. Least absolute deviations estimation for the censored regression model. *Journal of Econometrics*, 25(3):303–325, 1984.

[176] RL Prentice. Linear rank tests with right censored data. *Biometrika*, 65(1):167–179, 1978.

[177] RL Prentice, JD Kalbfleisch, AV Peterson Jr, N Flournoy, VT Farewell, and NE Breslow. The analysis of failure times in the presence of competing risks. *Biometrics*, 34(4):541–554, 1978.

[178] C Proust-Lima, P Joly, JF Dartigues, and H Jacqmin-Gadda. Joint modelling of multivariate longitudinal outcomes and a time-to-event: a nonlinear latent class approach. *Computational Statistics & Data Analysis*, 53(4):1142–1154, 2009.

[179] C Proust-Lima and JMG Taylor. Development and validation of a dynamic prognostic tool for prostate cancer recurrence using repeated measures of posttreatment PSA: a joint modeling approach. *Biostatistics*, 10(3):535–549, 2009.

[180] H Putter, M Fiocco, and RB Geskus. Tutorial in biostatistics: competing

risks and multi-state models. *Statistics in Medicine*, 26(11):2389–2430, 2007.

[181] G Qin and BY Jing. Censored partial linear models and empirical likelihood. *Journal of Multivariate Analysis*, 78(1):37–61, 2001.

[182] AM Richardson and AH Welsh. Asymptotic properties of restricted maximum likelihood (REML) estimates for hierarchical mixed linear models. *Australian Journal of Statistics*, 36(1):31–43, 1994.

[183] Y Ritov. Estimation in a linear regression model with censored data. *The Annals of Statistics*, 18(1):303–328, 1990.

[184] D Rizopoulos. Dynamic predictions and prospective accuracy in joint models for longitudinal and time-to-event data. *Biometrics*, 67(3):819–829, 2011.

[185] D Rizopoulos. *Joint Models for Longitudinal and Time-to-Event Data: With Applications in R*. CRC Press, 2012.

[186] D Rizopoulos and P Ghosh. A Bayesian semiparametric multivariate joint model for multiple longitudinal outcomes and a time-to-event. *Statistics in Medicine*, 30(12):1366–1380, 2011.

[187] D Rizopoulos, G Verbeke, and G Molenberghs. Multiple-imputation-based residuals and diagnostic plots for joint models of longitudinal and survival outcomes. *Biometrics*, 66(1):20–29, 2010.

[188] J Robins and AA Tsiatis. Semiparametric estimation of an accelerated failure time model with time-dependent covariates. *Biometrika*, 79(2):311–319, 1992.

[189] JM Robins, A Rotnitzky, and LP Zhao. Analysis of semiparametric regression models for repeated outcomes in the presence of missing data. *Journal of the American Statistical Association*, 90(429):106–121, 1995.

[190] GJM Rosa, CR Padovani, and D Gianola. Robust linear mixed models with normal/independent distributions and Bayesian MCMC implementation. *Biometrical Journal*, 45(5):573–590, 2003.

[191] J Roy and X Lin. Analysis of multivariate longitudinal outcomes with nonignorable dropouts and missing covariates: changes in methadone treatment practices. *Journal of the American Statistical Association*, 97(457):40–52, 2002.

[192] J Roy and X Lin. Missing covariates in longitudinal data with informative dropouts: Bias analysis and inference. *Biometrics*, 61(3):837–846, 2005.

[193] DB Rubin. Inference and missing data. *Biometrika*, 63(3):581–592, 1976.

[194] DB Rubin. *Multiple Imputation for Nonresponse in Surveys*, volume 81. John Wiley & Sons, 2004.

[195] A Sancho, A Ávila, E Gavela, S Beltrán, J Fernández-Nájera, P Molina,

J Crespo, and L Pallardó. Effect of overweight on kidney transplantation outcome. In *Transplantation Proceedings*, volume 39, pages 2202–2204. Orlando, FL: Grune & Stratton, 2007.

[196] JL Schafer. *Analysis of Incomplete Multivariate Data*. CRC press, 1997.

[197] R Schall. Estimation in generalized linear models with random effects. *Biometrika*, 78(4):719–727, 1991.

[198] DA Schoenfeld. Sample-size formula for the proportional-hazards regression model. *Biometrics*, 39(2):499–503, 1983.

[199] X Song, M Davidian, and AA Tsiatis. A semiparametric likelihood approach to joint modeling of longitudinal and time-to-event data. *Biometrics*, 58(4):742–753, 2002.

[200] X Song and CY Wang. Semiparametric approaches for joint modeling of longitudinal and survival data with time-varying coefficients. *Biometrics*, 64(2):557–566, 2008.

[201] C Srinivasan and M Zhou. Linear regression with censoring. *Journal of Multivariate Analysis*, 49(2):179–201, 1994.

[202] R Stiratelli, N Laird, and JH Ware. Random-effects models for serial observations with binary response. *Biometrics*, 40(4):961–971, 1984.

[203] L Sue. Linear models, random censoring and synthetic data. *Biometrika*, 74(2):301–309, 1987.

[204] J Sun, DH Park, L Sun, and X Zhao. Semiparametric regression analysis of longitudinal data with informative observation times. *Journal of the American Statistical Association*, 100(471):882–889, 2005.

[205] J Sun, Ln Sun, and D Liu. Regression analysis of longitudinal data in the presence of informative observation and censoring times. *Journal of the American Statistical Association*, 102(480):1397–1406, 2007.

[206] L Sun, X Song, J Zhou, and L Liu. Joint analysis of longitudinal data with informative observation times and a dependent terminal event. *Journal of the American Statistical Association*, 107(498):688–700, 2012.

[207] DP Tashkin, R Elashoff, PJ Clements, J Goldin, MD Roth, DE Furst, E Arriola, R Silver, C Strange, M Bolster, et al. Cyclophosphamide versus placebo in scleroderma lung disease. *New England Journal of Medicine*, 354(25):2655–2666, 2006.

[208] DR Thomas and GL Grunkemeier. Confidence interval estimation of survival probabilities for censored data. *Journal of the American Statistical Association*, 70(352):865–871, 1975.

[209] AB Troxel, SR Lipsitz, and DP Harrington. Marginal models for the analysis of longitudinal measurements with nonignorable non-monotone missing data. *Biometrika*, 85(3):661–672, 1998.

[210] AB Troxel, G Ma, and DF Heitjan. An index of local sensitivity to nonignorability. *Statistica Sinica*, 14(4):1221–1238, 2004.

[211] C Tseng, R Elashoff, N Li, and G Li. Longitudinal data analysis with non-ignorable missing data. *Statistical Methods in Medical Research*, 22(1):205–220, 2012.

[212] YK Tseng, F Hsieh, and JL Wang. Joint modelling of accelerated failure time and longitudinal data. *Biometrika*, 92(3):587–603, 2005.

[213] A Tsiatis. A nonidentifiability aspect of the problem of competing risks. *Proceedings of the National Academy of Sciences*, 72(1):20–22, 1975.

[214] AA Tsiatis. A large sample study of Cox's regression model. *The Annals of Statistics*, 9(1):93–108, 1981.

[215] AA Tsiatis. Estimating regression parameters using linear rank tests for censored data. *The Annals of Statistics*, 18(1):354–372, 1990.

[216] AA Tsiatis and M Davidian. A semiparametric estimator for the proportional hazards model with longitudinal covariates measured with error. *Biometrika*, 88(2):447–458, 2001.

[217] AA Tsiatis and M Davidian. Joint modeling of longitudinal and time-to-event data: an overview. *Statistica Sinica*, 14(3):809–834, 2004.

[218] AA Tsiatis, V Degruttola, and MS Wulfsohn. Modeling the relationship of survival to longitudinal data measured with error. applications to survival and CD4 counts in patients with AIDS. *Journal of the American Statistical Association*, 90(429):27–37, 1995.

[219] R Tsonaka, G Verbeke, and E Lesaffre. A semi-parametric shared parameter model to handle nonmonotone nonignorable missingness. *Biometrics*, 65(1):81–87, 2009.

[220] I Van Keilegom and MG Akritas. Transfer of tail information in censored regression models. *Annals of Statistics*, 27(5):1745–1784, 1999.

[221] I Van Keilegom and N Veraverbeke. Estimation and bootstrap with censored data in fixed design nonparametric regression. *Annals of the Institute of Statistical Mathematics*, 49(3):467–491, 1997.

[222] K Van Steen, G Molenberghs, G Verbeke, and H Thijs. A local influence approach to sensitivity analysis of incomplete longitudinal ordinal data. *Statistical Modelling*, 1(2):125–142, 2001.

[223] G Verbeke, G Molenberghs, H Thijs, E Lesaffre, and MG Kenward. Sensitivity analysis for nonrandom dropout: a local influence approach. *Biometrics*, 57(1):7–14, 2001.

[224] AP Verbyla and BR Cullis. Modelling in repeated measures experiments. *Applied Statistics*, 39(3):341–356, 1990.

[225] A Verdonck, L De Ridder, G Verbeke, JP Bourguignon, C Carels, ER Kühn, V Darras, and F de Zegher. Comparative effects of neonatal and prepubertal castration on craniofacial growth in rats. *Archives of Oral Biology*, 43(11):861–871, 1998.

[226] WT Vetterling, BP Flannery, WH Press, and SA Teukolski. Numerical

recipes in fortran-the art of scientific computing. 1, 1989.

[227] S Viviani, D Rizopoulos, and M Alfó. Local sensitivity to non-ignorability in joint models. *Statistical Modelling*, 14(3):205–228, 2014.

[228] CY Wang. Corrected score estimator for joint modeling of longitudinal and failure time data. *Statistica Sinica*, 16(1):235, 2006.

[229] QH Wang and G Li. Empirical likelihood semiparametric regression analysis under random censorship. *Journal of Multivariate Analysis*, 83(2):469–486, 2002.

[230] Y Wang and JMG Taylor. Jointly modeling longitudinal and event time data with application to acquired immunodeficiency syndrome. *Journal of the American Statistical Association*, 96(455):895–905, 2001.

[231] C Waternaux, NM Laird, and JH Ware. Methods for analysis of longitudinal data: blood-lead concentrations and cognitive development. *Journal of the American Statistical Association*, 84(405):33–41, 1989.

[232] C Waternaux, J Ware, J Dwyer, M Feinleib, P Lippert, and H Hoffmeister. Unconditional linear models for analysis of longitudinal data. *Statistical Models for Longitudinal Studies of Health, Oxford University Press, New York*, 1992.

[233] GCG Wei and MA Tanner. A Monte Carlo implementation of the EM algorithm and the poor man's data augmentation algorithms. *Journal of the American statistical Association*, 85(411):699–704, 1990.

[234] LJ Wei, Z Ying, and DY Lin. Linear regression analysis of censored survival data based on rank tests. *Biometrika*, 77(4):845–851, 1990.

[235] DA Williams. Extra-binomial variation in logistic linear models. *Applied Statistics*, 31(2):144–148, 1982.

[236] R Wolfinger and M O'connell. Generalized linear mixed models a pseudo-likelihood approach. *Journal of Statistical Computation and Simulation*, 48(3-4):233–243, 1993.

[237] GY Wong and WM Mason. The hierarchical logistic regression model for multilevel analysis. *Journal of the American Statistical Association*, 80(391):513–524, 1985.

[238] L Wu, XJ Hu, and H Wu. Joint inference for nonlinear mixed-effects models and time to event at the presence of missing data. *Biostatistics*, 9(2):308–320, 2008.

[239] L Wu, W Liu, and X Hu. Joint inference on HIV viral dynamics and immune suppression in presence of measurement errors. *Biometrics*, 66(2):327–335, 2010.

[240] MC Wu and RJ Carroll. Estimation and comparison of changes in the presence of informative right censoring by modeling the censoring process. *Biometrics*, 44(1):175–188, 1988.

[241] MS Wulfsohn and AA Tsiatis. A joint model for survival and longitu-

dinal data measured with error. *Biometrics*, 53(1):330–339, 1997.

[242] Y Yang and J Kang. Joint analysis of mixed Poisson and continuous longitudinal data with nonignorable missing values. *Computational Statistics & Data Analysis*, 54(1):193–207, 2010.

[243] Z Ying. A large sample study of rank estimation for censored regression data. *The Annals of Statistics*, 21(1):76–99, 1993.

[244] M Yu, NJ Law, JMG Taylor, and HM Sandler. Joint longitudinal-survival-cure models and their application to prostate cancer. *Statistica Sinica*, 14(3):835–862, 2004.

[245] M Yu, JMG Taylor, and HM Sandler. Individual prediction in prostate cancer studies using a joint longitudinal survival–cure model. *Journal of the American Statistical Association*, 103(481):178–187, 2008.

[246] Y Yuan and G Yin. Bayesian quantile regression for longitudinal studies with nonignorable missing data. *Biometrics*, 66(1):105–114, 2010.

[247] SL Zeger and KY Liang. Longitudinal data analysis for discrete and continuous outcomes. *Biometrics*, 42(1):121–130, 1986.

[248] D Zeng and J Cai. Asymptotic results for maximum likelihood estimators in joint analysis of repeated measurements and survival time. *The Annals of Statistics*, 33(5):2132–2163, 2005.

[249] D Zeng and J Cai. Simultaneous modelling of survival and longitudinal data with an application to repeated quality of life measures. *Lifetime Data Analysis*, 11:151–174, 2005.

[250] D Zeng and D Lin. Efficient estimation of semiparametric transformation models for counting processes. *Biometrika*, 93(3):627–640, 2006.

[251] H Zhang, Y Ye, P Diggle, and J Shi. Joint modeling of time series measures and recurrent events and analysis of the effects of air quality on respiratory symptoms. *Journal of the American Statistical Association*, 103(481), 2008.

[252] Z Zheng. A class of estimators of the parameters in linear regression with censored data. *Acta Mathematicae Applicatae Sinica*, 3(3):231–241, 1987.

[253] M Zhou. Asymptotic normality of the "synthetic data" regression estimator for censored survival data. *The Annals of Statistics*, 20(2):1002–1021, 1992.

[254] M Zhou. M-estimation in censored linear models. *Biometrika*, 79(4):837–841, 1992.

[255] M Zhou and G Li. Empirical likelihood analysis of the Buckley–James estimator. *Journal of Multivariate Analysis*, 99(4):649–664, 2008.

Index

Accelerated failure time, 11
Accelerated failure time model, 120,
    121, 160, 169
Adaptive Gauss–Hermite
    quadrature, 104
Adaptive Gaussian–Hermite
    quadrature, 72, 99, 102
Adaptive rejection sampling (ARS),
    154
Akaika information criterion (AIC),
    113, 155, 175

Balanced, 17
Baseline survival function, 120
Bayes Information Criterion (BIC),
    174, 175
Bayesian approach, 73, 89, 108, 115,
    137, 157, 187, 201
Bernoulli distribution, 109, 205
Best linear unbiased predictor
    (BLUP), 22
Bootstrap, 73, 83, 122, 123

Canonical link, 28
Cause-specific competing risks
    model, 155
Cause-specific hazards model, 138,
    156
Cholesky decomposition, 23, 151, 152
Class-specific proportional hazard
    model, 173
Class-specific recurrent event model,
    183
Competing risk, 5, 137, 148, 152, 156
Complete-data likelihood, 143
Complete-data log-likelihood, 144
Conditional independence, 128
Conditional linear model, 82

Conditional score approach, 108, 111
Conditional score approach (CS),
    114, 115
Cook-type distance, 201
Corrected score approach, 119
Covariate-dependent dropout, 79
Cox proportional hazards model,
    105–107, 119, 154, 167, 169
Cox regression, 69, 125
Cox's proportional hazards model, 1

Deviance Information Criterion
    (DIC), 155, 156, 160, 170
Dirichlet process, 168
Dirichlet process (DP) prior, 205
Disease-free survival (DFS), 184, 187
Dummy variable, 26

Eigenvalue, 193
Expectation-Maximization (EM)
    algorithm, 71, 74, 80, 89,
    101, 108, 112, 113, 121, 127,
    140, 143, 144, 148, 174, 179,
    183
Exponential family, 20, 26–28

Fixed effect, 20–22, 28, 39, 206

Gamma distribution, 127
Gaussian distribution, 144
Gaussian process, 70, 71, 75, 95, 107,
    178, 198, 199
Gaussian quadrature, 28, 29, 72, 90,
    101
Gaussian–Hermite quadrature, 102
Generalized autoregressive
    parameters (GARP), 152,
    153, 155

Printed and bound by CPI Group (UK) Ltd, Croydon, CR0 4YY

24/10/2024

01778278-0008